Thoracic Surgery

Thoracic Surgery for Nurses

K. Moghissi
B.Sc., M.D., F.R.C.S.(Ed.), Académie de Chirurgie (Paris)
Consultant Cardio-Thoracic Surgeon, Humberside Cardio-Thoracic Surgical Centre,
Castle Hill Hospital, Cottingham, North Humberside

with contributions by
M. Clarke
S.R.N., R.N.T., B.Sc., M.Phil.
Director of the Institute of Nursing Studies, Hull University, North Humberside

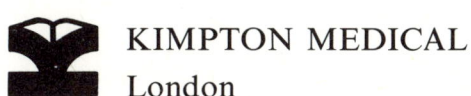

KIMPTON MEDICAL
London

A division of Teviot Scientific Publications Ltd., Edinburgh, London and New York

NOTICE

Medicine is an ever-changing science. As new research and clinical experience broaden our knowledge, changes in treatment and drug therapy are required. The editors and the publisher of this work have made every effort to ensure that the drug dosage schedules herein are accurate and in accord with the standards accepted at the time of publication. Readers are advised, however, to check the product information sheet included in the package of each drug they plan to administer to be certain that changes have not been made in the recommended dose or in the contraindictions for administration. This recommendation is of particular importance in regard to new or infrequently used drugs.

© 1982 Kimpton Medical
205 Great Portland Street
London
W1N 6LR
United Kingdom

British Library Cataloguing in Publication Data
Moghissi, K.
    Thoracic surgery for nurses.
    1. Chest—Surgery.   2. Surgical nursing
    I. Title
    617'.54059'024613   RD536

ISBN 0-85313-811-7 (soft back)

Filmset by Advanced Filmsetters (Glasgow) Ltd
Printed and bound in Great Britain by Cambridge University Press

To my patients

Contents

Foreword

Thoracic surgery has emerged as one of the most dramatic developments in the history of modern medicine. In a few decades it has emerged from infancy into full and robust adult life and though it is based on the general principles of medicine it has certain features that have rendered to segregate it into special units or contours. Apart from operative treatment of empyema the first real demand for surgery came from the treatment of pulmonary tuberculosis and though happily and hopefully control of that dreaded disease has been largely achieved many of the sanatoria have continued to treat chest disease and developed into important units.

Chest surgery is a multidisciplinary subject. Many individuals—physicians, surgeons, nurses, physiotherapists and ancillary services—cooperate to form a team in a manner that is not always seen in other branches, and here the nursing profession plays a vitally important role in ensuring that the patient is guided through hospital towards recovery and rehabilitation

In this book Mr. Moghissi gives a clear account of the principles and practices involved. Mr. Moghissi is a highly accomplished surgeon who has worked in several units in this country and abroad and is a recognised authority on thoracic surgery. He is now in charge of an admirably equipped unit in Humberside which serves a large population.

The plan of the book starts with a clear account of the anatomy and physiology of the chest and proceeds to descriptions of the disorders and operations that involve the intrathoracic contents. Surgery of the heart, which has become a subject of its own is not considered as it has received a good deal of attention in other works, but the theme of the whole book is towards a practical understanding of the problems involved and it should not only be of great value to nurses but to students and doctors who wish to be more fully acquainted with the subject.

> T. Holmes Sellors,
> D.M., M.Ch., F.R.C.P., F.R.C.S.
> Past President Royal College of Surgeons
> Consultant Surgeon: Middlesex, London
> Chest, National Heart and Harefield Hospitals

Preface

The history of organised nursing since the early days of the Kaiserwerth Deaconesses and the Nightingale school for nurses has seen many developments, of which two have been seminal in the conception of this book. Firstly, nurses have become involved to an ever-increasing degree, not only in nursing care, but more particularly in the total management of patients. Secondly, there has been a trend towards specialisation in nursing, reflecting a similar trend in medicine and surgery: an inevitable consequence of expanding knowledge. My chief objectives in writing this book have been therefore to present an up-to-date volume on thoracic surgery for nurses, embracing the afore-mentioned developments.

In attempting to fulfil these aims I have been led to enter more fully than I believe has been the case hitherto, into the principles and the practice of thoracic surgery as applicable to present-day nursing. Cardiac surgery is not included in this volume. Not that I believe it to be an entirely separate speciality, but because publications on the subject are numerous and because cardiac surgery for nurses requires a volume of its own.

The book is designed primarily for practising thoracic surgical nurses and styled to be understandable to all grades. Nurses in general medicine or surgery will also find this book helpful when dealing with chest patients. In thoracic surgery a number of people in para-medical professions share in the care and treatment of patients; it is hoped that this book will equally be of assistance in the expansion of their understanding of thoracic surgical problems. Finally, for those in training it is hoped that this volume will in Florence Nightingale's own words 'enable the nurse to see what she sees' when observing thoracic surgical patients.

Keyvan Moghissi
1982

Acknowledgements

I wish to express my gratitude to Miss M. Clarke, Director of the Institute of Nursing Studies, Hull University, for writing the chapter on the physiology of respiration, as well as for reading the whole book and making many suggestions and amendments.

My thanks also go to Dr. J. Dyet, Consultant Radiologist, Dr. G. Murtagh, Consultant Anaesthetist and Mrs. E. Johnson, Head of the Physiotherapy Department, all at Castle Hill Hospital, Cottingham, for their respective contributions on radiology, anaesthesia and physiotherapy.

The photographs were prepared by Mr. G. Whitehead, Medical Illustrations Department, Hull Royal Infirmary and Mr. M. Whitlock, Castle Hill Hospital.

The late Mrs C. Lutley was a great stimulus to me in starting the book and she also drew some of the illustrations. I can only acknowledge with sadness her help and encouragement.

It is no exaggeration to say that this book would never have been finished without the constant and painstaking efforts of Mrs. F. M. Strugnell-Roy. Not only has she drawn most of the illustrations and prepared the artwork, but she has also read and corrected the text and supervised the typing of the manuscript.

Many nurses in the Department of Cardio-Thoracic Surgery at Castle Hill Hospital have given me useful practical advice. I am grateful to them all.

Finally, I wish to acknowledge my appreciation of the editorial advice and assistance given to me by Miss Pat Pembroke of Kimpton Medical Publications.

Keyvan Moghissi
1982

Introduction

Thoracic surgery deals essentially with the pathological conditions of the thoracic wall and structures within the thoracic cavity; namely the lungs, heart, great vessels and oesophagus. However, thoracic surgery can at times, extend upwards to the neck and downwards to the abdominal cavity. To illustrate this point, the oesophagus extends from the neck to the stomach, therefore oesophageal surgery may involve the neck, thorax and abdomen.

In considering this and the inclusion of related subjects in a volume of thoracic surgery, this book comprises four parts. The first three deal with thoracic surgery proper. The first part concerns the respiratory system which includes the chest wall, pleura, lungs and the general principles of thoracic surgical nursing. The second part concerns the oesophagus, the third part the diaphragm, mediastinum and its contents. Finally the fourth part comprises several unrelated topics, knowledge of which is indispensable for the practice of thoracic surgery.

Part 1
The Lung and Pleura

This section deals primarily with surgery of the lung and pleura. It appeared reasonable, however, to include a brief anatomical description of the thorax as a whole and the physiology of respiration. The chapters on operations on the lungs, post-operative care and complications of lung surgery contain details relevant to thoracic surgery as a whole. This fact should be borne in mind when reading Parts 2 and 3.

1 Structure of the Thorax

The thoracic walls consist of a bony framework and soft tissues. The sternum in front and the vertebral column behind form the two pillars of this framework held in position and joined by a series of arcuate (bow-shaped) bridges, the ribs. This bony framework forms the anterior, posterior and lateral walls of the thoracic cavity (Fig. 1.1a,b). The inferior surface, or outlet, is formed by a musculo-tendinous structure, the diaphragm, separating the thorax from the abdominal cavity. The superior surface, or inlet, is closed by a fascia separating the thoracic cavity from the neck.

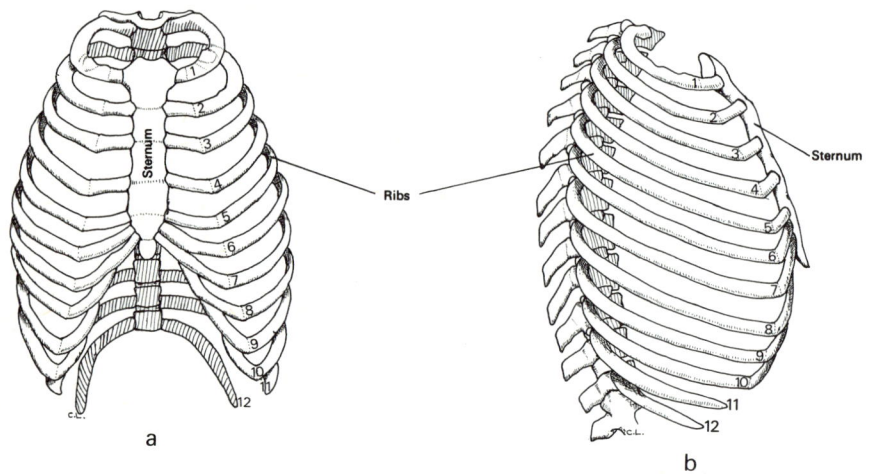

Figure 1.1 Bony framework of the chest: (a) anterior and (b) lateral aspects.

The vertebrae and their intervertebral discs, the ribs and their articulation with the sternum in front and the vertebral column behind provide a thorax well suited to its function. The many pieces of bone and the number of joints involved give a firmness that can withstand external pressure and yet allow changes in volume and movements required for ventilation.

The thoracic cavity is almost oval in shape, somewhat flattened in the middle due to the forward projection of the thoracic vertebrae. There are two lateral compartments enclosed by the ribs on either side and containing the lungs. The middle portion, called the mediastinum, accommodates the heart and the great vessels that emerge from it, the trachea and its division, the thymus and the lymphatic glands (Fig. 1.2a,b).

2

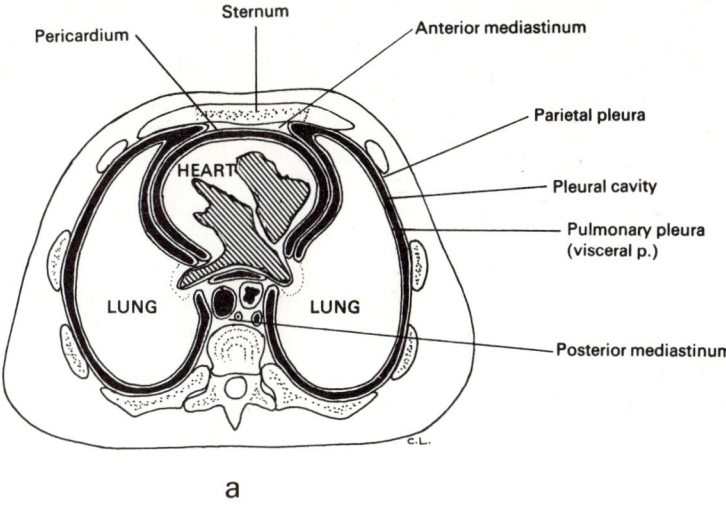

a

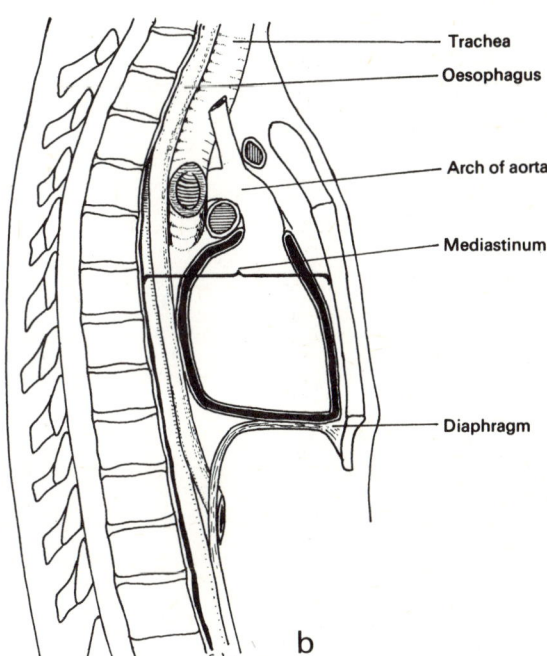

b

Figure 1.2 (a) *Cross-section of the chest illustrating general arrangement of the thoracic cavity.* (b) *Vertical section of the chest showing general arrangement of the mediastinum.*

THE STERNUM

The sternum, or breast-bone, is a flat bone consisting of three parts, the manubrium, the body and the xyphoid process (Fig. 1.3a,b).

The junction of the manubrium and the body is indicated anteriorly by a prominence easily palpable (Angle of Louis). This is an important land mark corresponding laterally to the 2nd costal cartilage. More laterally and slightly lower is the 2nd intercostal space. On the supero-lateral aspects of the manubrium there is one articular surface on each side for the clavicles, forming the sterno-clavicular joints. Between them the supra-sternal notch forms the superior surface of the manubrium. Laterally the manubrium provides articular surfaces for the first, and half of the second, costal cartilages. There are further articular surfaces on the lateral aspects of the body for half of the second and third, to the seventh costal cartilages inclusive. The xyphoid process is the lower part of the sternum and provides an attachment for the diaphragm.

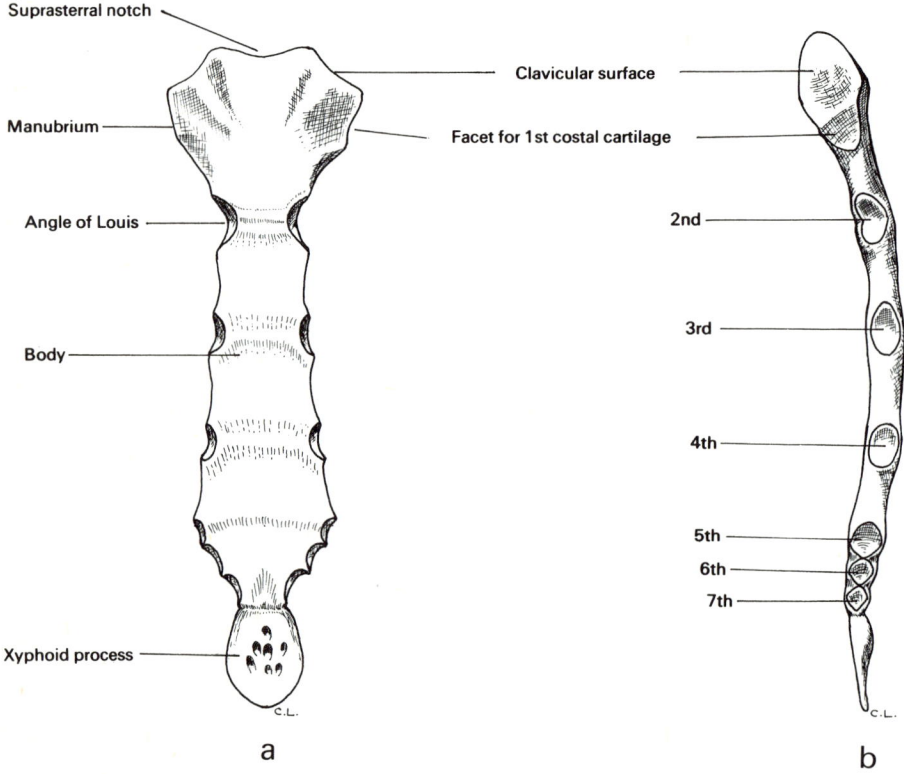

Figure 1.3   Sternum: (a) anterior and (b) lateral aspects.

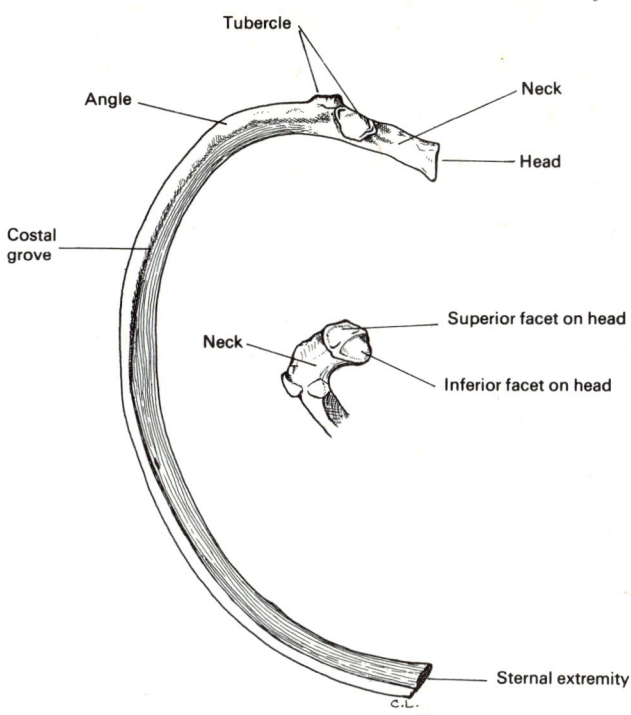

Figure 1.4   Inner aspect of a 'true' rib. Inset illustrates the head and neck.

THE RIBS

There are twelve pairs of ribs (see Fig. 1.1a). The first seven pairs are individually attached to the sternum by costal cartilage; they are known as true ribs. The next three pairs have their costal cartilage inserted into the one above and not directly to the sternum: they are known as false ribs. The remaining two pairs of ribs do not have any anterior attachment, hence their name of floating ribs. The junction between the central cartilage and the sternum is called the costo-chondral joint. It is a synovial joint except for the first pair of ribs where there is a primary cartilaginous joint.

Each rib consists of a head, neck and shaft (Fig. 1.4). The head is situated posteriorly and articulates with the vertebral bodies. Below the head lies a slightly constricted portion called the neck. Connecting the neck with the shaft is the tubercle which has two facets: a medial facet forming a joint with the transverse process of the vertebra and a lateral facet for the attachment of a strong ligament. (This does not apply to the first pair of ribs which articulate with the upper border of the first thoracic vertebra.)

The shaft forms the main body of the rib and has an outer convex inner concave surface, and upper and lower borders. On the lower part of the inner surface there is the costal groove which accommodates the intercostal vein, artery and nerve. Anteriorly the shaft becomes flatter and cartilaginous for its attachment to the sternum.

THE VERTEBRAL COLUMN

The vertebral column forms the central axis of the body. Owing to its structure it has great strength and flexibility and protects the spinal cord contained within the spinal canal. Each vertebra has a body and a posterior vertebral arch (Fig. 1.5a,b). The vertebral body is a thick rounded mass of bone, flat above and below and separated from the adjacent vertebrae by an intervertebral disc. On each side of the body two pairs of costal facets provide articulation with the heads of the ribs. Projecting backwards from the body are two bars of bone, the pedicles. They are connected by the laminae which meet in the midline and terminate as a single backward projection, the spinous process. Above and below the pedicles are two pairs of projections which articulate with the pedicles of adjacent vertebrae. Between the body and the pedicle there is a notch: adjacent notches make the intervertebral foramina through which the spine nerves pass.

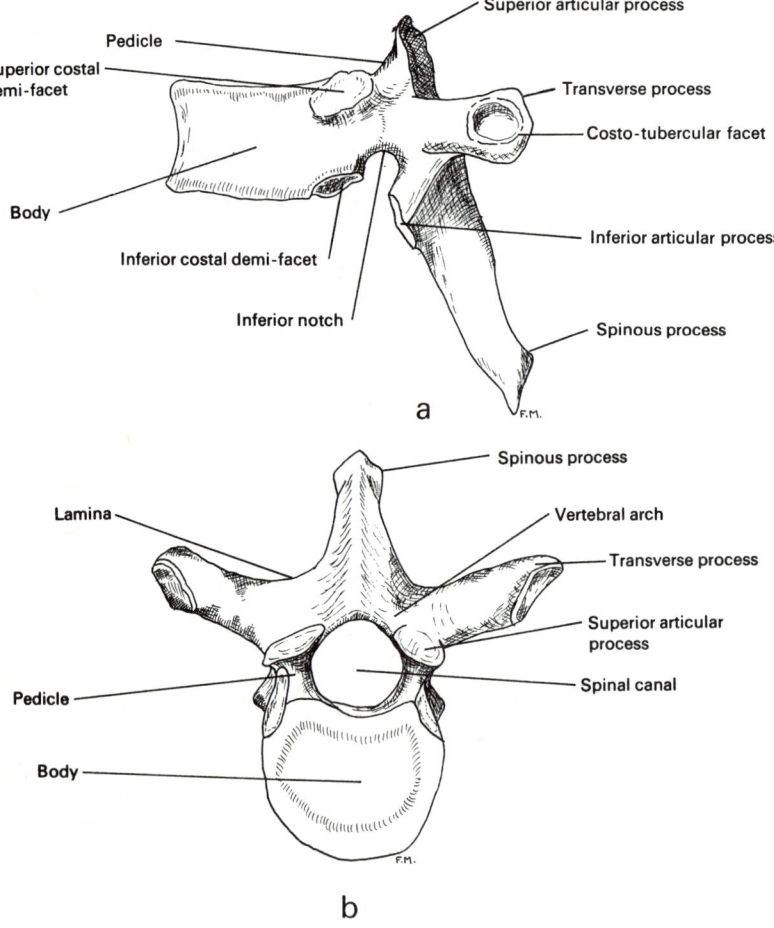

Figure 1.5   Thoracic vertebra: (a) lateral and (b) superior aspects.

THE MUSCLES OF THE THORAX

The main muscles of the thorax are the intercostal muscles and the larger muscles of the body wall. They are anteriorly the pectoralis, the rectus abdominis, the interdigitating serratus anterior and the external oblique muscle (Fig. 1.6a). Posteriorly the trapezius, latissimus dorsi and the rhomboids (major and minor) (Fig. 1.6b).

The intercostal muscles are a series of short muscle fibres running between the edges of adjacent ribs forming a musculo-osseous wall for the thoracic cavity.

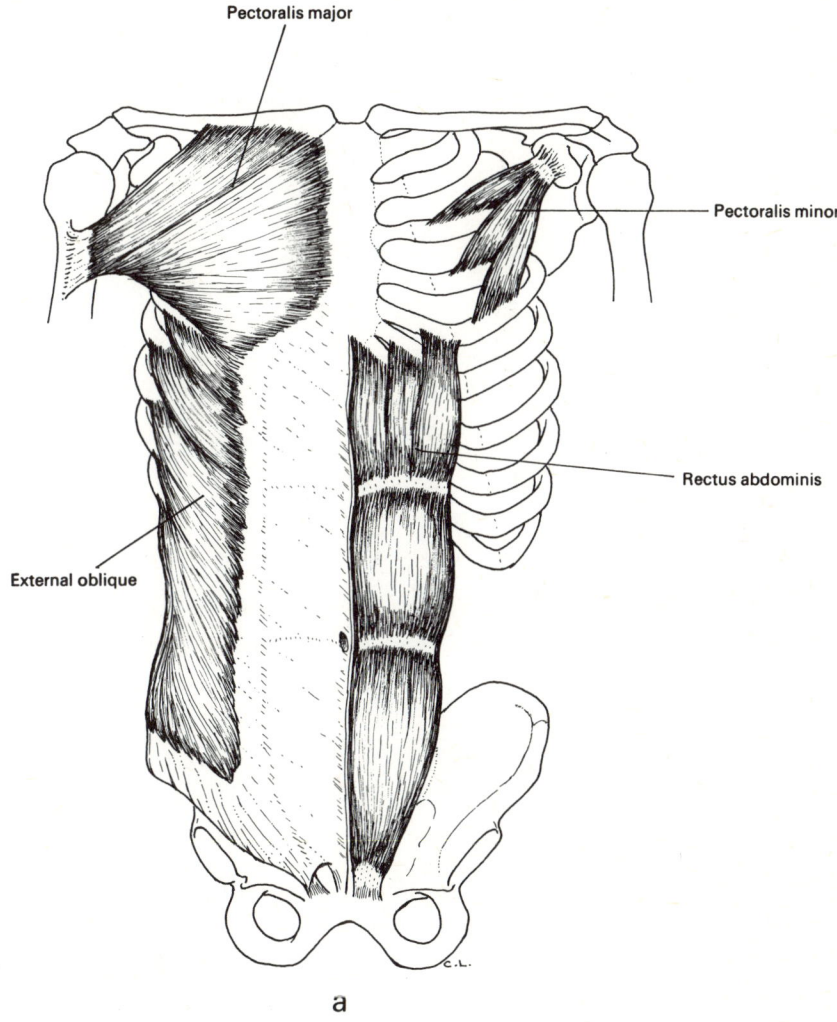

Pectoralis major

Pectoralis minor

Rectus abdominis

External oblique

a

Figure 1.6   Chest muscles: (a) anterior aspect.

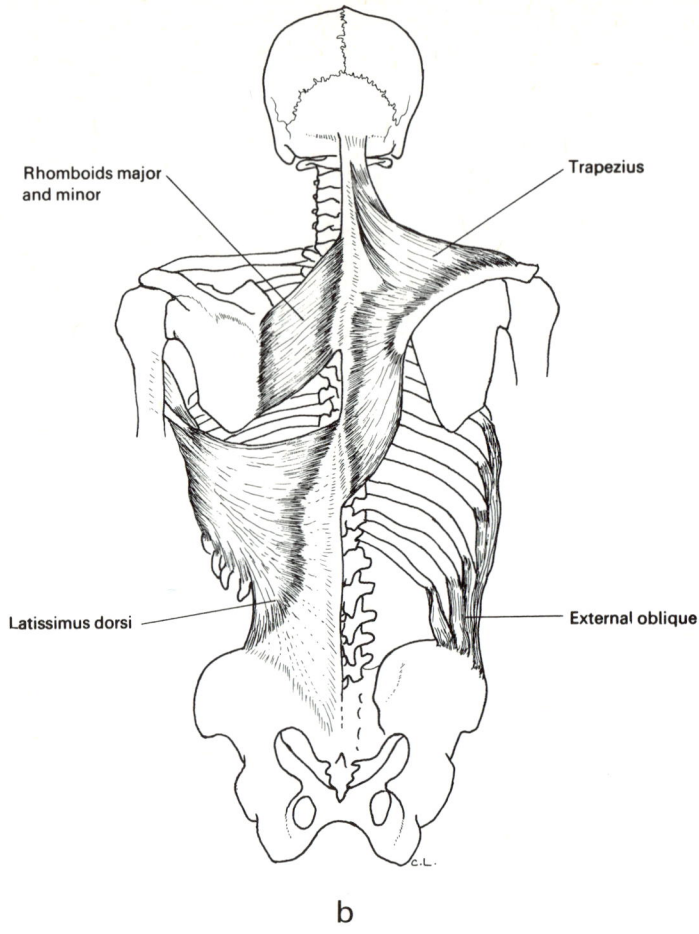

Rhomboids major
and minor

Trapezius

Latissimus dorsi

External oblique

b

Figure 1.6   Chest muscles: (b) posterior aspect.

There are three layers of intercostal muscles forming three sheets of muscles and called the inner layer, the internal layer and the external layer (Fig. 1.7). The external intercostal muscles are directed downwards and forwards from the rib above to the rib below; the internal intercostal muscles are directed downwards and backwards from the rib above to the rib below. Therefore contraction of the external intercostal muscles elevates the anterior end of the rib and carries the sternum forwards while contraction of the internal intercostal muscles pulls the ribs and sternum downwards and backwards.

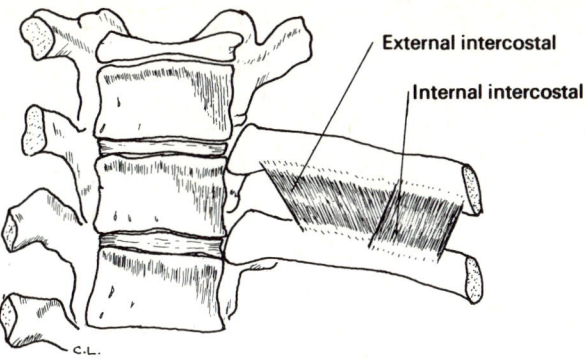

Figure 1.7   Intercostal muscles. (Inner layer not shown.)

2 Respiratory System

The respiratory system is formed by a series of air-conducting tubes leading to the lungs as the main respiratory organs. The air-conducting structures consist of the nose, mouth, larynx, trachea and bronchi.

THE NOSE

The external meatus leads into two nasal cavities which posteriorly open into the naso-pharynx via the internal meatus. The nasal conchae are bony projections on the lateral walls of the nasal cavities. They are covered by a very vascular respiratory mucous membrane which warms, moistens and filters the incoming air.

THE MOUTH

This cavity extends from its external opening on the face to the oro-pharyngeal isthmus behind, where it opens into the pharynx.

THE PHARYNX

Although the pharynx is usually associated with the alimentary tract, it forms part of the respiratory tract in that it is an air duct as well as a food passage. The posterior wall of the pharynx is complete and lies against the vertebral column. Its anterior wall is incomplete and communicates with the nose, mouth and the larynx. The pharynx is therefore usually thought of as naso-pharynx, oro-pharynx and laryngeal pharynx (Fig. 1.8).

Structurally the pharynx is a musculo-membranous tube lined with a mucous membrane, covered by ciliated columnar epithelium (respiratory type) in the naso-pharynx, and stratified squamous epithelium in the oral and laryngeal pharynx. The muscles are striated in type and consist of three constrictors on either side, forming a median raphe on the posterior wall. It is to be noted that the lower portion of the inferior constrictor forms a muscular ring called the crico-pharyngeal muscle acting as a muscular sphincter for the oesophageal inlet. Nerves of the muscles are derived from the vagus and the glossopharyngeal nerves.

THE LARYNX

The larynx is a cylindrical tube formed by a number of cartilages articulating with each other and are covered by small muscles and a mucous membrane (Fig.

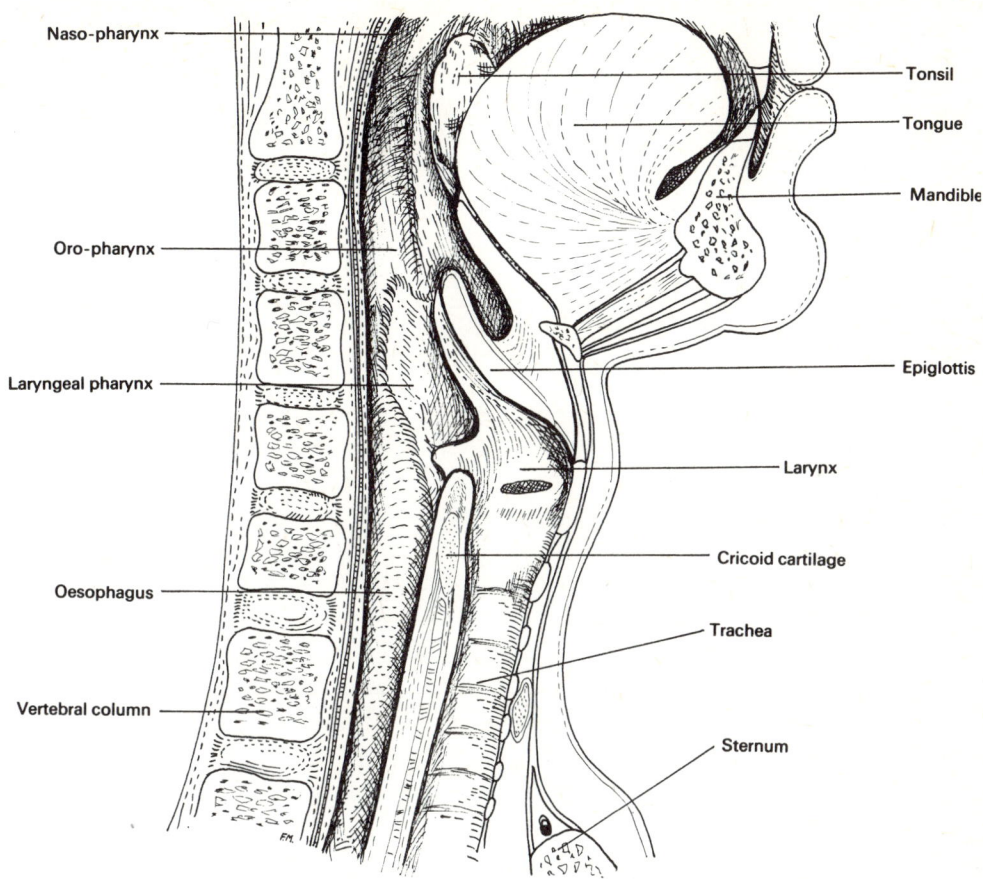

Naso-pharynx

Oro-pharynx

Laryngeal pharynx

Oesophagus

Vertebral column

Tonsil

Tongue

Mandible

Epiglottis

Larynx

Cricoid cartilage

Trachea

Sternum

Figure 1.8   Vertical section of the neck.

1.9a). It opens above into the pharynx through which it communicates with the nose and the mouth. Below, it continues with the trachea. On the inside of each lateral wall there is a shelf-like projection: the vocal cords. Approximation (adduction) of the vocal cords reduces the lumen to a narrow slit, while their retraction (abduction) produces a widening of the opening (Fig. 1.9b). Adduction and abduction of the vocal cords are effected by muscles supplied by the recurrent laryngeal nerves. The cartilaginous foundation of the larynx is the cricoid cartilage, above and in front of which lies the thyroid cartilage forming the Adam's apple. Behind and above the thyroid cartilage is a leaf-shaped cartilage, the epiglottis, which protects the laryngeal opening by folding back over the lumen.

The arytenoids are a pair of small cartilages which articulate with the postero-superior part of the cricoid and to whose vocal processes the vocal cords are attached.

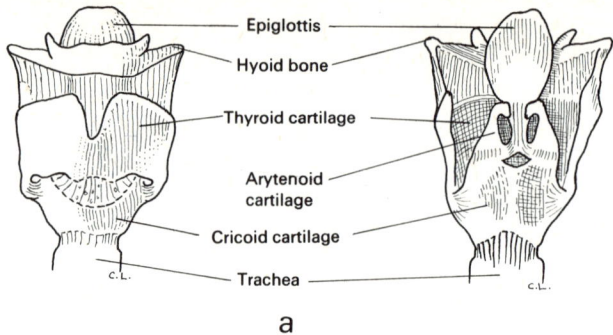

a

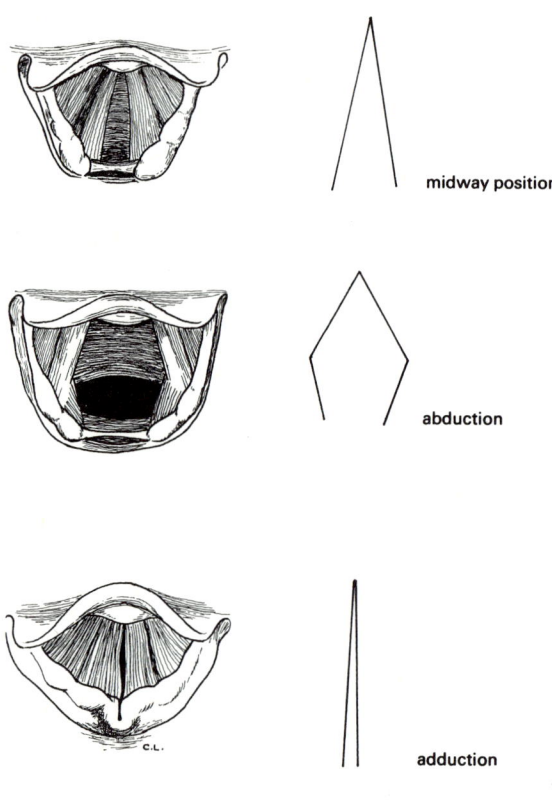

midway position

abduction

adduction

b

Figure 1.9   (a) Anterior (left) and posterior (right) aspects of the larynx. (b) Movement of the vocal cords.

The functions of the larynx are:

1. To protect the trachea and bronchial trees from food and other particles.
2. To moisten and filter inspired air and to allow effective coughing.

In addition the larynx plays an important role in the production and quality of the voice.

THE TRACHEA

The trachea (Fig. 1.10) extends from the base of the larynx to its division into the left and right bronchi. The division is shown internally by a mid-line ridge known as the carina. Externally the trachea ends behind the sternum at the junction of the manubrium and the body. It is a 12 to 14 cm long fibro-cartilaginous tube whose patency is maintained by 16 to 20 C-shaped rings of hyaline cartilage interfaced with fibro-muscular tissues. The gap in the cartilage is posterior. The trachea is lined with ciliated columnar epithelium.

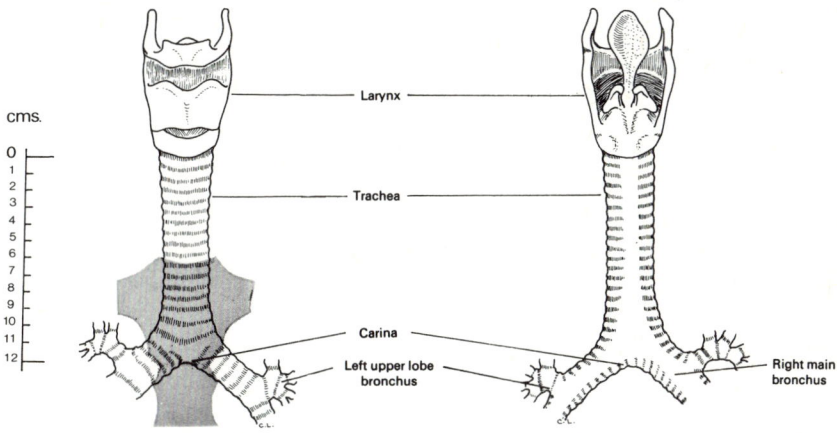

Figure 1.10   Anterior (left) and posterior (right) aspects of the larynx and trachea.

THE BRONCHI

The bronchi (Fig. 1.11) extends from the carina to the hilum of the lung. Basically their structure is similar to that of the trachea except that the cartilage rings are complete. The left bronchus is longer and more horizontal than the right, therefore inhaled foreign bodies are more likely to enter the right bronchus. The right main bronchus subdivides into the upper middle and lower bronchi for the upper, middle and lower lobes of the right lung. The left main bronchus subdivides into an upper and lower lobe bronchus for the upper and lower lobes of the left lung. The upper lobe bronchus on the left also subdivides into a lingular bronchus. Each lobar bronchus subdivides into segmental bronchi, as illustrated in Figure 1.11.

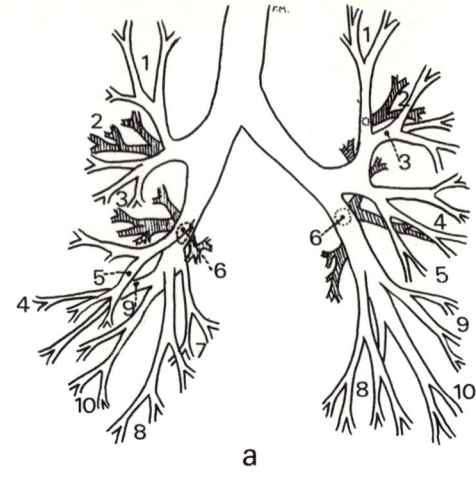

a

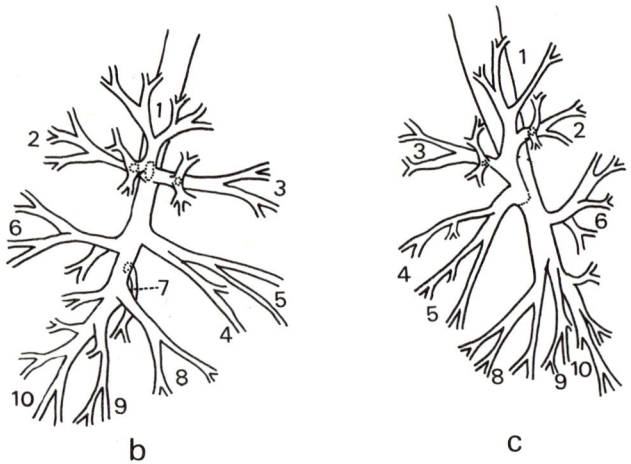

b   c

Figure 1.11   (a) Anterior, (b) right lateral and (c) left lateral aspects of the bronchial tree. (1) = Apical segmental bronchus; (2) = Posterior segmental bronchus; (3) = Anterior segmental bronchus; (4) = Lateral segmental bronchus; (5) = Medial segmental bronchus; (6) = Apical bronchus; (7) = Medial basal segmental bronchus; (8) = Anterior segmental bronchus; (9) = Lateral segmental bronchus; (10) = Posterior segmental bronchus.

LEFT BRONCHIAL TREE: Left upper lobe *bronchus subdivides into* (1), (2) *and* (3); Lingular *bronchus subdivides into* (4) *and* (5); Lower *bronchus subdivides into* (6), (8), (9) *and* (10).

RIGHT BRONCHIAL TREE: Right upper lobe *subdivides into* (1), (2) *and* (3); Middle lobe *subdivides into* (4) *and* (5); Lower lobe *bronchus subdivides into* (6), (7), (8), (9) *and* (10).

The bronchi divide into the bronchioles, the larger of which have the same structures as the bronchi and the trachea. As the bronchioles decrease in size, so does the amount of cartilage until there is only a muscular tube lined with ciliated epithelium. The bronchioles finally divide into several alveolar ducts leading to the alveoli. The alveoli are made of a single layer of epithelium and are surrounded by capillaries from the pulmonary circulation. The air containing oxygen and the capillaries containing blood are thus separated by a thin membrane called the alveolo-endothelial membrane.

THE LUNGS

They are two cone-shaped organs (Figs 1.12 and 1.13) occupying the lateral compartments of the thoracic cavity. They extend from 2 to 3 cm above the first rib to the diaphragm. Anteriorly they are bound by the sternum, the first five pairs of ribs and intercostal muscles. The ribs and intercostal muscles also form the lateral and posterior boundaries around the lung. The heart, the great vessels and oesophagus lie medially, the diaphragm inferiorly. Superiorly a fascial membrane separates the lungs from the neck structures. The main bronchus, pulmonary vessels, lymphatics and nerves enter the lungs medially on the inner surface. This area is known as the hilum and is the root of the lung.

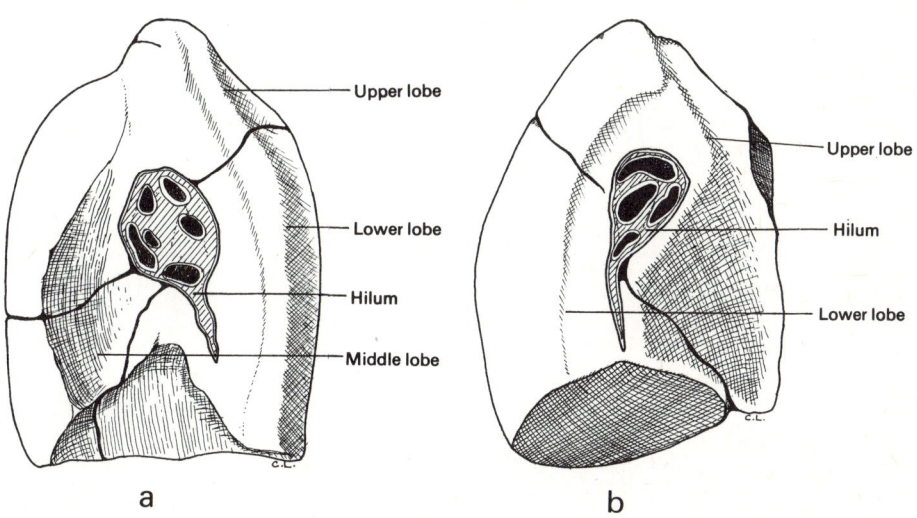

Figure 1.12   Mediastinal (medial) aspect of the (a) right and (b) left lung.

The lungs are covered with a serous membrane, the pleura, which reflects back on itself at the hilum to line the interior wall of the chest. This reflection forms a sac known as the pleural cavity (Fig. 1.2a, p. 3). The layer adherent to the external surface of the lung is called the visceral pleura, while the reflected layer which covers the chest wall and upper diaphragmatic surface is called the parietal pleura.

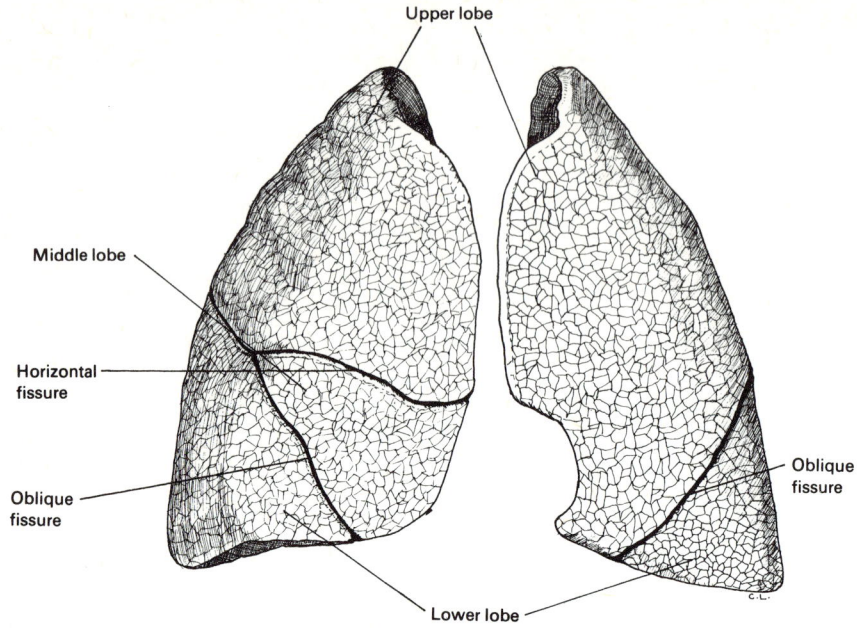

Figure 1.13   Anterior aspect of the lungs.

Fissures divide the lungs into lobes. A fissure is a deep cleft whose walls are lined by visceral pleura. The left lung has one fissure, namely the oblique fissure, separating the upper and the lower lobe. The right lung has an oblique fissure which separates the upper and the lower lobe and a horizontal one lying between the upper and the middle lobe. The latter is often incomplete. Each lobe is supplied by its own bronchus (see Fig. 1.11). The right lung has three lobes while the left has two. Lobes are then subdivided into segments. Both upper lobes have an apical, anterior and posterior segment. The left lung has no middle lobe, but the left upper lobe has an additional lingular segment divided into a superior and an inferior segment. The right lung has a middle lobe which in turn contains a medial and a lateral segment. Each lower lobe has an apical, posterior, anterior, medial and lateral segment. On the left side the medial segment is absent because of the position of the heart.

Blood supply to the lungs has a dual purpose:

1. The pulmonary arterial supply, with a total flow equal to cardiac output (4 to 5 litre/min), carries venous blood from the right ventricle. This blood flow does not supply the lung parenchyma but is exposed to the alveolo-endothelial membrane and thus passes through the lung to be oxygenated. The main trunk of the pulmonary artery divides into right and left pulmonary arteries directed to each lung respectively. In each lung the artery gives off branches to supply each segment.

2. The bronchial arteries supply the bronchial tree with oxygenated blood.

Lymphatic drainage from the lungs reaches the hilar glands. They are nodes in the path of the lymphatics which continue along the bronchi and trachea to the

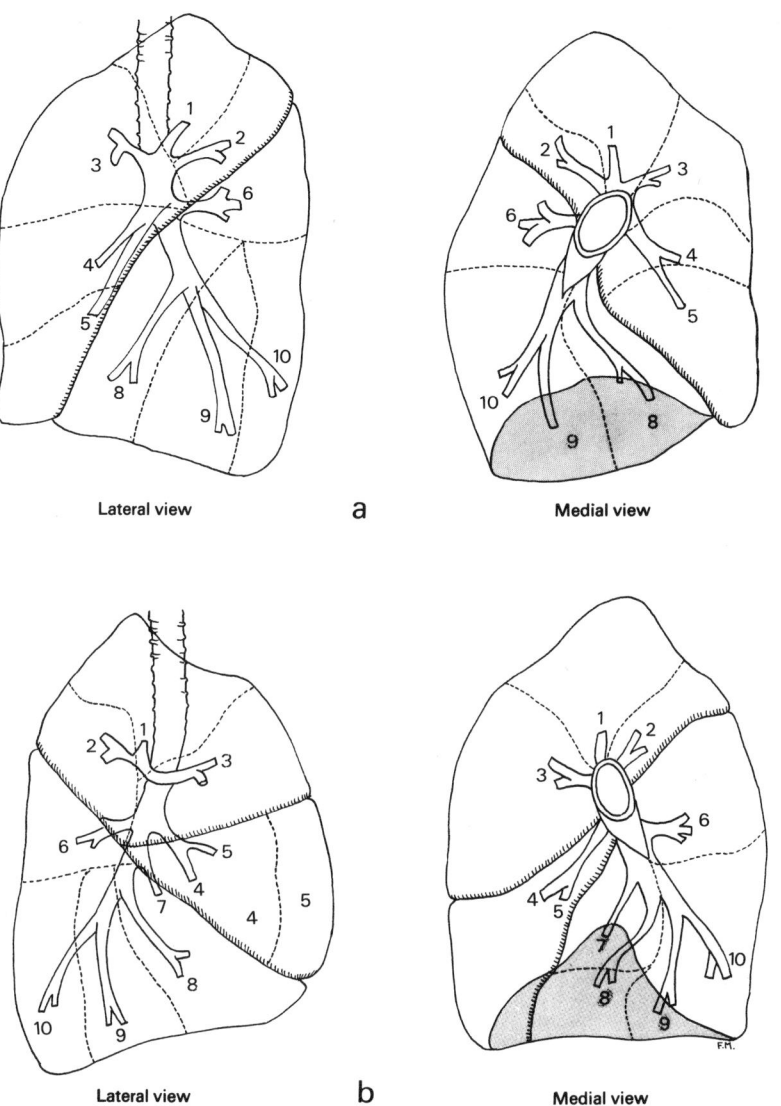

Figure 1.14 (a) Left and (b) right broncho-pulmonary segments.

tracheo-bronchial nodes, then to the paratracheal glands (around the trachea). The lymph is then drained upwards to reach the scalene nodes (groups of glands in the supra-clavicular fossa).

In the description of the anatomy of the airways and the lungs (p. 15), reference is made to the branching of the bronchi and the division of the lung parenchyma into lobes and segments. A portion of the lung receiving a segmental bronchus and segmental vessels is known as a broncho-pulmonary segment (Fig. 1.14). In clinical work it is customary to indicate the precise site of the pathology in an area of the lung. This is important as some diseases appear to have a preferential site (e.g. pulmonary tuberculosis in the apical and posterior segment of the upper lobes, lung abscesses in the apical segment of the lower lobe). Each lung is divided into ten segments receiving:

1. A branch of the pulmonary artery, referred to as a segmental artery.

2. A bronchial division, called segmental bronchus and providing ventilation. (N.B. The final branchings of the segmental bronchus are the terminal bronchi and alveoli.)

3. One or two branches of the pulmonary veins, called segmental veins. They converge to form lobar veins which then join to form two major pulmonary veins on each side, which deliver the oxygenated blood to the left atrium.

The lungs are made of bronchial tubes, blood vessels, connective tissues and a mass of alveoli. The functional unit of the lungs is the alveolus with its capillaries derived from the ramifications of pulmonary arteries and veins. The air-conducting system (respiratory tract) carries the air to and from the interior of the alveoli while the pulmonary vessels carry the blood to and from the exterior of the alveoli. It is at the alveolar level that air and blood are in close contact separated only by the thin alveolo-endothelial membrane which allows the exchange of gases (oxygen and carbon dioxide). This exchange is the essence of respiration.

3 Physiology of Respiration

Tissue cells depend upon energy to (1) maintain their structural integrity, (2) carry out their specialised functions and (3) replicate themselves. The energy they use is obtained from the combination of oxygen with a food substance such as glucose, glycerol or a fatty acid during a series of chemical transformations which ensure that energy is released gradually. The end products of this process, which is called internal respiration, are water and carbon dioxide. It is dependent upon a constant level of oxygen and carbon dioxide both within the cell itself and within its environment. As intracellular oxygen is used up so it must be replaced by a continuing supply to the cell. Similarly, carbon dioxide must be continually removed as it is produced in order to maintain constant levels of these gases. These important gases are carried in the bloodstream.

External respiration is the process by which interchange of gases takes place between the blood and the air within the alveoli of the lungs. The act of breathing ensures an interchange of gases between the alveolar air and the atmospheric air. Table 1 shows the composition of atmospheric air and alveolar air. It can be seen from this that whilst the two are similar in composition the relative proportion of constituent gases differs slightly, there being slightly less oxygen (O_2) and more carbon dioxide (CO_2) in the alveolar air. The composition of the alveolar air is affected by the diffusion of gases into and out of the pulmonary capillaries.

Table 1 Composition of atmospheric and alveolar air

	Atmospheric air* (mm. Hg)	Alveolar air (mm. Hg)
N_2	597.0 (78.62%)	569.0 (74.9%)
O_2	159.0 (20.84%)	104.0 (13.6%)
CO_2	0.3 (0.04%)	40.0 (5.3%)
H_2O	3.7 (0.50%)	47.0 (6.2%)
Total	760.0 (100.00%)	760.0 (100.0%)

* On an average cool, clear day.

RESPIRATORY TRACT

A column of air within the respiratory tract separates the alveolar air from the atmospheric air and acts to keep the composition of alveolar air remarkably constant in spite of the different composition of inspired and expired air (see

Table 2 Composition of inspired and expired air

	Humidified air (mm. Hg)	Expired air (mm. Hg)
N_2	563.4 (74.09 %)	566.0 (74.5 %)
O_2	149.3 (19.67 %)	120.0 (15.7 %)
CO_2	0.3 (0.04 %)	27.0 (3.6 %)
H_2O	47.0 (6.20 %)	47.0 (6.2 %)
Total	760.0 (100.0 %)	760.0 (100.0 %)

Table 2). On inspiration the air becomes warm and is saturated with water vapour due to contact with the mucous membrane of the respiratory tract. By the time the air reaches the alveoli, it has acquired the temperature of the blood and is freed from all contained large particulate matter. Hairs in the nostrils strain out most of the particles which are larger than $10\,\mu$ in diameter. Particles between 10 and $2\,\mu$ in diameter fall on the lining of the trachea and bronchi where they initiate bronchial constriction and coughing. Such particles are moved away from the lung toward the oropharynx by the action of the cilia which beat 600–1000 times per minute in a co-ordinated way, moving particles at a rate of $16\,mm/minute$. Small particles of less than $2\,\mu$ in diameter reach the alveoli and are ingested by macrophages. Irritants such as cigarette smoke can increase mucus production from the lining of the respiratory tract. This can drain into the lower respiratory tract and cause obstruction or interfere with the diffusion of gases.

The alveoli form the gas-exchanging surface of the lung. Each alveolus is lined with epithelium in which there are phagocytes and cells which secrete surfactant. Outside the epithelium lies the endothelium lining the capillaries of the pulmonary circulation. In some of the alveoli the basement membrane of the epithelium and the endothelium are fused together, but in most there is interstitial tissue containing fibrils, elastic fibres and fibroblasts. Pores or openings in the alveolar walls connect the lumen of adjacent alveoli and allow direct movement of gases, liquids and infection. Alveoli have a very large surface area allowing diffusion of gases in and out of the pulmonary circulation.

BREATHING

During inspiration, when the thoracic cavity increases in volume, the alveoli expand. The detergent-like surfactant helps the alveolar expansion by reducing the surface tension of the lining of the alveolus which would otherwise resist this 'ballooning'. During expiration, the thoracic cavity is reduced in volume and the walls of the alveoli collapse down, helped by the elastic fibres in the wall. Surfactant helps to prevent complete collapse of the alveoli and also helps to prevent pulmonary oedema.

Breathing comprises inspiration and expiration. Inspiration consists of the expansion of the volume of the chest cavity brought about by the contraction of the external intercostal muscles and the diaphragm. The external intercostals lift the ribs and expand the anterior–posterior diameter of the chest. Contraction of the dome shaped diaphragm, which separates the thoracic and abdominal cavities, causes it to flatten down into the abdominal cavity acting like a piston to draw air into the thoracic cavity. In quiet respiration the action of the diaphragm accounts for 75 % of the change in intrathoracic volume. Expansion of the thorax brings about the expansion of the volume of the lungs because of the intimate relationship between the chest wall and the lungs. Increasing the volume of the lungs reduces the pressure of gas within them to a level below atmospheric pressure (i.e. negative pressure) and so air flows from the atmosphere into the lungs.

Expiration follows due to relaxation of the respiratory muscles, elastic recoil of tissue and upward pressure of the abdominal contents. A more active process, in asthma for example, may involve the contraction of the internal intercostal muscles. The volume of the chest and lungs is reduced, increasing the pressure of gas within the lungs to above atmospheric pressure and air is forced from the respiratory tract into the atmosphere.

The intimate relationship between the lungs and the chest wall is maintained by the two pleural membranes, the visceral pleura which invests the lungs and the parietal pleura which lines the thoracic cavity. These are serous membranes which in health are in contact with one another and slide smoothly over one another during breathing. This is due to reduced surface tension which is brought about by the serous fluid which acts in a similar way to that of water between two glass slides (i.e. one can slide them together but it is difficult to pull them apart). There is a potential space between the two membranes called the pleural cavity, and there is negative pressure in this cavity which is essential for the expansion of the lungs on inspiration.

The pleural fluid is a filtrate from capillaries in the parietal pleura. Drainage of this fluid is into the visceral capillaries and the lymphatics of the visceral and parietal membranes. Excessive pleural fluid (a pleural effusion) can be caused by changes in capillary pressure relationships which would cause oedema elsewhere; heart failure is an example. Pneumothorax or air in the the pleural cavity leads to collapse of the lung, since it breaks the airtight seal around the lung and leads to positive pressure within the pleural cavity (see also Chapters 6 and 9).

RESPIRATORY GAS VOLUMES

The volume of air which is breathed in and out during normal quiet breathing is known as the tidal volume and it averages about 500 ml in a normal adult. If the individual breathes in as deeply as possible after a normal breath, the amount taken in is known as the inspiratory reserve volume. By asking an individual to exhale as much air as possible after a normal expiration we can obtain a volume of air known as the expiratory reserve volume. Inhaling as deeply as possible, followed by forcible exhalation, gives us the vital capacity. It is impossible to remove all the air from the lungs and the amount left after complete forcible expiration is known as the residual volume. These relationships are shown in Table 3 and further explained on p. 29. The respiratory rate is the number of breaths per minute and the minute volume is the amount of air inhaled in one minute. Not all air which is inspired during breathing is available for gas exchange within the alveoli. Approximately 150 ml of the 500 ml tidal volume lies in the 'anatomical dead space', i.e. within the nose, pharynx, larynx, trachea and

Table 3 **Relationship between inspiratory reserve volume (IRV), tidal volume (TV) expiratory reserve volume (ERV), residual volume (RV)**

		Volume (litres) Men	Women	
Vital capacity	IRV	3.3	1.9	Inspiratory capacity
	TV	0.5	0.5	
	ERV	1.0	0.7	Functional residual capacity
	RV	1.2	1.1	
Total lung capacity		6.0	4.2	

Respiratory minute volume (rest): 6 litres/min.
Alveolar ventilation (rest): 4.2 litres/min.
Maximal voluntary ventilation (BTPS): 125–170 litres/min.
Timed vital capacity: 83 % of total in 1 sec; 97 % in 3 sec.
Work of quiet breathing: 0.5 kg⁻m/min.
Maximal work of breathing: 10 kg⁻m/breath.

bronchi, where no exchange of gases with the blood takes place. Other important functions do, however, take place in these structures. The 'physiological dead space' is a term used in disease states where there may be no gas interchange between some alveoli and the bloodstream. The alveolar ventilation volume is the volume of air reaching the alveoli in one minute. It is calculated by subtracting the dead space volume from the tidal volume, giving us the alveolar exchange volume in one breath and then multiplying that by the respiratory rate. For example:

	Minute volume	*Alveolar ventilation volume*
Individual A	500 ml × 16 = 8000 ml	(500 − 150) × 16 = 5600 ml
Individual B	250 ml × 32 = 8000 ml	(250 − 150) × 32 = 3200 ml

It is possible to take so many shallow breaths that air is never exchanged in the alveoli, i.e. panting, and can be seen in a dog who pants not to exchange gases but to cool himself.

ACTIVITIES WHICH ALTER THE RESPIRATORY PATTERN

The oropharynx is a structure which is common to both the respiratory and the alimentary tract. Below the oropharynx the two tracts separate, as it is vital that food, drink and vomitus are prevented from entering the respiratory tract. On swallowing, respiration is inhibited. The larynx is brought upwards and forwards so that it is closed off by the epiglottis. Reflex contraction of the adductor muscles within the larynx closes the vocal cords thus closing the glottis. When patients are unconscious, the muscles controlling the vocal cords may be paralysed allowing vomit or excessive secretion to enter the trachea. This may cause aspiration, pneumonia or oedema. If the abductor muscles are paralysed but the adductors are not, the latter contract unopposed, closing the vocal cords and causing inspiratory stridor.

Voice production occurs during slow expiration and is caused by the controlled expulsion of air through the contracted, vibrating vocal cords. Its pitch is determined by the length and tension of the cords. The voice is also affected by resonance in the air passages of the nose and the sinuses, whilst the different sounds we make in speech (phonemes) are determined by the shape of the mouth, lips and the position of the tongue. Loudness is controlled by the force of expired air.

Coughing consists of forced expiration of air against the glottis, which is initially closed. Strong contraction of the abdominal and respiratory muscles increases the intrathoracic pressure. The glottis suddenly opens, producing an explosive outflow of air under high velocity. Sneezing is the forced expiration of air with an open glottis. It is a reflex response to irritation of the nasal mucosa as we realise when we have a cold. Coughing is the response to irritation of receptors in the mucosal wall of the trachea or large bronchi.

Warning of the act of vomiting consists of nausea and salivation. The glottis closes and the breath is held in mid-inspiration. Muscles of the abdominal wall contract and with the chest held in a fixed position, this increases the intra-abdominal pressure and vomiting occurs.

PROPERTIES OF GASES

Before discussing the exchange of gases within the lungs, it is necessary to mention some of the properties of gases. Unlike liquids, gases always expand to fill the volume of the container. An identical number of molecules of a gas will exert greater pressure in a small rather than large container. As with liquids and solids, the volume occupied by a gas at a constant pressure expands as its temperature increases, but if the volume is held constant then its pressure increases as the temperature rises. Therefore in referring to gas pressures in relation to respiratory physiology there is always an implicit assumption that temperature is held constant. The volume occupied by a given number of gas molecules at a particular temperature and pressure is the same whether it is one gas or a mixture of gases.

In order to understand respiratory physiology we need to know the pressure exerted by oxygen (O_2) and carbon dioxide (CO_2) within a mixture of gases. This is called the partial pressure (P) of the gas and it is equal to the pressure exerted by the total mixture × the percentage volume which the gas of interest occupies within the gas mixture. As an example we can calculate the partial pressure of oxygen and carbon dioxide in air. The composition of dry air at sea level is given in Table 1, p. 19. At sea level, the pressure exerted by air is 760 mm Hg. Therefore the partial pressure of oxygen (PO_2) is $0.21 \times 760 = 160$ mm Hg, whilst the PCO_2 is $0.004 \times 760 = 0.3$ mm Hg.

Gas molecules always diffuse or move from an area of high to low pressure, evenly distributing themselves. Suppose we placed two gases separated from one another by a barrier within a container. If the two gases were different from one another (e.g. one being oxygen and the other carbon dioxide) when the barrier between the two was removed we would eventually obtain a gas in which the carbon dioxide and oxygen molecules were evenly distributed throughout. Diffusion of a gas, i.e. the movement of molecules of a gas, can take place through a semi-permeable membrane such as a capillary wall.

EXTERNAL RESPIRATION AND GAS TRANSPORT
TO AND FROM THE TISSUE

In the alveoli, because the partial pressure of O_2 (PO_2) in the alveolar air is greater than the PO_2 in the plasma of the pulmonary capillaries, O_2 molecules diffuse down the pressure gradient from the alveolus into the plasma. Carbon dioxide molecules diffuse in the opposite direction, since the PCO_2 in the plasma is greater than the PCO_2 in the alveolar air.

For the diffusion of gases it is the partial pressure exerted by the gas in simple solution within the plasma which is of prime importance although the quantity of gas carried in this form is totally inadequate to cope with tissue needs. In the blood, O_2 combines with haemoglobin (Hb) and CO_2 goes through a series of chemical reactions. This increases the total amount of these gases which can be carried in the blood seventy-fold in the case of oxygen and seventeen-fold in the case of carbon dioxide.

ALVEOLAR DIFFUSION OF OXYGEN
AND ITS CARRIAGE IN THE BLOOD

The partial pressure of oxygen in the alveolar air is 100 mm Hg, whilst the PO_2 in the venous blood arriving at the alveolar capillary is 40 mm Hg. O_2 diffuses across the alveolar and capillary membrane into the plasma. It dissolves in the plasma but most of it diffuses through the membrane of the red blood cells where it combines with haemoglobin, in a process called oxygenation. Most of the O_2 from the plasma combines with haemoglobin, but the residual dissolved gas in arterial blood leaving the lungs is at a pressure of 100 mm Hg, i.e. in equilibrium with alveolar PO_2. At standard temperature and pressure (760 mm Hg and 0°C) there are about 20 ml of O_2 bound to Hb and 0.3 ml O_2 in solution in every 100 ml of blood. Haemoglobin has an affinity with O_2 which it carries in a fairly loose combination, readily giving it up to the plasma as the plasma PO_2 falls on reaching tissues which are being supplied with O_2. An increase in dissolved CO_2 or hydrogen ions (H^+) in the vicinity of haemoglobin reduces its capacity to carry O_2 as does an increase in temperature. Actively metabolising tissue which is using O_2 will not only be releasing CO_2 and hydrogen ions (see p. 25), but will also have an increased temperature. Oxygen is therefore readily given up to such tissue from the Hb. The affinity of Hb for O_2 and its combination with it and release of O_2 is normally described by means of an oxygen dissociation curve (Fig. 1.15).

At the tissue, the PO_2, in the tissue fluid is low compared with that in arterial blood. O_2 diffuses from the plasma into the tissue and from the red cell into the plasma in a reversal of the process which took place in the lungs.

DIFFUSION OF CARBON DIOXIDE
AND ITS TRANSPORT IN THE BLOOD

The carriage of CO_2 in the blood is rather more complex than the carriage of O_2. At the tissues the partial pressure of dissolved CO_2 in the plasma is lower than that in the tissue fluid. CO_2 molecules therefore diffuse down the concentration gradient from the tissue fluid into the plasma. They also diffuse into the red

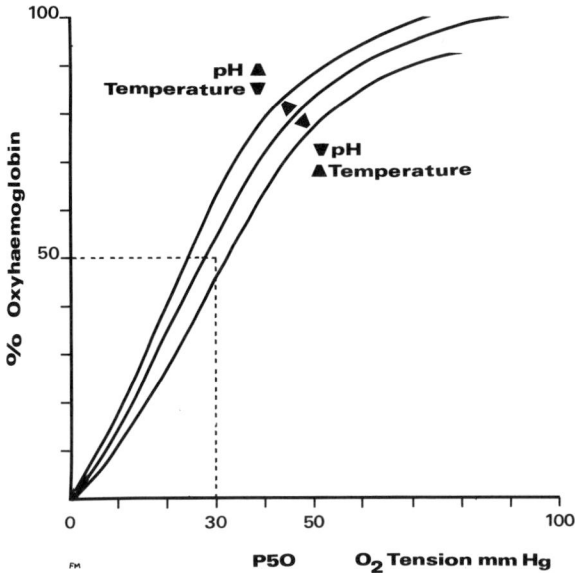

Figure 1.15   Normal oxygen-haemoglobin dissociation curve showing the effects on oxygen affinity of changes in pH and temperature.

blood cell. Within the red blood cell, CO_2 combines chemically with water (H_2O) under the influence of the enzyme carbonic anhydrase to form carbonic acid (H_2CO_3). Carbonic acid then tends to dissociate into a hydrogen ion (H^+) and a bicarbonate ion (HCO_3^-). Carbonic anhydrase is essential to this reaction which takes place very rapidly if the enzyme is present but much too slowly to be physiologically important in the absence of the enzyme. If all the hydrogen ions were allowed free they would alter the pH of the blood considerably, rendering it highly acid. Therefore most of the ions are either combined with a part of the haemoglobin molecule within the red blood cell (RBC), or with protein molecules in the plasma (i.e. the plasma proteins which act as buffers). The removal of the O_2 molecules from the Hb is aided by the combination of H^+ and Hb. The bicarbonate ions HCO_3^- are alkaline, and they diffuse from the RBC into the plasma. Chloride ions (Cl^-) tend to diffuse into the red blood cell (the so-called chloride shift) maintaining the balance of negatively charged ions inside and outside the red blood cell. Some of the CO_2 which diffuses into the RBC combines with the amino part of the haemoglobin and of the protein molecules in the plasma, forming carbamino compounds.

In each 100 ml of venous blood we find 52.7 ml of CO_2, of which 3.0 ml is in simple solution, 3.4 ml is carried as carbamino compounds and 46.3 ml are carried as HCO_3^-.

In the alveolar air the PCO_2 is 40 mm Hg whilst the PCO_2 in the venous blood arriving at the lungs is 46 mm Hg. CO_2 therefore diffuses from the plasma to the alveolar air. O_2 entering the red blood cell recombines with Hb and a reverse of the reactions which occurred in the tissue takes place under the action of carbonic anhydrase. The chemical equation describing this process is:

$$HCO_3^- + H^+ \rightleftharpoons H_2CO_3 \rightleftharpoons H_2O + CO_2$$

Deep respirations cause a reduction in alveolar PCO_2. In turn this is reflected by a decrease in plasma bicarbonate. A build up of tissue or alveolar PCO_2 leads to an increase in plasma bicarbonate and hydrogen ions. These two conditions are called hypocapnia and hypercapnia respectively. Short-term changes which maintain the pH homeostasis of the blood can be brought about by changes in alveolar ventilation rates, but long-term adjustment to maintain the constant pH of the blood is a function of the kidney.

PERFUSION (Pulmonary circulation)

The (venous) blood from the right ventricle is ejected into the pulmonary artery and eventually reaches the pulmonary arterial capillaries. The cardiac output of 5 litres per minute (in adults) allows sufficient blood to go through the pulmonary circulation for oxygenation.

Oxygenation occurs at alveolo-capillary level. The oxygenated blood is then transported by the pulmonary veins to the left atrium. The circulating blood transports the oxygen in the form of oxyhaemoglobin to all tissues and organs. The oxygen is then released from the haemoglobin and the reduced haemoglobin is returned to the heart and thence to the lungs to be re-oxygenated.

CONTROL OF RESPIRATION BY THE NERVOUS SYSTEM

Respiratory centres in the brain stem control respiration (Fig. 1.16), acting through motor nerves to the effector organs, which are in this case the muscles of respiration. Control is based upon information received from receptor organs through sensory nerves. Influences from the cerebral cortex also act upon the brain stem, modifying the action of the respiratory centres.

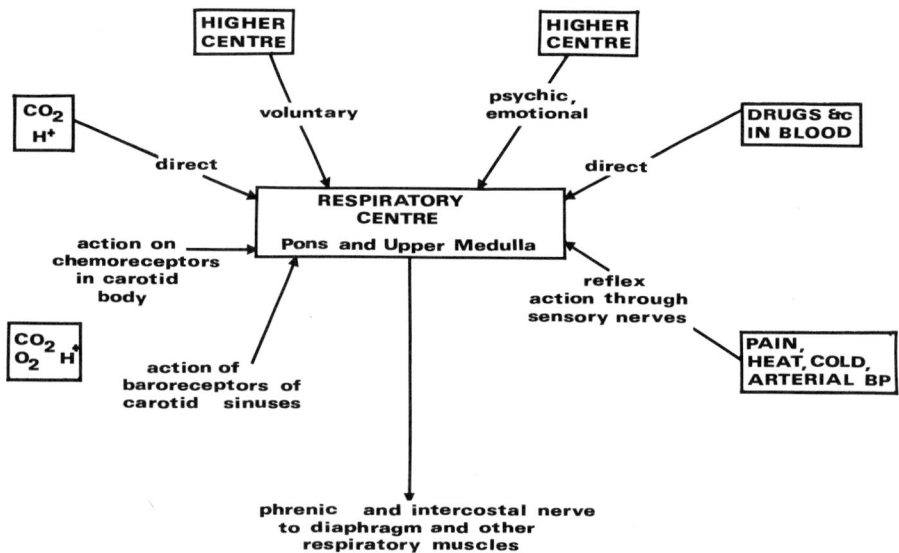

Figure 1.16   Control of respiration.

Inspiration and expiration depend upon rhythmic contraction and relaxation of the respiratory muscles. The diaphragm is innervated by the phrenic nerve and the intercostal muscles by the intercostal nerves. Control is exerted by neurones in the medulla which are said to form an inspiratory and an expiratory centre. The inspiratory centre has the dominant effect. The neurones of the inspiratory centre fire rhythmically to initiate contraction of the inspiratory muscles, at the same time causing inhibition of the expiratory muscles and of the expiratory centre. In turn the expiratory centre inhibits the inspiratory centre when it fires.

Neurones in the pons also participate in the control of respiration, influencing the medullary neurones. There seem to be two sets of neurones within the pons, one set is called the apneustic centre and it acts to smooth and regularise the firing of the inspiratory neurones of the medulla. The other centre is the pneumotoxic centre which influences the rate of firing of the medullary neurones and thus the rate of respiration.

In order to maintain homeostatis these centres are responsive to information about blood gas levels, lung inflation and exercise.

Receptors which respond to stretch within the visceral pleura, the bronchioles and the alveoli, send impulses via the vagus nerve to the respiratory centre which results in inhibition of inspiration, thus controlling the depth of respiration. This feedback loop is called the Hering-Breuer reflex and it prevents overstretching of thoracic structures. In a similar way sensory endings responding to deflation in the lungs serve to inhibit expiration once it is under way.

HUMORAL INFLUENCES UPON RESPIRATION

The important function of respiration is the maintenance of steady concentrations of oxygen, carbon dioxide and hydrogen ions in the tissue environment. Neurones controlling respiration are highly responsive to information concerning the level of these substances within the bloodstream. Their response is by a change in the rate of firing. There are two sets of receptors which are affected by humoral factors, these are in the region of the medulla and more peripherally in the carotid and aortic bodies.

The respiratory centre itself is responsive to the concentration of dissolved CO_2 and hydrogen ion concentration in the fluids of the respiratory centre. In addition there is a chemosensitive area on the surface of each side of the medulla which is sensitive to the hydrogen ion concentration of the cerebro-spinal fluid (CSF). Hydrogen ions do not pass through the blood/brain barrier into the CSF but dissolved CO_2 does. Therefore it follows that the hydrogen ions in CSF come from the hydration of CO_2 when once it is in the CSF and reflects the PCO_2 of blood. A rise in PCO_2 or H^+ concentration causes an increase in alveolar ventilation. A fall in PO_2 does not affect the humoral receptors of the medulla itself.

More peripheral receptors in the carotid and aortic bodies are responsive to an increase in PCO_2 and hydrogen ion concentration and to a fall in PO_2. These stimuli cause an increase in alveolar ventilation.

The most powerful stimulus to respiration is a rise in PCO_2. An increase in hydrogen ion concentration is also a strong stimulus and it is difficult to separate the effects of an increase in PCO_2 from the effects of an increase in hydrogen ion concentration. A fall in PO_2 is only a minor stimulus to respiration, since under most circumstances a rise in PCO_2 stimulates respiration long before a fall in PO_2 becomes apparent. Nevertheless the stimulus from a fall in PO_2 is important in disease and at high altitudes.

FACTORS INFLUENCING RESPIRATION

DRUGS
Morphine derivatives and barbiturates have a direct depressant effect upon the neurones of the respiratory centre. They also depress the action of the chemoreceptors which normally respond to the levels of CO_2 and hydrogen ion in fluids. Anaesthetic drugs have a similar effect.

CONSCIOUS FACTORS
An individual can consciously increase his respiratory rate and tidal volume. He can also hold his breath for a period, although anyone who has tried this knows that there comes a point when respiration takes place automatically. Cerebral connections to the respiratory centre to allow voluntary control over respiration are important during speech and singing.

EXERCISE
There is an increase in respiration (both depth and rate) during exercise, before the increase in PCO_2 and hydrogen ions can have an effect. It is thought that stretch receptors in muscles and joints exert an influence on the respiratory centres.

VASOMOTOR INFLUENCE
There are sensory or afferent fibres from the blood pressure sensitive receptors (baroreceptors) in the carotid sinuses, aortic arch, atria and ventricles which send impulses to the respiratory centre. Impulses indicating a rise in blood pressure inhibit respiration but the effect is slight and of little physiological importants.

Factors influencing respiration are summarised in Figure 1.16.

LUNG VOLUMES AND CAPACITIES

Pulmonary functions may be assessed by a group of tests designed to evaluate the basic trio of pulmonary physiology, viz. ventilation, diffusion and perfusion.

The pulmonary ventilation tests rely on the determination of lung volumes and capacities in an individual and their assessment by comparison with 'normal' subjects. It is therefore useful to define some of the terminology concerning lung volumes and capacities (Fig. 1.17):

Tidal volume: Volume of air inspired or expired during a quiet respiration, that is at rest.
Inspiratory reserve volume (IRV):   Maximum volume of air which can be inspired over and above the resting inspiratory volume (tidal volume).
Vital capacity (Forced Expiratory Volume) (FEV):   Total volume of expired air after a maximal inspiration.

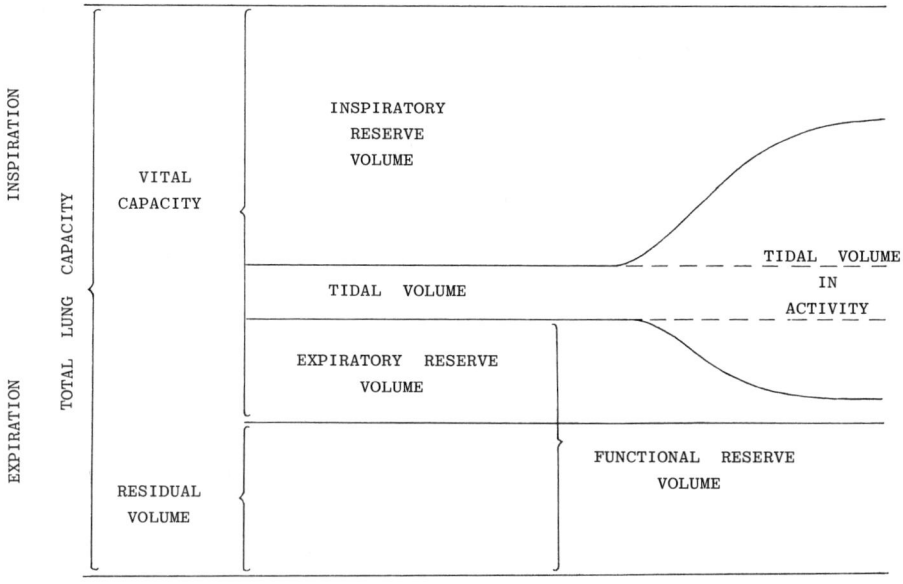

Figure 1.17 Lung volumes and capacities.

Residual volume: Volume of air remaining in the lungs after forced expiration.
Expiratory reserve volume (ERV):   Volume of air expired over and above the tidal expiratory volume.
Functional residual capacity: Volume of air remaining in the lungs after expiration of the tidal (resting) reserve volume (ERV) and residual volume.
Total lung capacity: Sum total of the vital capacity and residual volume.
Maximum breathing capacity (MBC):   Maximum and total volume of air which can be taken in or out of the lungs in one minute.

It is customary to describe two types of pulmonary function abnormality.

In one group, referred to as restrictive diseases, total lung capacity and vital capacity are reduced. In another group, referred to as obstructive diseases, the residual volume is increased.

All volumes and capacities, with the exception of FRC and RV can be determined by spirogram.

For the determination of FRC and RV a more sophisticated method of inert gas (helium) dilution is used.

PULMONARY FUNCTION TESTS

As the name implies these tests are designed to investigate lung function rather than lung pathology. They are useful in as far as they reveal, although indirectly, the effect of pathological conditions on lung function. They also provide objective criteria in the pre-operative assessment of patients.

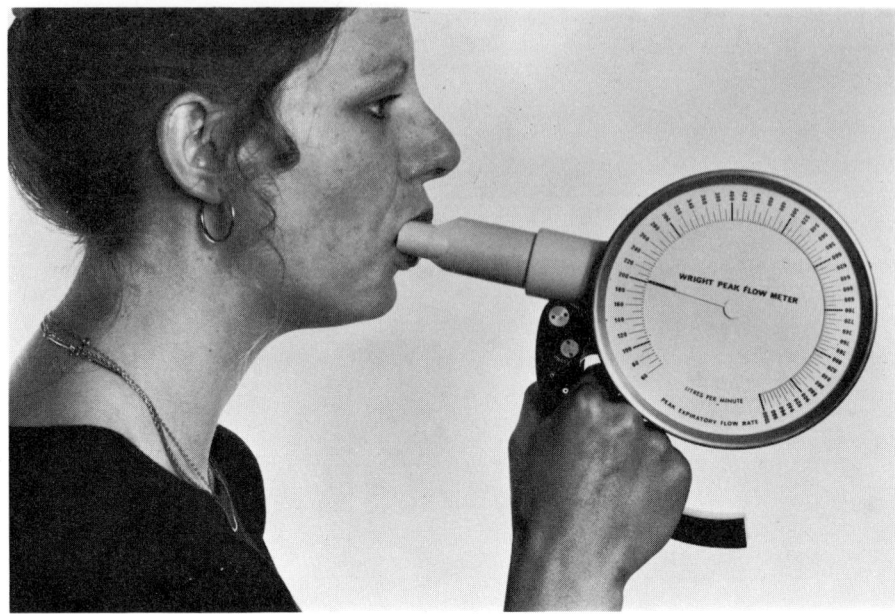

Figure 1.18   Wright Peak Flow Meter.

There are a number of tests which can give information on the ventilation, diffusion and circulation of the lungs. In the majority of surgical cases, clinical and simple laboratory tests are sufficient.

Clinically, the exercise tolerance of the patient can be judged easily (though roughly) by asking him to walk on a level surface and climb upstairs at different paces: slowly, normally and quickly. Snider's match blowing test can be used as a bedside method. The patient is asked to blow out a lighted match from a distance of 7 to 8 cm or more. Inability to do so indicates ventilatory impairment. Peak expiratory flow rate is another simple test which can be performed using a Wright Peak Flow Meter (Fig. 1.18). The patient breathes in fully and then breathes out forcibly through the flow meter which records the volume expired.

Lung volumes and capacities can be precisely determined with the use of sophisticated apparatus. However, total lung volume, forced vital capacity (FVC) and timed forced expiratory volume (FEV) are measured with the conventional spirometer or a dry spirometer (Vitalograph, Fig. 1.19). The patient breathes in deeply and then blows into the mouth piece of the spirometer. The vital capacity and the volume of air expired in one second are recorded. Important information can be obtained by calculating the ratio of the volume of the forced expiratory volume in one second over the total forced vital capacity i.e.:

$$\frac{\text{FEV 1 sec}}{\text{FVC}} \quad \frac{\text{(Forced Expiratory Volume in one second)}}{\text{Forced Vital Capacity}}.$$

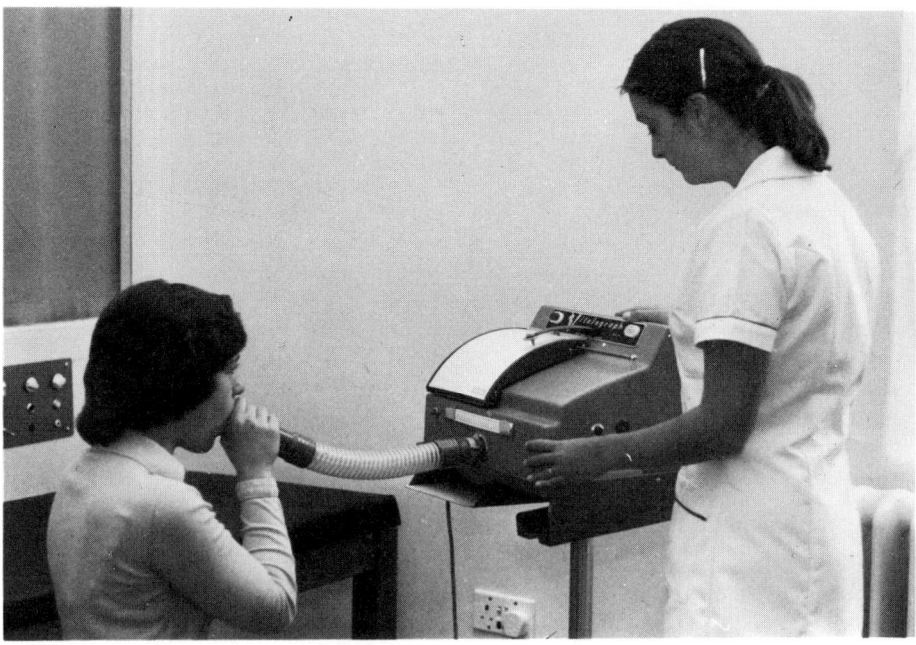

Figure 1.19   Vitalograph.

In a normal individual it should be over 80%. In effect, it means that a normal subject can expire 80% of his vital capacity in one second. An emphysematous patient can expire only a small fraction of his FVC in a second.

BLOOD GAS ANALYSIS

This test determines the pH, oxygen pressure (PO_2), carbon dioxide pressure (PCO_2) in the arterial blood and shows an overall picture of pulmonary function. Only 2 to 3 ml of arterial blood are needed for blood gas estimation.

4 The Pleura and the Pleural Space

The bony chest wall gives the thorax the firmness and strength necessary for the protection of intrathoracic viscera and offers resistance against the external atmospheric pressure. The inner surface of the thoracic cavity is lined by a thin serous membrane, the parietal pleura, which reflects at the hilum to cover the outer surface of the lungs as the visceral pleura. The visceral and parietal layers are separated by a potential space called the pleural space (or cavity). Collection of air, fluid, pus or blood causes the pleural space to enlarge by further separation of the visceral and parietal layers at the expense of the lung which collapses. The degree of collapse depends on the amount of abnormal collection. The parietal pleura has sensory nerves and is sensitive to pain stimuli. The visceral pleura has no such nerves and is insensitive to pain.

The lungs are elastic structures with a tendency to recoil and collapse. Because they are enclosed within the thoracic cavity with its bony frame the pressure in the pleural space is lower than the atmospheric pressure. The chest wall is well adapted to allow this differential pressure. Normal atmospheric pressure is about 760 mm Hg, normal intrapleural pressure is 750–755 mm Hg and therefore subatmospheric. It is referred to as negative pleural pressure. Intrapleural

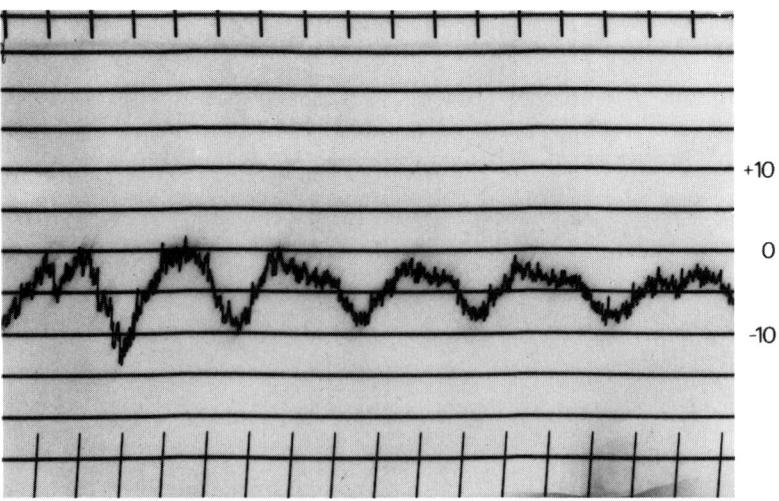

+10

0

-10

Figure 1.20   Recording of intra-pleural pressure.

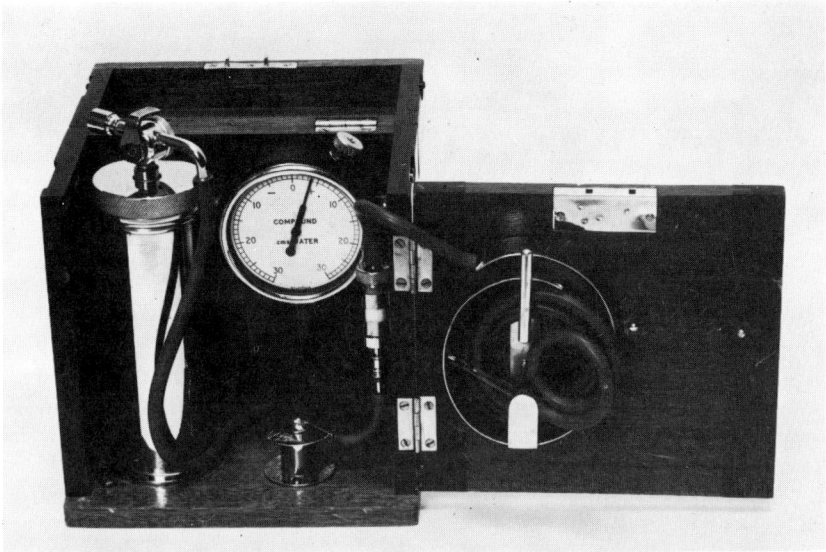

Figure 1.21   Maxwell box.

pressure can be measured by introducing a needle or a fine cannula into the pleural space connected to a manometer, calibrated to read zero for atmospheric pressure. This can be done using a transducer and an electronic pressure recorder (Fig. 1.20). Alternatively, pleural pressure can be measured by connecting the needle inserted into the pleural space to a manometer, such as the Maxwell Box (Fig. 1.21).

During inspiration the volume of the chest increases with consequent further reduction in pleural pressure. During expiration the volume of the chest reduces and intrapleural pressure returns to pre-inspiration level.

It is also important to realise that even at the end of the expiratory phase, the volume of the lung is not at its minimum, which would be its full relaxation volume, as the lung, owing to its elasticity, could still collapse further. Were it not for the firm thorax enclosing it, the lung would collapse along with the chest wall.

Abnormal communication between the pleural space and the atmospheric air surrounding the chest wall results in air moving from the high to the low pressure zone with consequent collapse of the lung.

PLEURAL EFFUSION

This term is used to indicate an accumulation of fluid in the pleural space (clinically and radiologically demonstrable). A wide variety of pathological conditions can cause pleural effusion. They can be classified as follows:

1. Pleural effusion in heart failure.
2. Traumatic pleural effusion.
3. Inflammatory effusion (pleurisy with effusion).
4. Neoplasms (e.g. mesothelioma).
5. Pleural effusion in a systemic disease.

CLINICAL MANIFESTATIONS OF PLEURAL EFFUSION
Although pleural effusion may be a manifestation of a primary pleural disease, it is however important to appreciate that it can be caused by an underlying lung condition and, therefore, the manifestations of pulmonary lesions may dominate the clinical picture. The more specific manifestations of pleural effusion are:

1. *Pleural pain*: The parietal pleura is highly sensitive and derives its nerve supply from the spinal nerves (through the intercostal nerves) and the phrenic nerve. The latter supplies the central tendon of the diaphragm. Pleuritic pain is characteristically related to breathing, and refers to the area of skin overlying the pleura and the tip of the shoulder.

2. *Dyspnoea*: The accumulation of fluid causes a corresponding degree of pulmonary collapse and dyspnoea.

3. Clinical signs of pleural effusion are related to the absence of breath sounds on auscultation in the area of the thorax occupied by the fluid, and dullness on percussion over that area. In cases of pleural effusion caused by an infection the general signs and symptoms of the latter are also present.

INVESTIGATIONS OF PLEURAL EFFUSION
They can be classified as general and specific investigations.

General investigations
They include a general clinical examination and appropriate laboratory studies of a general nature, such as full blood count and sedimentation rate.

Specific investigations
They include many of the special investigations for pulmonary disease, since in many conditions there is not only pleural but a pleuro-pulmonary involvement.

Investigations, as described on pages 54–65 should be carried out. It is obvious that pleural aspiration and pleural biopsy are extremely important and informative in the diagnosis of pleural diseases.

EMPYEMA (synonym empyema thoracis)

Empyema is a purulent effusion in the pleural space. In practice the term includes several types of effusion ranging from a slightly turbid fluid with a few micro-organisms and polymorphs, to frank and thick pus containing a variety of organisms and fungi, with much necrotic tissue as well as blood corpuscles.

AETIOLOGY
The majority of cases of empyema develop as an extension of pulmonary infection. In some cases, however, empyema follows an intra-abdominal infection, a perforating injury of the chest or septicaemia.

At an early stage empyema is widespread in the pleural space, though because of gravity the fluid accumulates mostly at the base of the lung. At a later stage, fibrin deposition leads to localisation of the empyema and walling off of the infection to smaller loculi.

CLINICAL FEATURES AND DIAGNOSIS

As the empyema follows infection, the presenting signs and symptoms can be those of pulmonary or other causative infections. Clinical features are related to (1) the severity and extent of the infection, (2) the nature of the infective organisms and (3) the condition of the underlying lung.

Pain in the chest, impaired respiratory movements, absence of breath sound on auscultation and dullness on percussion, which are characteristic of pleural inflammation and effusion, are also present. Laboratory examinations show the type of infecting organisms and the source of infection.

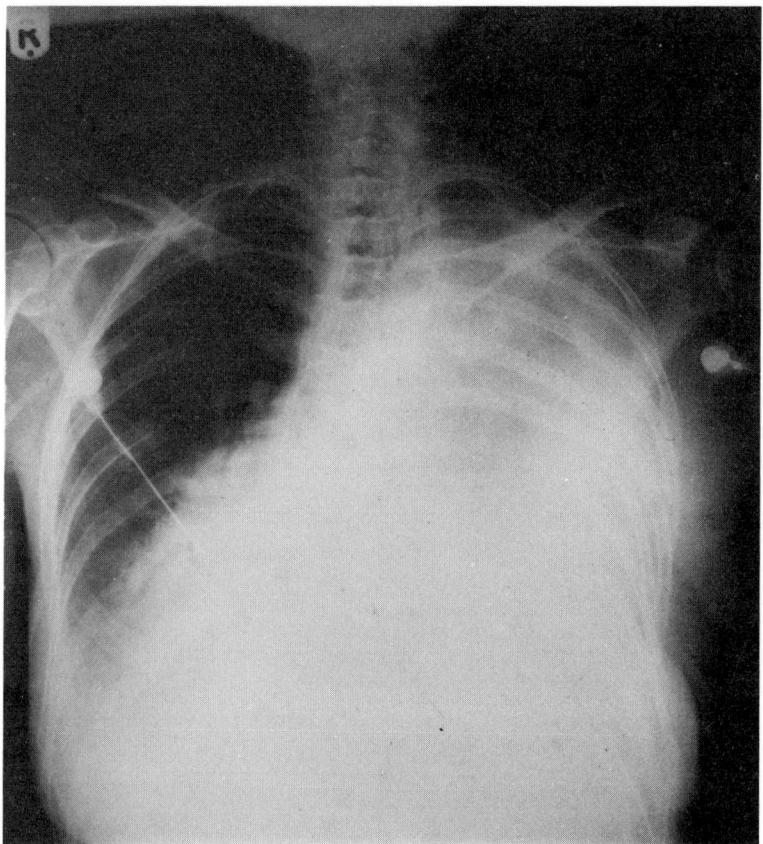

Figure 1.22   Radiograph of patient with left-sided empyema (pyothorax).

Chest radiograph

A chest radiograph indicates the presence and the extent of effusion and the pathological state of the underlying lung (Fig. 1.22).

Pleural aspiration

This provides important information regarding the pathogenic organisms and the cell type, including neoplastic ones.

Bronchoscopy

In almost all cases of empyema, particularly in older patients, it is necessary to bronchoscope the patient:

1. To eliminate neoplasia.
2. To diagnose bronchial obstruction and lung abscess which can be the primary cause of the empyema.
3. To carry out bronchial aspiration and disinfection.
4. To obtain a sample of bronchial secretions.

The outcome of an acute empyema as described depends on the promptness and effectiveness of treatment and the ability of the body to check the infection. In favourable cases there is a resolution (i.e. return to normal) leaving no detectable traces and with complete functional recovery. If unchecked the empyema extends or becomes chronic.

When an empyema is not diagnosed or is left untreated infection may spread and pus gradually finds its way through the lung or the chest wall. In the former case, a broncho-pleural fistula is formed and the sufferer expectorates the purulent contents of the pleural space. In the latter case, referred to as 'empyema necessitatis', a fistulous communication is created between the pleura and the skin with purulent material discharging from the skin. The discharge of pus in both cases brings an improvement in the patient's condition.

MANAGEMENT OF EMPYEMA

The principles of management consist of (1) control of the infection, (2) total evacuation of purulent effusion and prevention of its recurrence, (3) complete expansion of the lung, and (4) treatment of the primary cause.

In practice prompt evacuation of the pus, appropriate antimicrobial chemotherapy, high protein diet, correction of anaemia and active and energetic physiotherapy are the best means of achieving cure.

In the early stages, repeated chest aspiration and intra-pleural and systemic antibiotics can bring about satisfactory control. This, however, fails when there is much air in the pleural space, as well as pus with long-standing pulmonary collapse, or when the evacuation of pus or effective antimicrobial chemotherapy are delayed. Surgical treatment is required for chronic empyemas and those not responding to adequate treatment by aspiration.

SURGICAL TREATMENT

The surgical treatment of empyema is intercostal tube drainage, rib resection and drainage, and thoracotomy—evacuation of pleural space and decortication.

Intercostal tube drainage

This is suitable for relative early cases, when there is no loculation and also for emergency cases. The drain is connected to an underwater sealed system (see Chapter 5).

Rib resection

The operation is performed under local or general anaesthesia. Many surgeons prefer local anaesthesia when the patient can sit on a stool and comfortably bend over, his head and arms resting on a pillow placed on the operating table. The site of drainage is decided by chest radiograph and preliminary chest aspiration. A portion of the rib over the most dependent part is resected and the cavity entered. The pus is evacuated by suction and a large tube is inserted. The tube is connected (in most cases) to the underwater sealed drainage system, at least for a few days before it is cut and used as open drainage.

Decortication
When fibrin deposition over the visceral pleura lining the collapsed lung is substantial, mere evacuation of the pus can hardly be expected to achieve lung expansion. In these cases the method of choice is to perform a thoracotomy to carry out decortication in addition to drainage of pus. This operation is carried out more and more frequently, particularly in younger subjects, as it allows quick discharge from hospital and return to work. The operation consists of (1) a thoracotomy, (2) evacuation of pus, (3) excision of the 'sac' containing the pus together with the parietal pleura, and (4) fibrin and fibrous tissues deposited over the visceral pleura. The latter is peeled off allowing the expansion of the underlying suppressed and collapsed lung. The chest is drained.

POST-OPERATIVE MANAGEMENT
For empyema the post-operative management aims at early pulmonary expansion, prevention of loculation or recurrence of pus within the pleural cavity, and full functional recovery of the lung and chest wall movements.

Prevention of loculated empyema is achieved by gradual withdrawal of the intercostal drainage tube. The following steps should be taken:

1. Drainage tube attached to underwater sealed (closed) system: this is applicable when the empyema is treated by intercostal tube, rib resection or thoracotomy (see p. 40 and 48).

2. In some cases of acute empyema treated by simple intercostal drainage or thoracotomy, it is possible to remove the drainage tube without progressive shortening, providing that complete evacuation and the abolition of residual space have been achieved.

3. In the chronic type of empyema the intercostal drainage tube is disconnected from the closed system, and then cut off short to open into the dressing when, and *only when*, it is certain that the pleural infection (empyema) has become localised (i.e. walled off from the rest of the pleural cavity by fibrous tissue) and that the drainage tube is situated within this limited space.

4. After a few days the amount of drainage diminishes and the tube is shortened. The aim is to obliterate the space as the tube is gradually withdrawn. The rate of discharge (as judged by the frequency of dressing) and radiographic demonstrations of continued lung expansion regulate the frequency at which the tube is shortened. In chronic cases it is necessary to monitor tube shortening by intermittent pleurograms, so that gradual healing takes place without loculation. Complete withdrawal can take considerable time.

PLEURAL ASPIRATION

Pleural aspiration (chest aspiration–paracenthesis thoracis) is a procedure in which a needle is introduced through an intercostal space into the pleural cavity

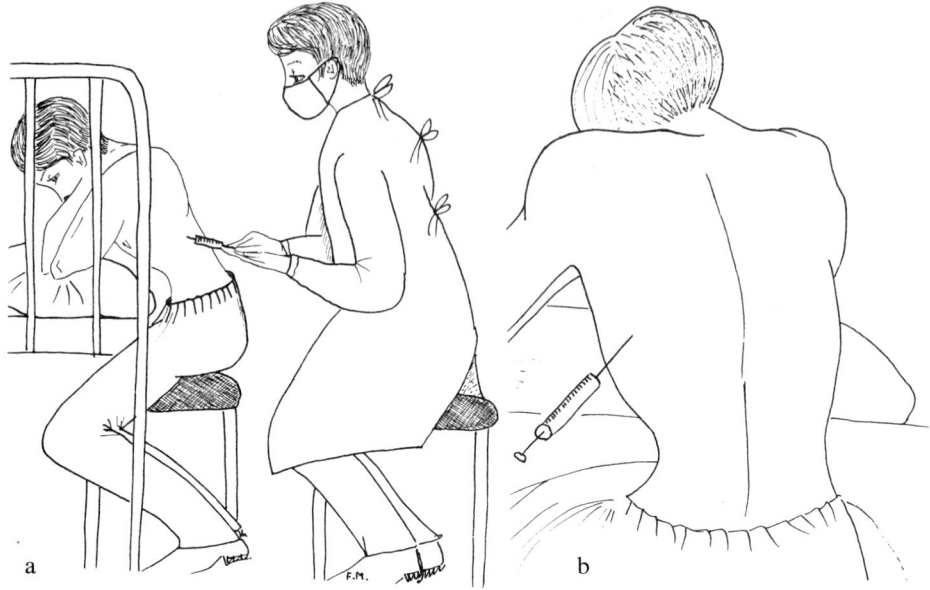

Figure 1.23   Position of patient for pleural aspiration: (a) out of bed and (b) in bed.

to aspirate air or fluid. The procedure is carried out for diagnostic purposes or for the relief of dyspnoea caused by the collapse of the underlying lung. It is usually carried out under local anaesthesia. In most cases the posterior aspect of the lower chest is the selected site for aspiration, because the fluid gravitates to the bottom of the thoracic cavity. When there is a pneumothorax, an antero-superior or a postero-superior site is chosen.

Before carrying out aspiration the procedure should be fully explained to the patient. It is also important to reassure him, and to provide a sedative 15–20 minutes beforehand.

When the patient is mobile the procedure is best carried out with the patient sitting out of bed as it is important for both patient and operator to be sitting in a comfortable position. The patient should sit on a stool bending down over 1 or 2 pillows placed on the side of the bed; the operator sits behind him (Fig. 1.23a). If the patient has to remain in bed, the aspiration is carried out with the patient bending forward over a pillow placed on the bed table (Fig. 1.23b). Alternatively, the mid-axillary line can be used. In all cases the nurse should provide the required set on a clean trolley and make sure that all necessary equipment and intruments are available.

APPARATUS

An aspiration set or pack for pleural aspiration contains the following (see also Fig. 1.24):

1. Towels, at least *two* of appropriate size to isolate the field of aspiration.
2. Swabs for cleansing skin and for applying after the procedure.

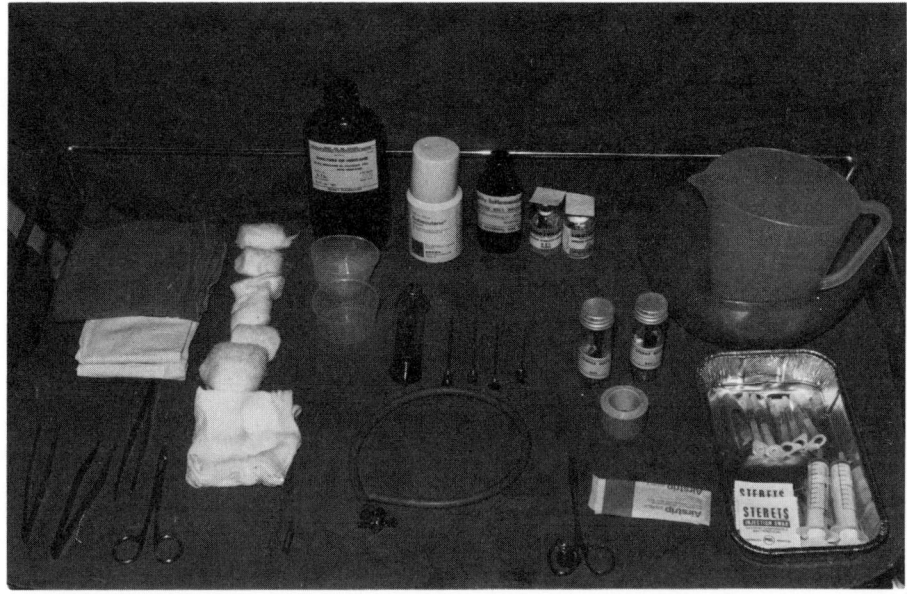

Figure 1.24   Pleural aspiration trolley. (See text for details.)

3. Two gallipots, one for antiseptic solution and a second one for local anaesthetic.

4. Local anaesthetic syringe with selection of matching needles. This is best provided by a standard local infiltration syringe and needles.

5. Aspiration syringe (20 ml), Luer lock or Martin's type, with matching two-way tap connector and selection of different bore needles (a selection of Martin's Trocars and Cannulae if Martin's syringe is provided), and a length of soft plastic or rubber tubing connected to fit the lateral side of the two-way tap.

6. Fine-pointed scalpel blade.

7. One pair of straight artery forceps.

8. At least one pair of non-toothed forceps for holding swabs.

In addition to this pack the nurse should provide:

9. Antiseptic solution, the one preferred by the operator.

10. A small dressing for covering the hole after aspiration.

11. Collodion solution of 'sealing' spray such as Nobecutane.

12. Some adhesive plaster.

13. Specimen jars for the collection of samples of fluid for bacteriology, cytology, and additional laboratory testing if required (chemistry, special bacteriology etc.).

14. An appropriate-sized container for the collection of the fluid. All fluid collected should be measured.

5 Pleural Drainage

UNDERWATER SEALED DRAINAGE SYSTEM

Because of the anatomical arrangement of the chest and the intrapleural pressure mechanism a special drainage system allowing the exit, (but preventing the entry) of air from the pleural space has been devised for chest drainage. It is called an underwater sealed drainage system.

To nurse the patient properly it is necessary to understand the equipment used (Fig. 1.25a,b). The drainage system consists of the following:

1. A large (Winchester) bottle containing 500 ml of sterile water or normal saline. The level of this fluid is marked by a piece of strapping. Alternatively a graduated bottle can be used or graduated marks can be used on the outer surface of the bottle indicating the volume.

2. A rubber cork or a metal screw top pierced by two rigid tubes of glass or plastic. One of the tubes dips into the water for 2–3 cm but does not touch the bottom of the bottle. The other tube enters the top of the bottle only, and is for the exit of air.

3. A length of rubber tubing is connected at one end to the underwater tube and the other end to a connector which joins it to the patient's intercostal drainage tube.

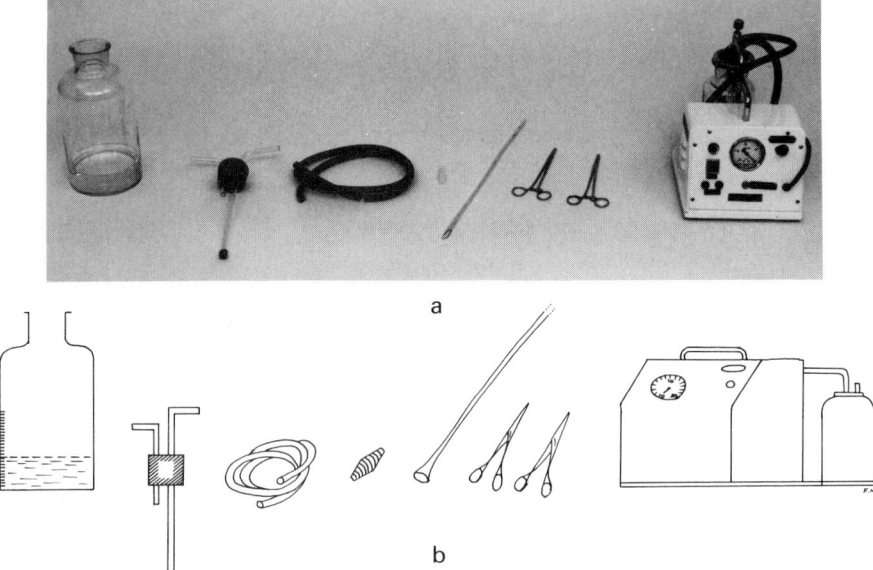

a

b

Figure 1.25   (a) and (b) Underwater sealed drainage equipment. (See text for details.)

4. Two pairs of tubing clamps, and a suction pump with adjustable suction power and digital display manometer

The system is assembled as follows: The patient's drain is connected to a length of tubing by a connector. This tube is in turn attached to the underwater glass or plastic tube. *The underwater tube passes through the same rubber bung which carries the air exit tube, and a mistake in connecting the patient's drain (with additional tubing) to the air exit tube is a serious one. If this happens the patient will have a pneumothorax and pulmonary collapse.* The patient's drainage tube must lead and be connected to the longer glass tube which dips into the water. The way to avoid mistakes is to stress carefully to the uninitiated the absolute necessity of connecting the patient's drain and tubing to the longer tube which goes into the water.

This simple system when assembled and connected to the pleural drain, allows the exit of air (and fluid) from the pleural space and prevents air from entering into the chest. The underwater tube acts as a one-way valve from the chest into the bottle. The reverse, that is the entry of air into the pleura from outside, is not possible as long as the end of the tube is truly underwater and the bottle is placed *below* the level of the patient's chest (e.g. on the floor at the side of the patient's bed).

During the inspiratory phase the negative intra-pleural pressure available acts as a suction force. If the drainage tube were free in the atmosphere, naturally the air would be sucked into the pleural space with consequent pneumothorax and collapse of the lung. When it is connected to the underwater system and the bottle is below the patient's chest, the inspiratory suction force can only push the column of water up into the underwater glass tube so that no air enters the pleural space. Furthermore, the lower the bottle is placed in relation to the patient's chest, the further away the column of water will remain from the chest.

During the expiratory phase, the column of water goes down because of the relative increase in the intra-pleural pressure (which is still subatmospheric). If there is a collection of air in the pleural space, with increased pleural pressure then expiration not only pushes the water column down but it also moves it completely out of the tube into the bottle, and then air is expelled in the form of bubbles. The next inspiration again pushes the water into the underwater glass tube. Deep expiration or the effort of coughing in these circumstances expels an even greater amount of air as it creates a temporary high positive pressure in the pleural space. During the following inspiration, air will not enter the pleural space; instead, a column of water will rise into the tube.

It is to be realised that any air expelled from the pleura must be ultimately expelled from the bottle and this can only be effected through the only outlet from the bottle which is the air exit tube. Therefore, this tube must be patent at all times and free in the atmospheric air or connected to a working suction pump capable of extracting air.

GENERAL CARE OF PLEURAL DRAINS

When a patient returns from the theatre to the ward the receiving nurse should enquire about (1) the nature of the operation, (2) the number and position of drains, and (3) whether the drains are on free drainage or clamped. Further

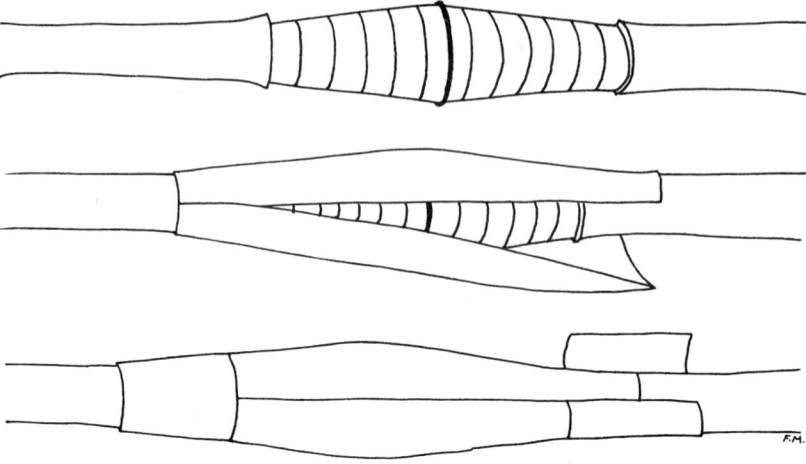

Figure 1.26   Securing the connector with tape.

instructions regarding the drains will concern their attachment to suction pumps.

During the transfer of the patient to his bed, the intercostal drain or the connecting tube should be clamped before lifting up the drainage bottle. All staff handling thoracic surgical cases should acquire a mental discipline and a reflex to check the component parts of the drainage system as soon as the patient is returned to his bed, and the whole of the system should be further inspected for possible air leaks and loose connections.

When the preliminary inspection is completed (and only then) the clamps are removed, allowing proper functioning of the drains to be resumed. The following additional points are relevant:

1. Connectors at the junction of the intercostal drain and the additional tube, and to the underwater tube, should be secured. One way to do this is as follows (Fig. 1.26).

(a) Apply two pieces of strapping, longitudinally, one on each side to cover the junctions, overlapping the connector itself and the adjacent tubes. (b) Place two pieces of strapping around, one at each end, covering the longitudinal pieces and the adjacent tubes.

2. Make sure the patient is not compressing or kinking the drain or the additional tubing attached to it, thus blocking the drainage system.

3. See that the drain and tubing from the patient to the underwater tube is of the correct length. Tubes must neither be too long nor too short. Take a sufficient length from floor to bed, then apply a large safety-pin (which must not pierce the tube), or strapping, fixing the tube to the bedclothes at that point. Leave an extra length in bed for easy movement and to prevent a great length and weight hanging from the patient's skin to which the intercostal drain is fixed (Fig. 1.27a,b).

4. The nurse in charge should instruct all junior nurses, domestics and cleaners not to lift the drainage bottle from the floor.

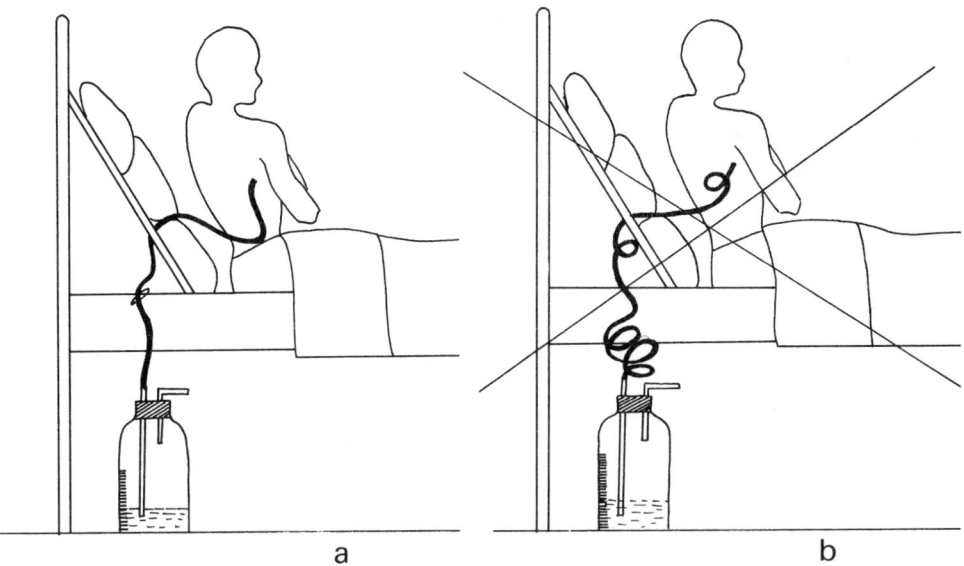

Figure 1.27 (a) *Correct and* (b) *incorrect method of securing the tubing.*

5. The quantity, rate and quality of drainage should be observed and recorded. It is easy to assess this when it consists of fluid or blood, and when graduated bottles are available. However, the amount of air leak cannot be assessed precisely, but it is possible to observe and record the air leak bubbling in descriptive terms such as 'enormous' (+ + +), 'large' (+ +) and 'slight' (+).

6. If the drainage bottle is to be connected to a suction pump, observe and record the amount and the type of drainage, and make a note of the air leak before attaching to the pump. Then set the pump to the required strength and connect the air exit tube to the pump. The following remarks should be noted: (a) a suction pump for this purpose must have a dial indicating the suction force and a centralised 'piped' suction (attached to wall) without a dial should not be used. (b) A suction pump for pleural drainage must provide adjustable degrees of suction force. It should be remembered that pumps available in hospitals are unfortunately variously graduated, some graduated in cm of water, other in mm, cm or inches of mercury. Therefore, when receiving instructions, the nurse should, according to the types of pump available in the ward, seek precise details regarding the strength and specific scale of suction required. Alternatively, a conversion table should be kept in the ward. (c) To set up a suction pump, connect it to the electricity supply and switch on before connecting it to the air-exit tube. With the adjusting knob turned down to the minimum and the dial indicating zero, clamp the suction tube of the pump and gently turn on the knob until the dial reads the required figure. Do not leave the clamp on the suction tube for too long.

7. In cases of an accident resulting in disruption of the pleural drainage system due to one of the following: (a) bottle breakage; (b) cork being dislodged; (c) underwater tube broken or dislodged out of the water; (d) connectors disconnected. Clamp the intercostal tube proximal to the point of disruption (that is, near the patient) and correct the fault, then remove the

clamps and reestablish drainage. Report the matter to the medical officer for further instructions.

8. When the drainage bottle is attached to a suction pump: (a) make sure the power and pump are switched on; (b) check the working of the pump. Pump or power failure cause the patient to develop a pneumothorax as the only exit for the air from the pleura is via the drainage system to the bottle with its ultimate extraction through the air exit tube by the suction pump. A functional failure of the pump causes a blockage in the system of air extraction leading to accumulation of air in the chest. If and when the suction pump is not operational, the suction tube should be disconnected from the air exit tube of the bottle.

It is worthwhile mentioning that in some hospitals there is only one electric point beside a patient's bed. Temporarily, the point may be required for another electrical appliance and an uninstructed member of staff may remove the suction pump's plug from the socket without disconnecting the suction tube from the air exit tube. This can result in irreparable damage and at times seriously endanger life. The practice of switching off electricity, or removing the pump's plug from the socket must be discouraged, and if it becomes inevitable, then the drainage bottle must stand without suction pump attachment.

PLEURAL DRAINAGE IN SPECIAL CASES

Following thoracic surgical procedures, patients are usually kept in bed for 24 hours. Thereafter they are mobilised to various degrees. It is the practice of many surgeons to mobilise patients with pleural drains *in situ* by getting them out of bed into a chair, and/or letting them walk about, particularly if they do not require suction pump attachment. In these circumstances, the pleural drain with all its attachments (except the suction pump), can be carried by the patient. This 'carrying bottle' is provided with an appropriate container, a basket, and is referred to as a 'walking bottle' (Fig. 1.28).

In some hospitals these baskets are made by the patients themselves as part of their occupational therapy.

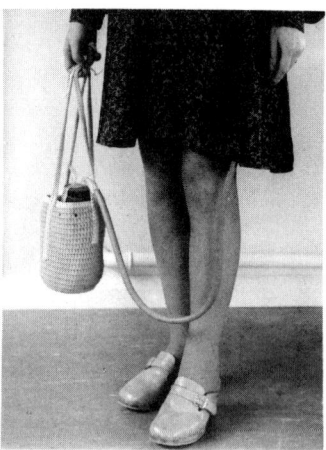

Figure 1.28   A 'walking' bottle.

AFTER PARTIAL PULMONARY RESECTION

Following pulmonary resection, the future of the residual part of the lung is dependent on its speedy expansion and the abolition of the space created by the disproportion between the size of the thoracic cavity and the volume of the remaining segments or lobes.

Expansion depends on several factors of which the following are particularly important:

1. The adequacy of ventilation assured by effective deep breathing and assisted by breathing exercises.
2. Clearing of the airways from excessive normal or abnormal secretions, achieved by chest physiotherapy and postural drainage, assuring the patency of the bronchial trees.
3. Removal of air from the pleural space (a constant air leak being present in the early post-operative period from the line of separation of lobes or segments) and re-establishment of the negative intrapleural space.
4. Drainage of serous and blood-stained fluid, the collection of which acts as a space-occupying mass and leads to lung collapse.

In most, if not all, cases of pulmonary resection, the pleural space is usually drained by two drainage tubes. One drain is placed at the apex, principally to drain the air, and the other at the base, principally to drain the fluid (Fig. 1.29a,b). Each drain is individually connected to its own underwater sealed system. The air exit tubes of the drainage bottles are usually connected to a suction pump.

The nurse should receive instructions as to the degree of suction. The pump or pumps should be checked before connecting them to the drainage bottles, both for their working order and the correct registering of the suction pressure. The rate of air leak or drainage should be noted.

The bottles, particularly the one receiving the basal drainage tube, usually require changing the day after the operation because of the quantity of drainage.

A record is made of the amount of fluid in the bottle subtracting 500 ml (originally water) from it to obtain the amount of drainage.

The procedure to be followed must be understood, taking care to prevent contamination. One method is to (1) prepare a fresh sterile drainage bottle containing the appropriate amount of sterile water, (2) double clamp the patient's intercostal tube, (3) disconnect the air exit tube from the pump, (4) change the bottle either by removing the cork (together with the two glass or plastic tubes through it) from the bottle, or by disconnecting the patient's tube from the underwater rod of the bottle to be changed and connecting it to the underwater rod of the new bottle, (5) remove clamps from the intercostal tube and (6) connect the air tube to suction pump.

There is no virtue in changing bottles every day after the first 24 to 48 hours unless drainage is high or there are other reasons for doing so.

An additional point of importance is that when both drainage bottles show evidence of free air leak, the two intercostal drains should not be clamped at the same time. They should be clamped individually before changing the bottle, otherwise the temporary accumulation of undrained air in the chest could result in pneumothorax.

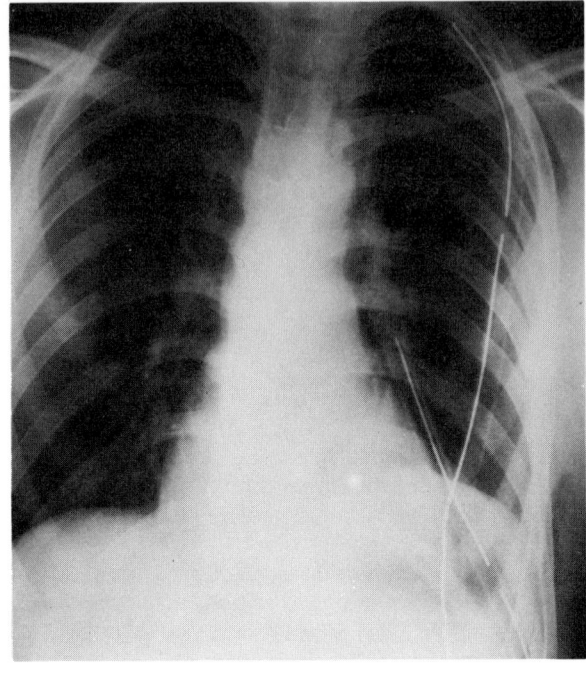

a

b

Figure 1.29   (a) and (b) Pleural drain in situ *after partial pulmonary resection.*

AFTER PNEUMONECTOMY

There is essentially no need to drain a 'clean' pneumonectomy space. This belief is not, however, universally accepted. Therefore either of the two methods can be adopted.

1. Surgeons who do not drain the pleural cavity use the Maxwell Box to measure the intrapleural pressure (on the pneumonectomy side) before the patient leaves the theatre. If the pressure is found to be above atmospheric pressure (over the zero line of the manometer during expiration) residual air is removed until a subatmospheric pressure of -5 mm Hg is recorded. Later the patient is observed and, if necessary, the pressure is measured and adjusted two, three or even more times during the post-operative period.

2. Surgeons who insert a drain in the pleural space connect the drain to an underwater sealed system (without a suction pump). It is desirable to remove the drain as soon as possible, usually after 24 hours. It is also important to allow intermittent access of atmospheric air into the pleural space so that the mediastinum does not shift too much to the pneumonectomy side.

This can easily occur through uninterrupted connection to the underwater drainage system, because each time the patient coughs, additional air is expelled from the drain and a lower intrapleural pressure is created and maintained by the very existence of the underwater sealed system. One way to alleviate this is to devise a system, as illustrated in Fig. 1.30, which allows the drain to be connected to the underwater sealed system by clamping tube C; or else to leave the drain

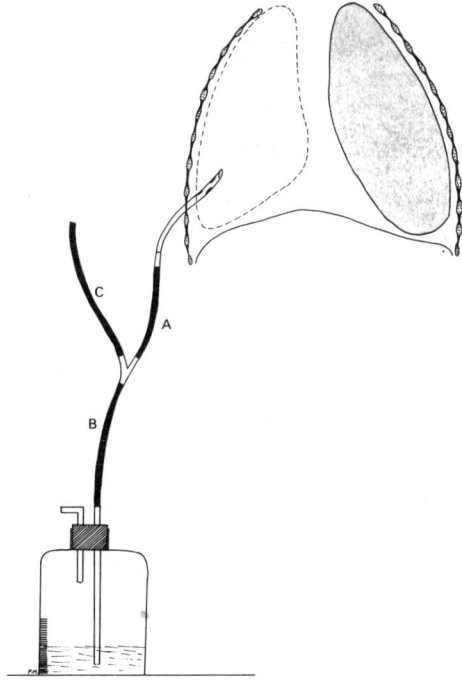

Figure 1.30   Pleural drain in situ *after pneumonectomy.*

connected to the air by clamping tube B and thus by-passing the underwater sealed system. Tube A draining the pleural space is joined by a connector to the underwater sealed system through one limb of the connector (B) and to the air through the other limb (C).

Instructions should be sought as to how long each tube should be clamped.

INTERCOSTAL DRAINAGE OF PNEUMOTHORAX

In many cases the chest is drained by inserting an intercostal drain connected to an underwater sealed system. Just after insertion of the intercostal tube the underwater sealed system shows a constant air leak in the form of bubbling on suction.

Later on there are no air bubbles on suction but there is a swing in the column of water during ventilatory movements showing the presence of residual air in the space between the visceral and parietal pleural indicating an increase in the size of the pleural space.

After a few days there is no swing in the column of the underwater tube. Clinically and radiologically the lung is expanded.

The patient should be mobilised as soon as possible either with a 'walking bottle', or by connecting the intercostal tube to a special one-way valve tube. When the 'bubbles' and the swing have stopped the intercostal tube is removed.

PLEURAL DRAINAGE IN CASES OF EMPYEMA

Drainage of empyema thoracis can be effected by means of intercostal drain. Often this is carried out by an operation in which a short segment of rib is excised; in this way space for an adequate-sized tube is provided. Management of these drains can be described as follows:

1. The drainage tube is connected to an underwater sealed system of drainage. This is because at this stage the empyema is connected to the general pleural space and the collection of pus has not as yet been walled off. A suction pump may be required to remove any air which may also be present (pyo-pneumo-thorax). The aim is to expand the lung as quickly as possible.

2. When the empyema is judged to be localised, that is when the collection of pus is walled off from the general pleural space, the intercostal tube can be disconnected from the underwater sealed system in either of two ways: (a) if drainage is still copious the intercostal tube can be connected to a bag; (b) if drainage is moderate or slight the intercostal tube is cut off near the skin (the original skin stitch inserted by the surgeon to fix the tube is removed). A large safety-pin is then passed through the tube and the tube is fixed by two strips of strapping to the skin (Fig. 1.31). The tube is then held in place and dressings applied over it.

3. After an appropriate time the tube is gradually shortened and eventually removed following full expansion of the lung and abolition of the empyema cavity as judged by pleurograms.

PLEURAL DRAINAGE FOLLOWING OTHER INTRATHORACIC PROCEDURES

Thoracotomy is carried out for lesions of the mediastinum, heart and great vessels, and oesophagus. In these and other transthoracic operations, there is usually no air leak. The pleura is often drained by one drain which has two

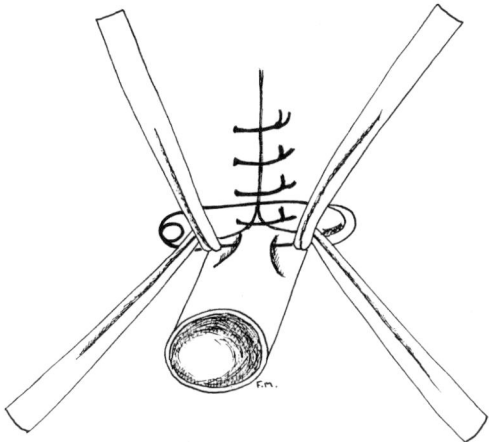

Figure 1.31   Method of fixing open pleural drain in case of chronic empyema.

purposes: first to remove any residual air which may remain in the chest after closure, and second to drain blood, serum and fluid. Such a drain is connected to an underwater sealed system and often does not require any suction pump. The rate of drainage has to be noted and recorded. The tube is removed 24 to 48 hours later.

INSERTION AND REMOVAL
OF INTERCOSTAL PLEURAL DRAINS

INSERTION OF INTERCOSTAL TUBE
The procedure is usually performed under local anaesthetic.

Equipment required
A medium or large-size dressing trolley (Fig. 1.32a) and a small dressing trolley is required (Fig. 1.32b).

Large trolley—Top shelf: A sterilised pack containing three material dressing towels (not paper as these slip too much); gauze swabs; a pair of sponge-holding forceps (Ramsey's sponge-holder); Martin's syringe—Luer lock or 20 ml disposable; syringe; a large bore aspirating needle; pair of medium size artery forceps; pair of fine curved artery forceps; Bard Parker handle; No. 11 Bard Parker blade; pair of scissors; four sutures 564 (skin); two pairs of tubing clamps (8″ straight artery forceps); two gallipots; trocar and cannula, there are usually three sizes (large, medium and small); catheters (or tubes) to fit in the appropriate cannula; tube connectors.

Large trolley—Bottom shelf: Skin cleaning solution; local anaesthetic; disposable syringe and large, medium and small needles for administration of local anaesthetic; mediswab (to clean top of local anaesthetic solution); sterile disposable intercostal tube of choice with or without trocar; antibiotic spray;

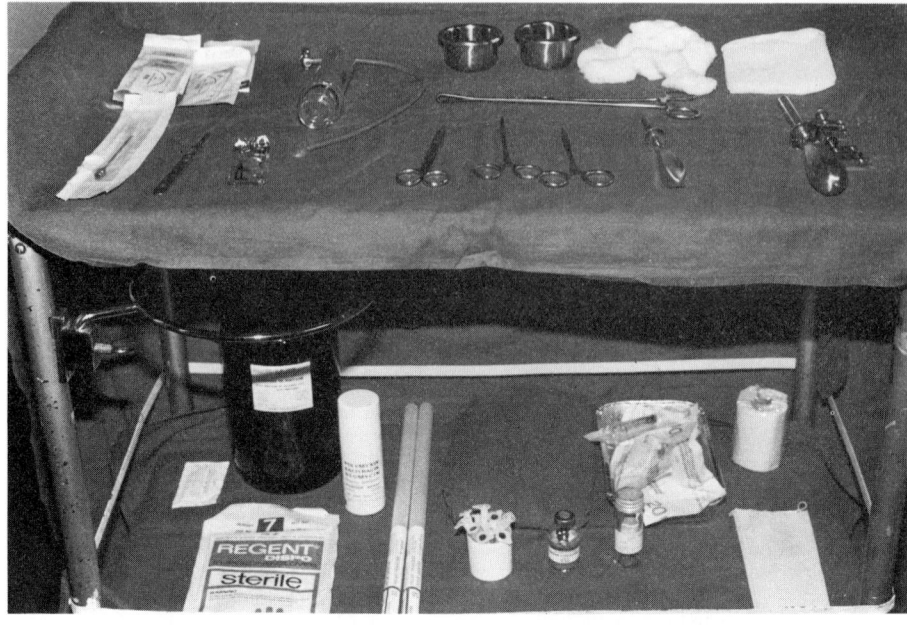

a

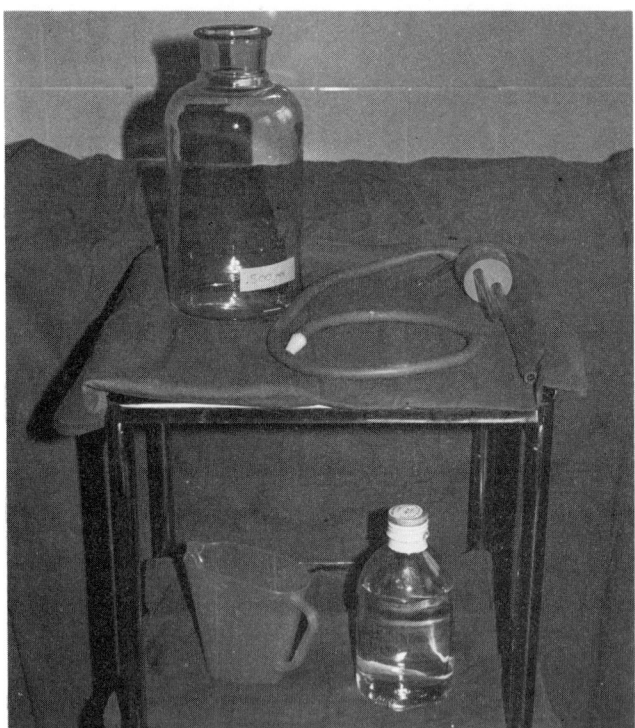

b

Figure 1.32   (a) Large trolley for insertion of intercostal tube. (See text for details.) (b) Small trolley.

specimen pot (for fluid if present); clean gown, mask and sterile gloves for operator; 3 inch elastoplast.

Small trolley— Top shelf: Sterilised pack containing drainage bottle and tubing.

Small trolley—Bottom shelf: Sterile jug and 500 ml sterile water; label to mark bottle with the level or volume of water. When checking the equipment it may be helpful to think in terms of (1) skin cleaning and drapes or towels, (2) local anaesthetic, (3) insertion of the tube, (4) underwater seal drainage systems.

PREPARATION AND POSITION OF PATIENT

The procedure must be explained to the patient who should be reassured. Simple explanations usually secure co-operation. If the patient is nervous, or in great pain (e.g. after an injury), a sedative and an analgesic are administered intravenously if necessary. The patient is best seated outside the bed on a stool, leaning over a pillow placed on the side of the bed or table. This position is especially suitable if the posterior aspect of the chest is the site for the insertion of the tube (e.g. when draining a haemothorax or an empyema).

If the patient cannot get out of bed, or if the anterior aspect of the chest is going to be the site of insertion, the patient can lean back in a sitting position on his own bed. An axillary or apical site can be used with the patient in or out of bed.

The second intercostal space anteriorly is generally favoured for draining a pneumothorax, but in our view this should not be used in female patients as the tube passes through mammary tissues leaving undesirable scarring. In such cases the axillary line is much preferred.

Following the cleansing and disinfecting of the skin, the proposed site of insertion is infiltrated with local anaesthetic. Exploratory aspiration is then carried out. This confirms diagnosis and indicates the depth of the pleural space from the skin. The operator then makes a skin incision 1.5 to 2.0 cm long over the intercostal space. The muscle layers are then split, and the trocar and cannula introduced in one thrust. The trocar is removed, leaving the cannula in the pleural space. The catheter is then introduced into the cannula. The latter is removed leaving the catheter in the pleural cavity: the catheter is then connected to the underwater system. The catheter may have to be adjusted before it is fixed to the skin with a stitch. A dressing is applied.

When a Trocar Catheter type of tube is used, no trocar and cannula are needed but the muscle and the extra-pleural tissue have to be split or divided more thoroughly, as this particular type of trocar is not sharp.

REMOVAL OF INTERCOSTAL (PLEURAL) DRAINS

Following thoracotomy or insertion of an intercostal pleural drainage tube, the drains (tubes) are left in the pleural space until drainage is completed. When this is achieved, when there is no air leak and when the lung is fully expanded the tube is removed.

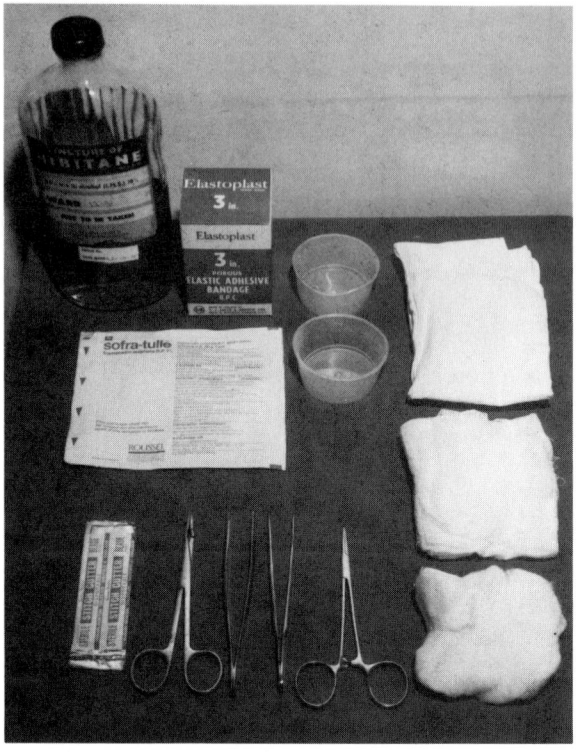

Figure 1.33   Equipment for removal of intercostal drains.

Equipment
For the removal of the drain a tray containing the following (or a pack provided by CSSD) is prepared for the operator (see also Fig. 1.33):

1. Sterile gloves, mask and gown.
2. Antiseptic solution (Hibitane in spirit).
3. One gallipot (for the antiseptic solution).
4. Cotton wool and swabs. A square of sofratulle.
5. A pair of non-toothed holding forceps.
6. A pair of scissors or a curved stitch-cutting scalpel.
7. Blade No. 11.
8. One or two pieces of adhesive elastoplast.

Procedure
The patient should be informed of the procedure. A nervous or apprehensive patient may require a mild sedative or an analgesic given 20 to 30 minutes beforehand.

The patient is requested to lie on the opposite side. The nurse removes or loosens the elastoplast. The operator (scrubbed and wearing gloves, mask and gown) removes the dressings and clears the skin around the tube. There are usually two stitches, one fixing the tube to the skin and the other loosely wrapped around the tube with a knot. This latter stitch is the one to be tied following removal of the tube to approximate the edges of the incision. The knot is cut to separate its two limbs. The stitch fixing the tube is then cut. The operator takes hold of the tube (connected to the underwater sealed drainage system) in one hand. In the other hand he takes some swabs. The patient is requested to breathe in and out on command. The tube is removed at expiration and the swabs are quickly applied. It is preferable to remove the tube whilst still connected to the suction machine (underwater seal interposed). The operator hands over the forceps to the nurse to press on the dressing over the hole, and then ties the stitch to close the incision.

The skin is cleaned. A layer of sofratulle and swabs is applied and covered with a short piece of elastoplast. The patient is made comfortable. The removal of the tube is entered in the Cardex or nursing notes.

6 Investigations of Pulmonary Diseases

INVESTIGATIONS OF LUNG DISEASES

Patients admitted to a thoracic surgical unit are investigated for two distinct purposes:

1. To establish diagnosis of their pathological condition.
2. To evaluate their suitability for proposed surgery and bring to light both related and unrelated coincidental pathology which may influence either the choice of treatment or the type and extent of operation.

The investigations undertaken may be classified as clinical investigations, non-specific laboratory investigations or special investigations.

CLINICAL INVESTIGATIONS
They include the patient's detailed medical history and recording of symptoms and signs. It is important to notice the clinical manifestations of respiratory diseases with particular reference to the following:

Cough
The outstanding symptom of many respiratory diseases is coughing. The cough can be dry, i.e. non-productive, or productive.

Sputum
A small volume of secretions from the bronchial tree is normally sufficient to moisten the mucosal surface. An increase in the amount of secretions and the addition of pus or other material constitutes sputum. In surgical cases it is important to notice the quantity and type of sputum which may be:

1. *Mucoid*: More viscous (less fluid, more sticky) than usual and clear in colour.
2. *Purulent*: Appears yellowish green colour and contains pus.
3. *Fetid*: Variously coloured with a peculiar smell.
4. *Blood-stained*: Containing streaks of blood.

Haemoptysis
This means expectoration of blood. The material is usually bright red and frothy. According to its severity, haemoptysis may be no more than streaks in the sputum or a complete replacement of sputum by blood (frank haemoptysis).

Chest pain
In many respiratory diseases, chest pain is present. It is one of the most distressing symptoms and can be produced by a wide variety of conditions

affecting the thoracic walls or viscera. The site, distribution and radiation of pain have to be noted in addition to its severity, quality and frequency.

Dyspnoea

It is usually defined as 'breathlessness', 'difficulty of breathing' and 'shortness of breath'. It is in fact an awareness of breathing requiring in addition some conscious effort.

Dyspnoea is not simply a manifestation of respiratory diseases. It can be present in patients suffering from other conditions, such as cardiac and metabolic diseases. The physiopathological bases of dyspnoea are in fact little understood. Mechanical and nervous disturbances of respiration can produce dyspnoea, but increased carbon dioxide tension, reduced oxygen tension, low pH in arterial blood do form, in many cases, the basis for dyspnoea. Although dyspnoea is a subjective phenomenon, it is important to assess it objectively and record it.

It is customary to grade dyspnoea according to its evaluation by the sufferer. Some patients have difficulty in assessing their disability because of sub-conscious adaptation and self-imposed restrictions. This can be unmasked in the course of questioning. Dyspnoea is graded as mild (Grade 1) when it only appears after a strenuous effort, such as running for a bus, in a subject who could do so previously. Moderate dyspnoea (Grade II) is present when everyday activities become an effort. Severe dyspnoea (Grade III) is diagnosed when an even minimal amount of physical activity becomes difficult. Gross dyspnoea (Grade IV) is present when the subject is completely disabled and practically bed-ridden.

The Medical Research Council Committee on Chronic Bronchitis (1966) suggests a useful guideline for the evaluation of dyspnoea:

1. Are you breathless when hurrying on level ground or walking up a slight hill?
2. Or when walking with people of your own age on level ground?
3. Do you stop for breath when walking at your own pace on level ground?

A negative answer to the first question means no dyspnoea. A positive answer means dyspnoea which varies in severity depending on a positive answer to the second and third questions.

Wheeze

This is an abnormal noise accompanying breathing, usually in its expiratory phase. It denotes airway obstruction caused by spasm, thick secretions, a foreign body or neoplasm.

Stridor

This is an extreme form of difficult breathing in which respiration is noisy and associated with much effort particularly in the inspiratory phase. It generally means severe obstruction to air entering the respiratory tract.

Cyanosis

A bluish tinge of the conjunctiva, mucous membrane, and skin can be defined as cyanosis.

It is to be noted that the normal colour of the skin is dependent on pigmentation which in turn is governed by the amount and distribution of the pigment melanin in the melanoblasts (the pigment cells of the skin) and the basal cells of the epidermis. The melanoblasts are capable of manufacturing pigment and passing it to the basal cells.

Discoloration of the skin in cyanosis is due to an abnormally high level of reduced haemoglobin (i.e. haemoglobin from which oxygen has been removed) in the blood circulating in the minute vessels (capillaries and sub-papillary plexus of skin and mucous membrane).

Cyanosis appears when a minimum of 5 g of haemoglobin in every 100 ml of blood is reduced. As each gram of haemoglobin takes up 1.34 ml of oxygen when fully saturated, 5 g will take up $5 \times 1.34 = 6.7$ ml of oxygen per 100 ml of blood, which is the minimum amount of oxygen deficiency necessary to produce cyanosis. Let us assume that each 100 ml of blood contain 15 g of haemoglobin. As each gram of haemoglobin takes up 1.34 ml of oxygen when fully saturated, the oxygen content of the fully saturated blood is about 20 ml per 100 ml. This has to fall to 13.3 ml of oxygen per 100 ml of blood $(20 - 6.7 = 13.3)$ before cyanosis becomes apparent.

Clubbing of finger and toe nails

This is a change in the shape of the nails and terminal portion of the fingers and toes (Fig. 1.34). The nails are excessively curved and the distal portions of the fingers are bulbous. Although clubbing is a common finding in some respiratory conditions, its cause is not clearly understood. When mild, only the nails are affected; but when severe, the fingers become mis-shapen and look like drumsticks.

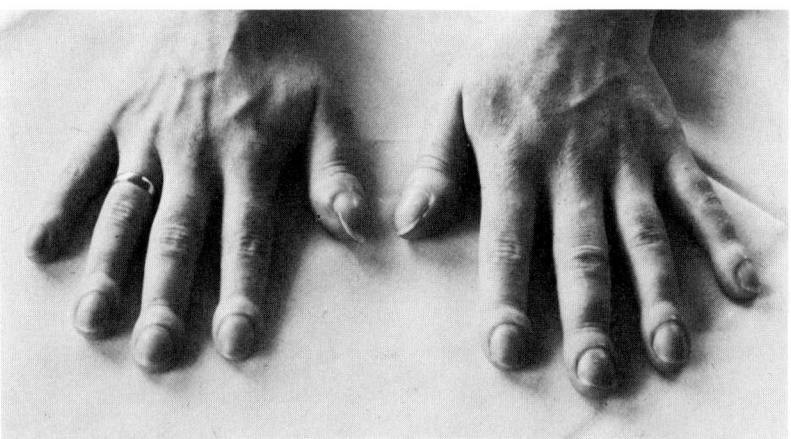

Figure 1.34　Fingernail clubbing.

CLINICAL EXAMINATION

In addition to the clinical history and manifestations of respiratory disease as indicated above, clinical investigations should cover a systemic examination. The medical officer is responsible for clerking patients and recording the relevant findings. Nurses, particularly those responsible for day-to-day care, are advised to read case notes and remember any abnormal findings. They should also carry out a limited examination of their own. The result of this examination should be attached to the nursing history. The purpose of this practice becomes obvious when later observations are made and compared with observations recorded on admission.

Systemic examination should take into account palpable lymphadenopathy, oedema and obvious skin lesions. Attention should be paid to the state of the teeth and mouth; dental sepsis and gum infections should be investigated. The cardio-vascular system is examined with regard to heart rate and rhythm, pulse volume and arterial blood pressure. The respiratory system is examined for chest expansion, rate and depth of breathing and abnormal physical signs. Abnormality of the alimentary tract such as the presence of pain or difficulty on swallowing should be noted together with bowel habits.

Particular attention should be paid to micturition. As many male patients with respiratory diseases are elderly and have prostatic enlargement, the quantity and quality of urine passed should be noted. Haematuria may be the first sign of renal secondaries of a bronchial tumour, or tuberculosis involving the kidneys.

In females, changes in the menstrual period and its abnormalities should be noted. Suspected pregnancies should be pointed out to the medical staff as it is important to be cautious with regard to medications and X-ray exposure.

Finally, abnormalities of the locomotor and central nervous system should be clearly noted.

NON-SPECIFIC LABORATORY INVESTIGATIONS
General laboratory investigations are carried out as follows:

Blood
Full blood count, biochemical profile and ESR are routinely examined and the patient's blood group is determined.

Urine
General ward examination of urine for the presence of sugar and protein should be carried out. The quantity of urine may be charted if required.

ECG
All patients should have an ECG taken pre-operatively.

SPECIAL INVESTIGATIONS
It is largely due to the development of special investigations that more precise diagnosis and earlier treatment of patients with respiratory conditions can be undertaken. These include:

Sputum
The quantity and the type of sputum should be recorded. A specimen is delivered to the laboratory for:

1. *Micro-biological studies*, that is identification of micro-organisms, their culture and sensitivity to antibiotics.

2. *Cytological examination*. It is based on the recovery and identification of abnormal neoplastic (malignant) cells shed in the tracheo-bronchial secretions. Neoplastic cells detach themselves and are shed more easily than their normal counterparts.

Collection of sputum for cytological examination should be carried out over three consecutive days.

In order to have accurate results, it is important to obtain a specimen of bronchial secretions by asking the patient to cough and expectorate. Spitting saliva is useless. An early morning fresh specimen of sputum is preferable and should be delivered to the laboratory within 2 to 3 hours of collection. Specimens of sputum for tubercle bacilli should be sent to the laboratory straight away, if ZN staining is to be carried out. Specimens of sputum for identification of fungi should also be fresh, correctly expectorated and delivered to the laboratory as soon as possible. In each hospital the guidance of the bacteriological laboratory should be sought.

Staining of organisms   The recognition of micro-organisms under microscope in pathological materials is only possible if they are stained, that is making them visible by differential colouring. The Gram technique is based on staining organisms with a dye like crystal violet or methyl violet and then with iodine solution. This stained preparation is submitted to discolouring by alcohol or acetone. Gram-positive organisms resist discolouring and retain the blue colour, whereas Gram-negative ones become red and resist discolouring even with strong acid or alcohol. For this reason an organism is referred to as AFB meaning Acid and Alcohol Fast Bacillus.

ZN (Ziehl-Neelsen)   Owing to their characteristic properties tubercle bacilli can be identified by microscopic examination. The staining method used is ZN. A smear is made and stained. The staining method is based on the knowledge that tubercle bacilli require prolonged exposure to the dye (with application of heat) before taking the stain. However, once the dye has taken they are resistant to the discolouring action of acid and alcohol. They are therefore called 'acid- and alcohol-fast bacilli'.

RADIOLOGICAL INVESTIGATIONS
Chest radiographs in the antero-posterior (or postero-anterior) and the appropriate lateral view are taken in all cases (see also Chapter 25).

Additional radiological investigations can be required and are set out below.

Tomography
It is based on sectional depth radiography of the chest. It gives a clearer delineation of the intrathoracic lesions normally obscured by overlying structures. Tomography is particularly helpful in demonstrating tuberculous cavities and solid tumours.

Bronchography

The bronchial trees can be outlined on an X-ray plate by filling the segmental and sub-segmental bronchial branches of each lung with a radio-opaque solution. Bronchography is particularly useful in the diagnosis of bronchiectasis and bronchial blocks.

Angiography

It consists of the injection of radio-opaque material into a blood vessel, followed by radiography.

Superior vena caval and inferior vena caval angiography shows the outline of these major veins and therefore their deformities reflecting mediastinal abnormalities.

Pulmonary angiography reveals the vascular pattern of the lungs and their anomalies (e.g. blockage by embolus).

Isotope scan

This test is designed to give information about perfusion through the lungs and the distribution of blood within the pulmonary parenchyma. The technique is based on the use of a radioactive trace (radio-isotope). Albumin is tagged with Technitium 99 m and distribution is recorded with a body scanner and a camera. The result (Fig. 1.35) shows the extent of perfusion in the form of multiple dots. Areas of poor or no perfusion are indicated by scanty dotting or a complete lack of dots.

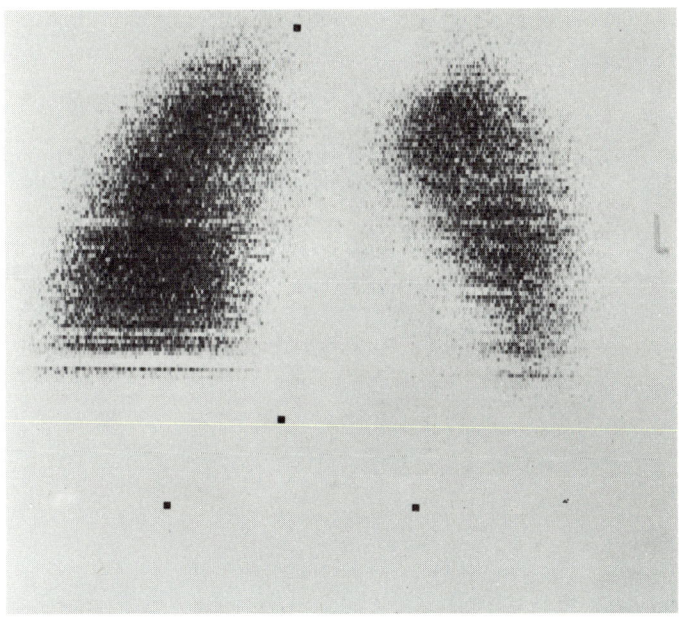

Figure 1.35   Normal pulmonary perfusion scan; anterior view.

Endoscopy

This involves procedures in which visual examination of the interior of an organ or a system is carried out using specially designed instruments. In lung diseases endoscopic examinations are of great diagnostic value and constitute an important investigation.

Bronchoscopy

In this procedure the airways are examined under vision. The scope of bronchoscopy extends from the back of the mouth to the larynx, trachea, main bronchi as far as the lobar and segmental bronchial openings. Traditionally the examination is made under direct vision through the lumen of an instrument called a bronchoscope (Fig. 1.36). In addition, magnification can be obtained by direct and angled telescopes. More recent flexible fibroptic instruments provide a telescopic view of the bronchial trees and of the pulmonary, segmental and sub-segmental orifices (Fig. 1.37).

Bronchoscopy can show anatomical abnormalities and pathological conditions affecting the walls or the lumen of the bronchi. It also provides a means of obtaining bronchial secretions for laboratory (cytological and micro-biological) studies and a biopsy sample. Finally, it allows the removal of foreign bodies and aspiration of abnormal bronchial secretions, particularly after an operation and when patients are not able to get rid of these by natural means, that is by coughing and expectorating. It also allows bronchial disinfection and lavage.

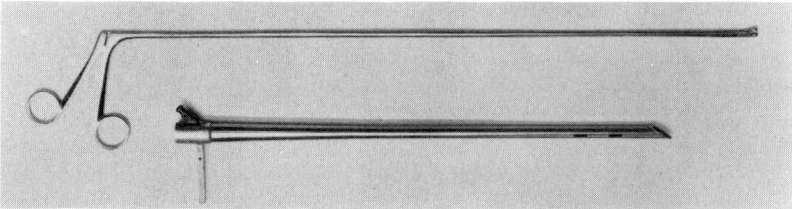

Figure 1.36   Negus bronchoscope and bronchial biopsy forceps.

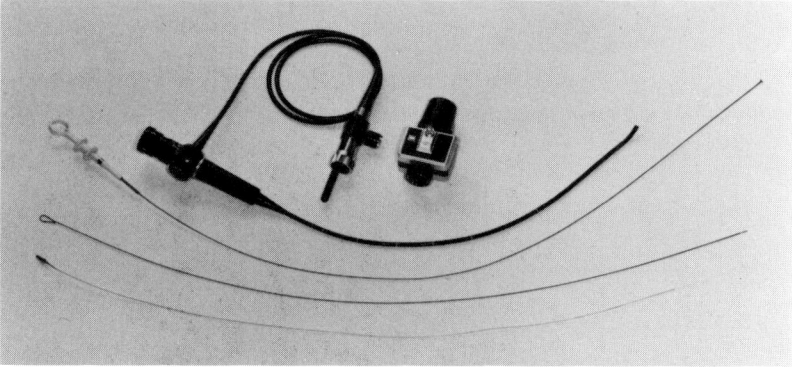

Figure 1.37   Flexible fibroptic bronchoscope.

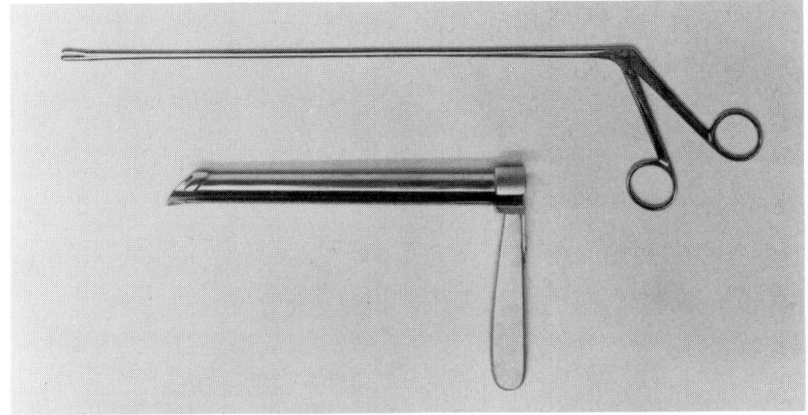

Figure 1.38   Mediastinoscope and biopsy forceps.

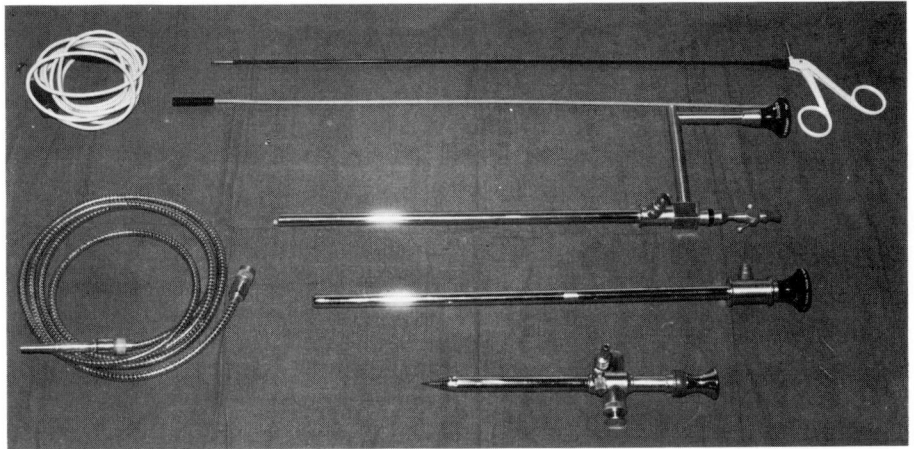

Figure 1.39   Thoracoscopes.

Mediastinoscopy
This is the visual exploration of the superior mediastinum through the mediastinoscope (Fig. 1.38). The instrument is introduced through an incision over the supra-sternal notch. Abnormalities of the superior mediastinum can be detected and lymph node samples obtained for biopsy material.

Thoracoscopy
The pleural cavity is inspected through an instrument called a thoracoscope (Fig. 1.39). Cases requiring this diagnostic procedure are rare. The prerequisite for the use of this instrument is the existence or the provision of a space between the lung proper and the parietal pleura (i.e. the chest wall) to allow the introduction of the instrument. Biopsy material can be obtained through the thoracoscope.

Biopsies

The Oxford dictionary defines biopsy as the 'examination of tissues cut from the living body'. The idea of a biopsy evolved from the development of the microscope and its routine use in medicine. In the field of chest diseases, biopsies enable us to obtain accurate diagnostic information. The biopsy specimen is preserved in formalin solution and then delivered to the laboratory.

Bronchial biopsy

A sample of tissue is obtained during bronchoscopic examination, taking into account the location and the extent of the disease. The sample is obtained using a pair of biopsy forceps passed through the lumen of the bronchoscope.

Gland biopsy

Lymphatic glands are involved sooner or later in the course of the development of pulmonary diseases such as tuberculosis, sarcoidosis and malignancies. In practice a lymph node sample is obtained by:

1. Surgical excision of a palpable enlarged node in the supra-clavicular fossa.
2. Excision of the scalenous pad of fat together with the uninvolved or obviously involved lymph nodes (scalene node biopsy). Scalene lymph nodes are situated over the scalenus anterior muscle at the root of the neck. They become involved at an early stage by pathological conditions of the lungs. Their biopsy is therefore useful in early diagnosis of lung diseases.
3. Obtaining a sample of a node in the superior mediastinum, viewed and removed through the mediastinoscope.
4. Excision of a group of glands in the thoracic cavity following thoracotomy.

Pleural biopsy

This is a biopsy of the parietal pleura covering the chest wall. In some cases of pleural effusion the parietal pleura is involved by pathological processes. In such cases a sample of parietal pleura is of obvious diagnostic value. Parietal pleura biopsy can be obtained essentially by either of the following techniques:

1. *Blind biopsy*—using a needle or a punch biopsy instrument, several types of which are in use. In this country Abram's needle and Moghissi's punch (Fig. 1.40) are most commonly used. With both instruments the biopsy is obtained blindly by the 'feel' of the pleura.

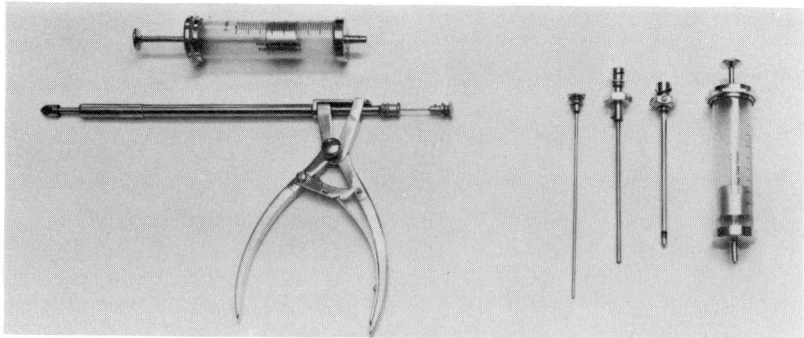

Figure 1.40   Moghissi's biopsy punch (left) and (right) Abram's needle.

2. *Thoracoscopic pleural biopsy*—the pleura is examined with the thoraco-scope and a suitable sample is obtained.

3. *Open pleural biopsy*—a suitable pleural sample is obtained through a limited thoracotomy.

IMMUNOLOGICAL INVESTIGATIONS

These tests are designed to determine the presence of special substances, the immune bodies, in the circulating blood and/or within the cells and tissues. Immune bodies are produced in response to specific micro-organisms or foreign proteins called antigens.

An antigen can be defined as a substance, usually a protein, foreign to the body whose presence is recognised and acknowledged by specialised tissues called collectively the reticulo-endothelial system (e.g. lymph nodes, liver and spleen). Recognition and acknowledgement are followed by the production of another protein called an antibody (or immune body) which tends to counteract or neutralise some of the effects of the antigen.

The immune response refers to this phenomenon of immune body production and plays an important part in defence mechanism and resistance to infection.

The causative agents of some respiratory diseases are antigenic, in which case the demonstration of their appropriate antibodies indicates the actual presence of or previous exposure to the antigen (i.e. the disease). The existence of immune bodies in the serum or tissues of a patient can be investigated by exposure to their antigens *in vitro* (i.e. in the test tube)—e.g. Wasserman test for syphilis—or *in vivo* (i.e. in the living body)—e.g. Mantoux test for tuberculosis. In thoracic diseases immunological investigations are of particular interest.

They can be described under:

1. Delayed-type skin hypersensitivity test in which the tissue (skin) is exposed to the antigen. The presence of antibodies, in this case attached to the cells, is revealed by a local inflammatory reaction at the site of entry of the antigen after 48 to 72 hours. Examples of these are: (a) Tuberculin test, which can be Mantoux test or Heaf Multiple Puncture, and (b) Kveim test.

2. Other-type sensitivity tests.

3. Serological tests.

DELAYED-TYPE SKIN HYPERSENSITIVITY TESTS

Tuberculine test
This test is based on exposing the skin to the protein derived from the tubercle bacilli (with its antigen properties). A positive reaction helps to confirm diagnosis or previous exposure and a negative one to exclude tuberculosis. Preparations used (as antigen) are (1) old tuberculin (OT) obtained from the culture of the tubercle bacilli and specially prepared, and (2) purified protein derivatives (PPD). As the name implies the purified protein is prepared from cultured tubercle bacilli. It is superior to OT because of the elimination of undesirable protein fraction.

Mantoux test   0.1 ml of 1/1000 (or stronger) tuberculin is injected intradermally through a fine needle usually on the anterior aspect of one forearm. On the opposite arm the same quantity of sterile water is injected intradermally. After 48 to 72 hours the injected area is inspected. A positive reaction is shown by swelling or inflammation with oedema over a circular area of 5 mm (or more) in diameter at the site of the tuberculin injection. The opposite site (injected with sterile water) shows no significant reaction.

Heaf Multiple Puncture   A drop or two of PPD is applied over the skin of the forearm. It is introduced into the skin by using the instrument (Fig. 1.41) which has a ring of six needles which can be released by pressing a catch on the handle. The result is read after 48 hours. A grading of 1–4 is made according to the presence of indurations, a ring of oedema, a large area of swelling, or necrosis at the site of the injection.

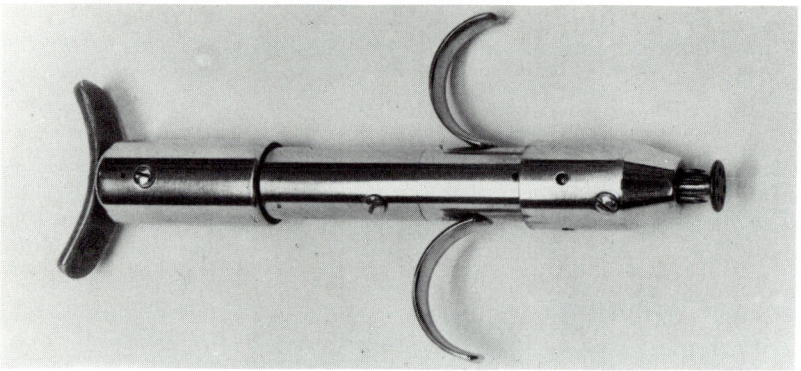

Figure 1.41   Heaf multiple puncture instrument.

Kveim test

This test used to confirm or exclude the diagnosis of sarcoidosis. Injection of 'sarcoid product' into the skin is followed by the appearance of a small nodule at the site of injection. Some particular points have to be mentioned:

1. The product injected is a suspension of an involved lymph node obtained from a patient (0.1 ml of 10% suspension).
2. The reaction becomes apparent slowly and a month or more is required before results can be read.
3. The nodule has to be excised and examined under the microscope.

OTHER-TYPE SENSITIVITY TESTS

In some conditions (e.g. hay fever and asthma) solutions of various incriminating and suspected material are injected, or placed over the skin and the skin scratched or pricked. Ten or fifteen minutes later the area is inspected. A positive reaction is noted by the presence of an inflammatory reaction with oedema, swelling and induration.

SEROLOGICAL TESTS

In the laboratory the patient's serum is exposed to the antigen from a specific micro-organism. A recognisable reaction (precipitation, flocculation) indicates the presence of the corresponding immune body in the serum and thus confirms the diagnosis beyond doubt. Serological tests are used in some fungal infections.

7 Congenital Abnormalities of Chest Wall and Lung

In this chapter conditions affecting the lungs, the pleura and the chest wall are discussed.

Of the many conditions affecting the lungs only a few are within the scope of surgery. The advent of antibiotics of increasing potency and spectrum have done much to reduce the necessity for surgery. At present the greatest number of patients requiring surgery are sufferers of neoplastic diseases and until a specific therapeutic agent is found surgery is the mainstay of treatment.

Before discussing diseases of the lung, it is appropriate to emphasise two points: (1) only conditions for which surgery is of therapeutic use either as a principal or as an accessory method of treatment are discussed here, and (2) some kind of working classification, even if pragmatic, has to be used in order to facilitate discussion and learning.

CHEST WALL DEFORMITIES

RIB ANOMALIES

Isolated rib anomalies are not infrequently found in the course of routine chest radiography. They do not usually cause any visible deformity. They need no treatment as they cause no symptoms or complications. Occasionally a prominent rib or a costal cartilage becomes noticeably deformed and unacceptable. It then requires excision.

ABSENCE OF A RIB

It is again more of a radiological curiosity than a clinical problem and needs no treatment. Sometimes rib anomalies are associated with vertebral anomalies and can cause scoliotic deformities.

PECTUS DEFORMITIES

These types of chest deformity are more complex and involve the sternum, costal cartilages and the ribs. They can be classified as pectus excavatum and carinatum, and mixed type deformities.

Pectus excavatum (Synonym Funnel Chest) (Fig. 1.42)   The lower sternum and the anterior ends of the ribs are depressed. The deformity may be mild and confined to a small area of the lower chest wall. It can be severe and extend from the level of the 2nd costal cartilage to the costal margin. Pectus excavatum can be a symmetrical or asymmetrical deformity (taking the midline as the middle of the sternum).

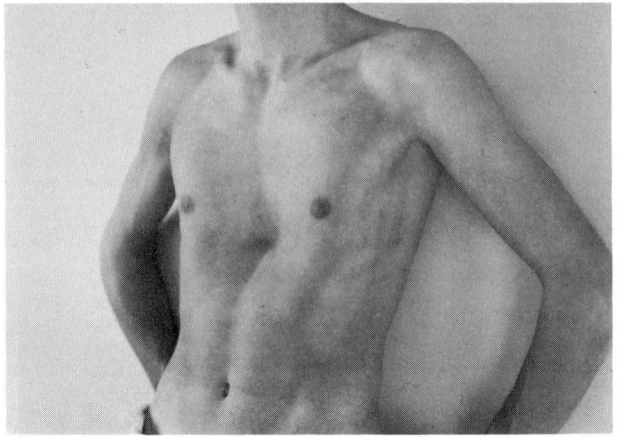

Figure 1.42   Pectus excavatum.

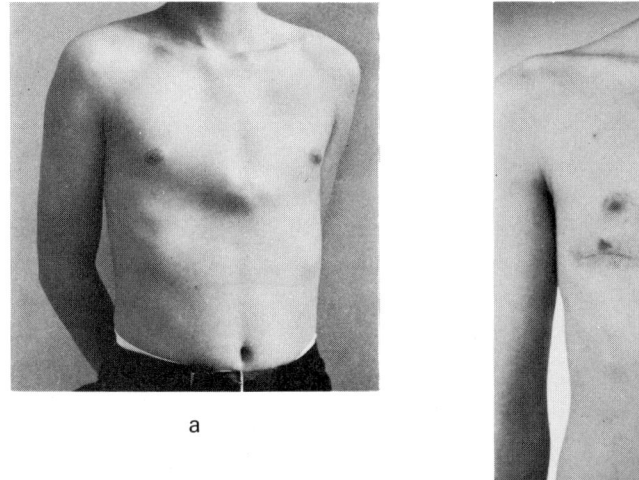

a

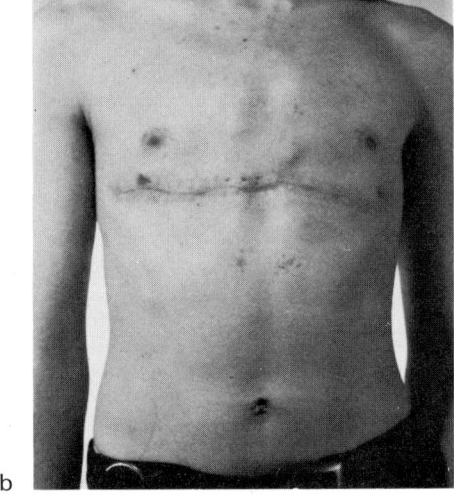

b

Figure 1.43   Pectus carinatum. (a) Before and (b) after correction.

Pectus carinatum (Synonym Pigeon Chest) (Fig. 1.43)   The lower sternum and the affected costal cartilages project forward and become prominent. Pectus carinatum can also vary in extent and be symmetrical or asymmetrical.

Mixed type deformities   Combined pectus excavatum and carinatum affect different areas of the anterior chest wall.

Clinical features

In most cases the condition is entirely asymptomatic and patients, or parents of a child, consult the doctor because of the peculiar shape of the chest or associated kyphosis in severe cases. Occasionally there can be associated respiratory or cardiac lesions with their respective symptoms and signs. Displacement of the heart and the unusual radiological appearance are generally of no physiological significance.

Management

In asymptomatic cases when the deformity is slight and when there are no associated psychological problems, reassurance is all that is needed.

In severe cases, or when the patient is psychologically disturbed by the deformity, surgical correction is undertaken. Full pre-operative investigations, including chest radiograph and ECG, are carried out. The patient is prepared and physiotherapy is given a few days beforehand. In many units a clinical photograph of the deformed chest is also taken for the records.

Surgical correction

There are several types of operation all consisting essentially of the excision of the deformed costal cartilage and the release of the sternum from its diaphragmatic and abdominal muscles attachments. The lower sternum is elevated by a transverse osteotomy. The elevation is maintained, usually by placing a stainless steel bar under its lower end. The soft tissues and skin incision are repaired, the mediastinum and the pleural cavities are drained (the latter only when they have been entered). The bar is removed six months later when the sternum and the corrected chest wall are stable.

Post-operatively the patient's ventilation should be watched carefully as the interference with the bony chest wall produces some degree of paradoxical breathing which can culminate in respiratory insufficiency requiring ventilatory assistance.

ABNORMALITIES OF THE LUNG

PULMONARY AGENESIS

Agenesis can be defined as complete absence at birth of an anatomical part (e.g. organ), as a result of lack of development during embryonic life. In pulmonary agenesis there are several types affecting different components of the lung.

HYPOPLASIA

Hypoplasia (under-development) is often associated with other congenital abnormalities such as congenital diaphragmatic hernia. Survival in these cases is dependent on the sum total of the normally functioning pulmonary parenchyma.

SEQUESTRATED LUNG (ectopic lung)

A mass of accessory lung tissues is either connected to an abnormal bronchus or attached to, but not communicating with, the bronchial tract. The abnormal lung tissue has an abnormal blood supply derived from the aorta. The condition is discovered either in the course of a routine chest radiograph or as a result of super-added infective complications leading to investigations of the patient. In

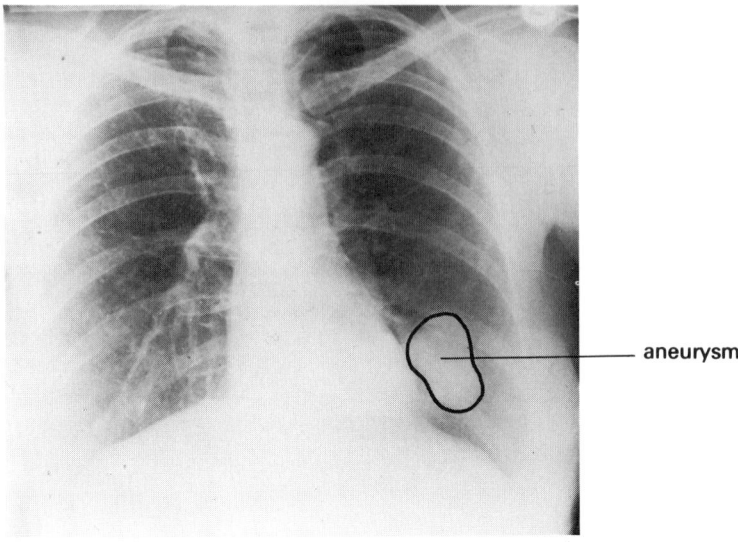

aneurysm

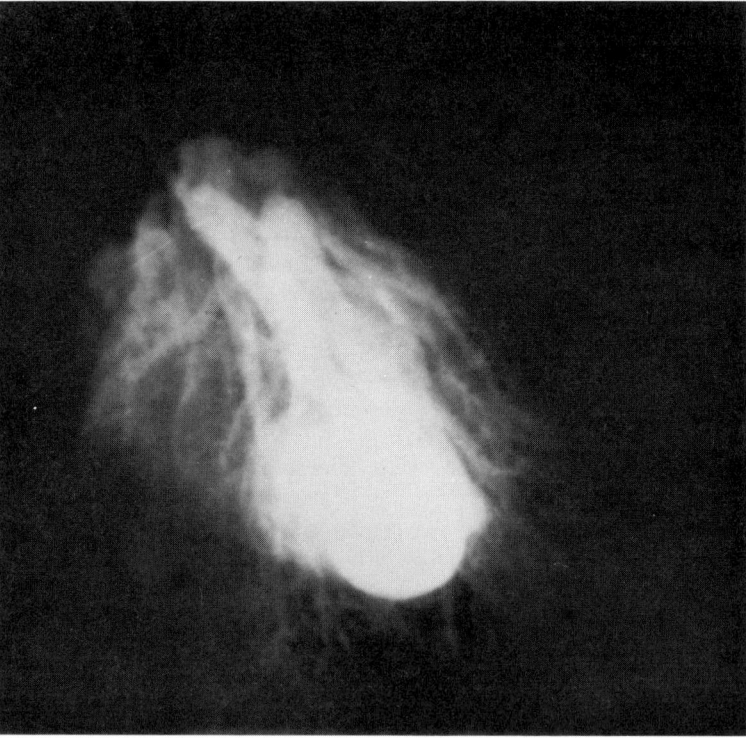

Figure 1.44   Pulmonary arteriovenous aneurysm (a) on chest radiograph and (b) injected with radio-opaque dye.

many instances, the ectopic tissue presents itself as an inter-lobar sequestrated mass which is excised.

CYSTS OF THE LUNG

Although most lung cysts are acquired some are congenital. In children the distinction may be difficult. Such cysts can be connected to the bronchi, in which case they contain air or fluid. They are discovered accidentally or through infective complications. Their management consists of their surgical exploration and excision.

PULMONARY ARTERIOVENOUS ANEURYSM

The condition has been variously described as pulmonary hemangioma, angiomatous hamartoma, pulmonary telangiectasis and pulmonary arterio-venous fistula. It consists of an abnormal formation of blood vessels in which there is essentially direct communication between the pulmonary arterial and venous branches (by-passing capillaries). The lesion consists of single or multiple arteriovenous communications, or there can be in addition a larger pool intervening between arterial and venous communications.

Presenting symptoms and signs depend on the size and the multiplicity of the lesions. When there are numerous or extensive lesions, cyanosis, dyspnoea and polycythaemia are present because of the high volume of arteriovenous mixing of the blood (constituting effectively a large arteriovenous shunt). When the lesion is single and limited in extent, it can be asymptomatic and discovered accidentally.

In many cases the increased density or a definite opacity on the chest radiograph (Fig. 1.44a) as an incidental finding or in course of investigations for haemoptysis, is the first indication of the lesion. Diagnosis is confirmed by pulmonary angiography showing the filling of the aneurysm with radio-opaque dye (Fig. 1.44b).

Treatment

Surgical excision of the lesion with its surrounding pulmonary parenchyma is, when possible, the curative treatment.

8 Chest Injuries

The majority of chest injuries in civilian life are caused by blunt trauma and are associated with road traffic accidents. A smaller number are caused by the penetration of sharp or blunt objects. In many casualties, there are multiple injuries, including those to the chest. The following classification can be adopted in describing the commonest types of chest injury.

1. *Blunt injuries*
   (a) Those resulting in a stable chest:
       (i) Chest wall injuries only.
       (ii) Chest wall and intrathoracic visceral injuries.
   (b) Those resulting in an unstable chest:
       (i) Chest wall injuries only.
       (ii) Chest wall and intrathoracic visceral injuries.
2. *Penetrating injuries*
    (i) Chest wall injuries only.
   (ii) Chest wall and intrathoracic visceral injuries.

This classification is based on the stability of the chest—an important consideration.

The distinction between stable and unstable chest is made on the presence or absence of paradoxical breathing (the term flail chest being synonymous with unstable chest). Paradoxical breathing is disharmonious and asymmetrical movements between the injured and healthy side of the chest. The injured side moves out of phase with the healthy one, so that when one is in the inspiratory phase the other is in the expiratory phase. Diagnosis of paradoxical breathing can be made by inspection and a simple manoeuvre consisting of placing the palm of each hand lightly over the anterior surface of the right and the left chest. Each hand will follow the movement of one side of the chest revealing the pattern of breathing.

GENERAL CONSIDERATION AND PHYSIOPATHOLOGY OF CHEST INJURIES

All but the simplest chest injuries have adverse effects on breathing and the respiratory function. The effect is more marked in individuals suffering from any form of respiratory or cardiac disease. Adverse effects are the results of one or more of the following:

1. Pain which prevents deep respiratory excursion.
2. Trauma to soft tissues (notably the intercostal and other muscles concerned with respiration) resulting in reduction of movement and expansion of the underlying lung.

3. Difficulty of expectoration.

4. Contusion of the lung with some degree of inflammation and oedema. At times this develops into major respiratory embarrassment known as 'wet lung', with an increase in bronchial secretions and pulmonary oedema.

5. Serious additional ventilatory problems in the case of chest wall injuries causing an unstable chest.

6. In visceral injuries, lung laceration, haematoma or simple pneumothorax directly impairing the function of the lungs.

Chest injuries lead to a disturbance of breathing ranging from temporary and trivial to longstanding and more important respiratory failure accompanied by hypoxia and carbon dioxide retention.

Pain and dyspnoea are usually present in all chest injuries. Haemoptysis and cyanosis, accompanied by surgical subcutaneous emphysema, usually indicate pulmonary injuries. Shift of the mediastinum can be diagnosed by the displacement of the trachea above the supra-sternal notch. It indicates differential pressure between the two sides of the chest. This is usually caused by air (pneumothorax) or blood (haemothorax) in the pleural space on one side pushing the mediastinum to the opposite side.

Radiological investigations are essential for precise diagnosis of injuries. Fractures of ribs, haemothorax, pneumothorax and various visceral injuries are detectable radiologically.

GENERAL MANAGEMENT OF CHEST INJURIES

This is considered under headings: (1) assessment of injuries, (2) early management and first-aid measures, and (3) specific treatment.

ASSESSMENT OF INJURIES

Before the type and severity of chest injury is assessed, the patient's general condition and the extent of injuries to other parts of the body are determined. It is important to record the state of consciousness and the coexistence of heart or abdominal injuries. It is also vital to ensure unobstructed airways, and to take appropriate and speedy measures against traumatic and hypovolumic shock.

The assessment of chest injuries itself involves clinical and radiological investigations.

EARLY MANAGEMENT AND FIRST-AID MEASURES

As already pointed out, even before assessing the precise nature of chest injuries, complete examination of the patient is essential in order to assess his general condition and injuries to other parts of the body, so that therapeutic measures essential to immediate survival may be taken.

Provision of clear airways must be the first priority in dealing with any serious injury, particularly chest injuries. This should be carried out at once and requires no more than a suction machine and few swabs. In practice, endo-tracheal intubation is performed in cases of severe injuries so that adequate ventilation is maintained during examination.

In penetrating wounds of the thorax causing direct communication between the pleural space and the atmospheric air, the opening must be sealed with swabs, towels or even the palm of a hand, thus preventing a sucking open pneumothorax (see Chapter 9).

Arrest of haemorrhage should be undertaken speedily.

A pleural drain should be inserted urgently when a haemopneumothorax is present.

An intravenous drip and a central venous pressure line (CVP) should be set up for all but the simplest injuries. When shock is present anti-shock measures should be undertaken (see *First-aid anti-shock measures*, p. 144).

In serious chest injuries with paradoxical breathing, it is usually necessary to carry out endo-tracheal intubation. A naso-gastric tube and a bladder catheter should also be inserted.

Emergency laboratory tests should be carried out on admission in serious cases. They include blood grouping and cross-matching, arterial blood gas analysis and urine testing for blood sugar and proteins.

In the course of early management and first aid, it is necessary to record initial observations such as:

1. Level of consciousness and all abnormal neurological findings.
2. Arterial and central venous pressure, and venous filling.
3. Body temperature.
4. Presence or absence of cyanosis, rate and depth of breathing as well as mode of respiration (regular, phasic and paradoxical respiration).
5. Abdominal distension, presence or absence of bowel sounds.
6. Presence of blood, sugar and proteins in the urine.

These initial observation recordings form a baseline against which subsequent recordings are placed and the patient's progress judged.

Further management of chest injuries depends on the nature and the severity of injuries.

SPECIFIC TREATMENT OF CHEST INJURIES

BLUNT INJURIES

Chest wall injuries
Isolated fractured ribs (Fig. 1.45) may not require hospital admission but in cases of multiple rib fractures admission is usually necessary even in the absence of paradoxical breathing. In the absence of paradoxical breathing or any other complication, ribs with a simple fracture only require relief of pain and prevention of lung collapse. Systemic analgesics have the disadvantage of depressing the nervous system including the respiratory centres. Therefore nerve block is preferred. A local anaesthetic is infiltrated around the intercostal nerves and near the area of fracture. It can be repeated 10 to 12 hours later. Mild analgesics and sedatives can be given.

Pulmonary collapse is prevented by active physiotherapy and early mobilisation.

When ribs are fractured in two or more places, the integrity and stability of the chest are lost and paradoxical breathing appears (Fig. 1.46). If the patient's condition is not too serious the same treatment applies as for simple fracture.

Severe cases of flail chest require complicated treatment, even when no other

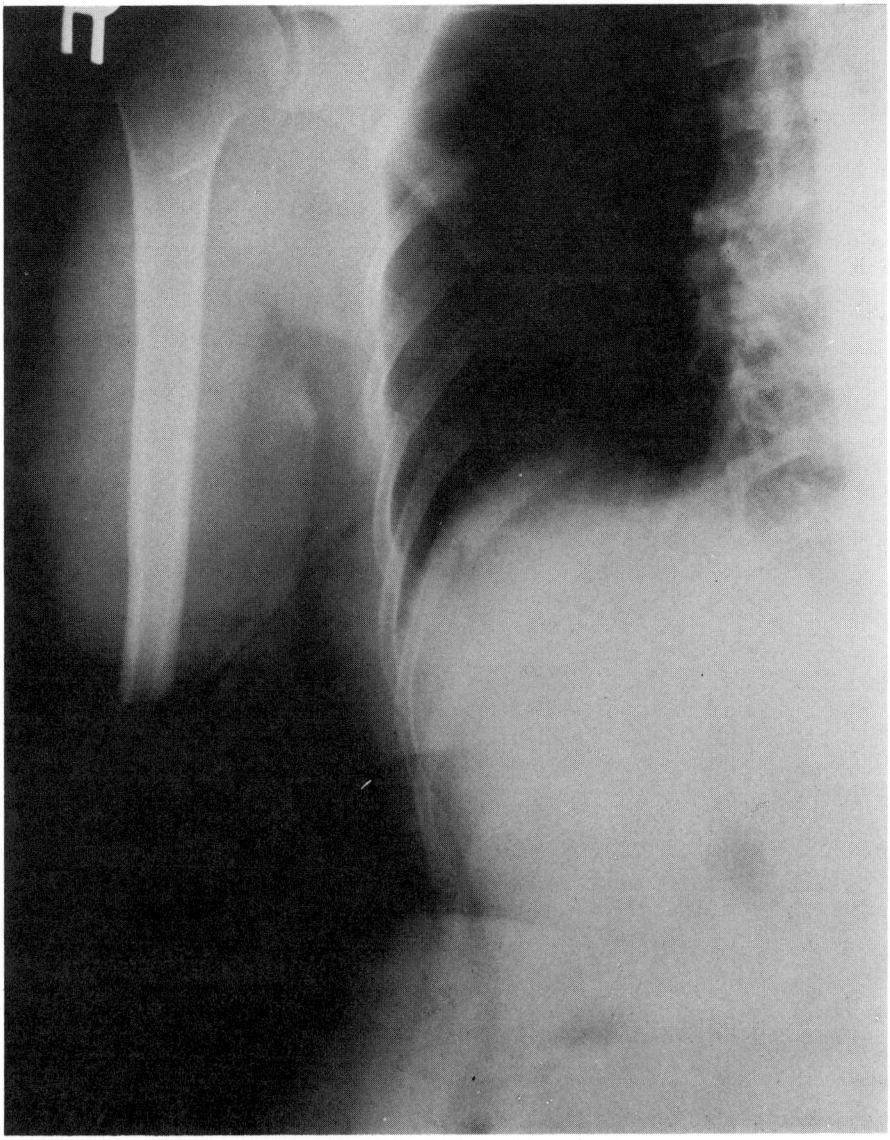

Figure 1.45   Simple rib fractures without displacement.

associated visceral injuries are apparent. Often the underlying lungs are contused and within the first 48 to 72 hours they become congested and oedematous. There are essentially two ways of treating the unstable chest with paradoxical breathing:

1. External splintage, consisting of:
    (a) Wiring and fixing of the fractured ribs during surgical exploration.
    (b) Fracture elevation by continuous traction of the depressed part of the ribs causing the flail chest.

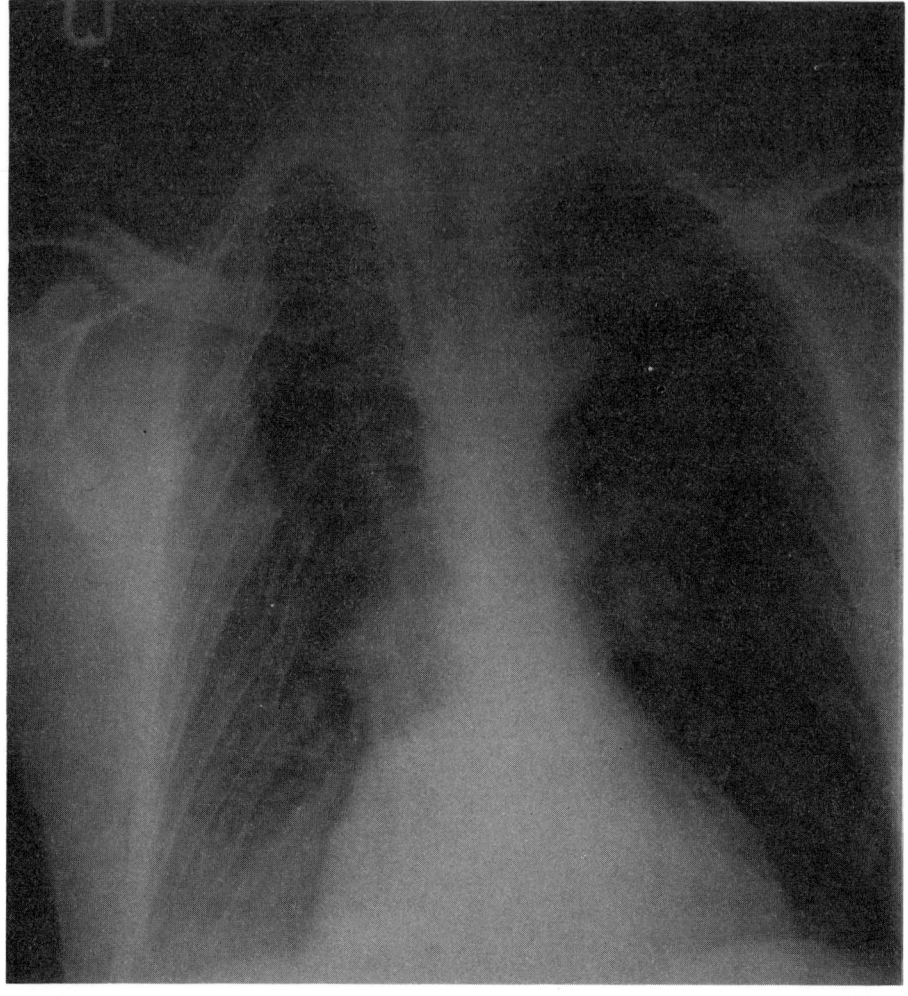

Figure 1.46 Multiple rib fractures with displacement of the segments causing paradoxical breathing.

2. Internal splintage consisting of endo-tracheal intubation (tracheostomy) and positive pressure ventilation.

The second method (internal splintage) is the most commonly used.

Fractured sternum
Fractured sternum occupies a special place, as it can occur with a stable or unstable chest.

Its management is similar to that of rib fracture. Particular attention must be paid to the fact that the pericardium and the heart are in direct anatomical contact with the sternum. Therefore extra care should be given to the diagnosis of pericardial/cardiac traumatic injuries.

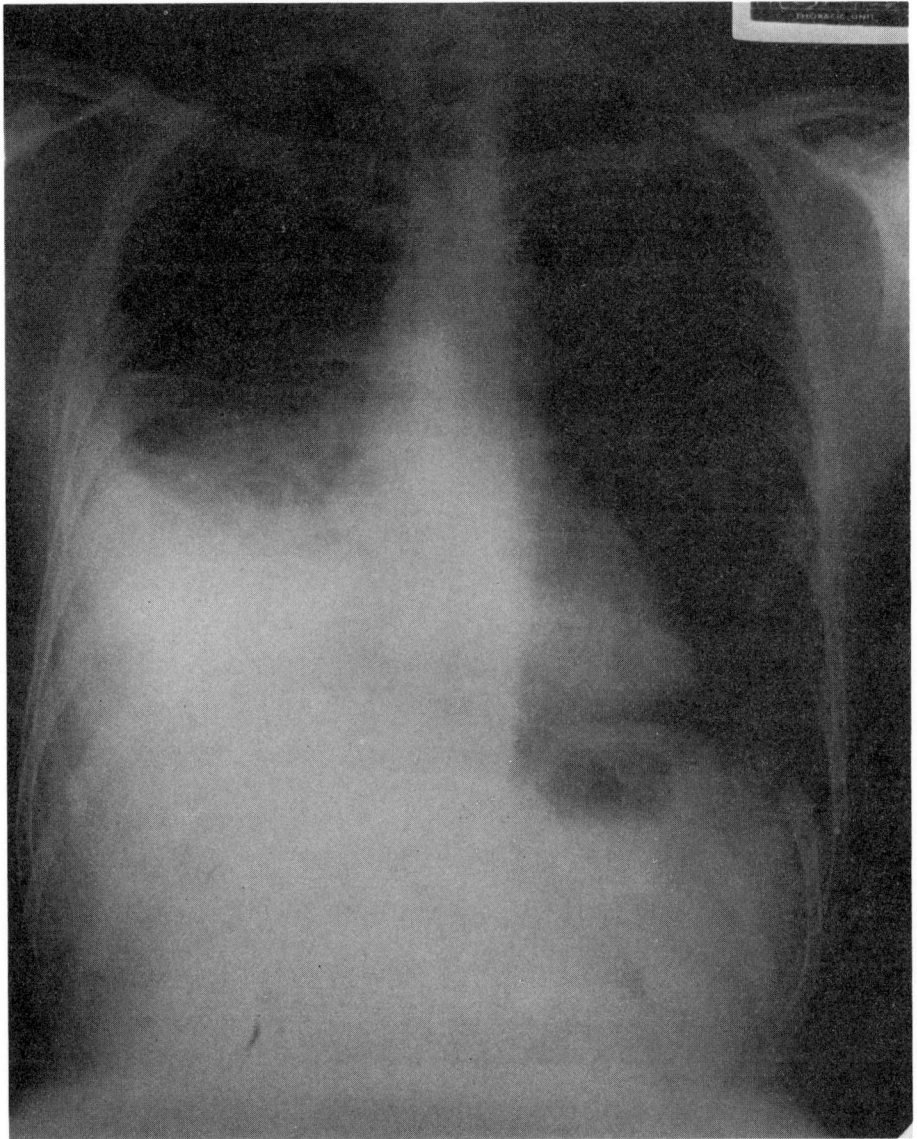

Figure 1.47   Traumatic haemo-pneumothorax on the right side.

Visceral injuries

Thoracic visceral injuries are in most cases associated with chest wall injuries.

Of all intrathoracic viscera, the lungs are the most frequently affected organs following trauma to the chest.

In minor pulmonary injuries a pneumothorax or a haemothorax can be present (Fig. 1.47). In cases of pneumothorax, the air may not be confined to the

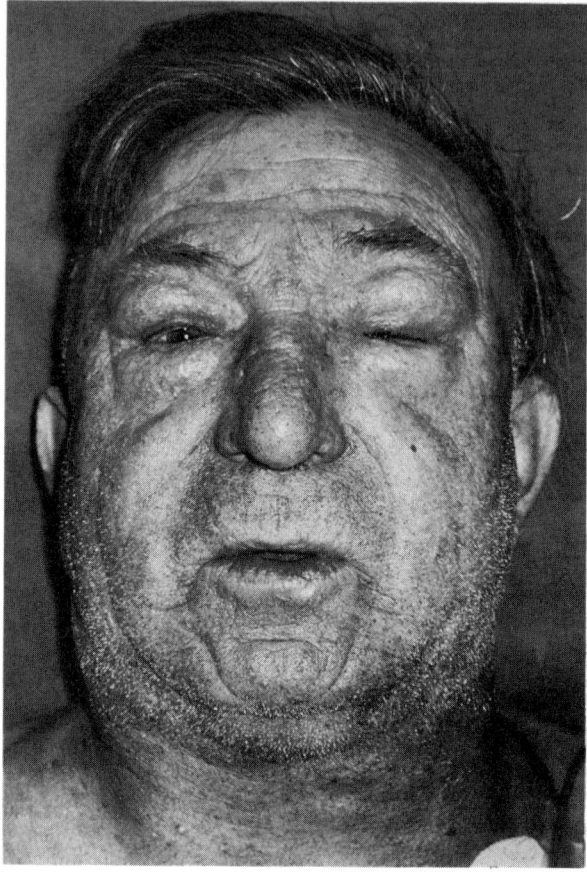

Figure 1.48   Surgical subcutaneous emphysema of the neck and face.

thorax. Escape into the soft tissues of the chest and neck causes surgical emphysema (Fig. 1.48). In a haemothorax the effects of lung collapse are added to those of haemorrhage and hypovolumia (Fig. 1.47).

Blunt trauma to the chest such as in road accidents can cause injuries to the heart or great vessels. Contusion and laceration of the heart with damage to valves or the intracardiac septum are occasionally found. Rupture of the thoracic aorta, usually just below the subclavian artery, is more common.

Such injuries require urgent accurate diagnosis, active resuscitation measures and carefully planned emergency surgical treatment in a department with facilities for all cardio-thoracic surgical procedures.

The general principles of the treatment consist of:

1. Drainage of the pleural space by an intercostal catheter connected to an underwater sealed system and low pressure suction (5 to 10 mm Hg). The volume

of drainage is measured and the blood loss replaced. The volume of drainage is monitored every 15 minutes. Continuous bleeding must be reported to the medical officer. Gross and uncontrollable air leak in the drain is often due to laceration of the lung or a ruptured bronchus. This should also be reported to the surgical team.

2. Frequent recordings of the pulse rate and volume, the arterial and the central venous pressures.

3. Chest radiograph taken after the intercostal drains have been inserted to check lung expansion.

When there is major pulmonary laceration with haemoptysis and extensive haemo-pneumothorax, or when a bronchus is ruptured, surgery is necessary. The patient is prepared for an emergency thoracotomy.

PENETRATING INJURIES

Chest wall injuries (superficial injuries)
Superficial wounds involving skin and soft tissues are managed in the same way as similar wounds in any other part of the body. Extensive lacerations need both local and general treatment. Locally the wound requires cleaning followed by surgical debridement and repair. Hypovolumic shock is prevented by administration of analgesics, plasma and blood. A suitable broad-spectrum antibiotic is given prophylactically.

Chest wall and visceral injuries (deep injuries)
In civilian life, injuries are caused by a variety of sharp weapons whose type varies according to social classes and customs. Knives of different sizes and shapes and broken bottles are the most common in this country. Shotgun wounds are occasionally encountered in farming communities (Fig. 1.49).

In cases of serious penetrating wounds, correct application of first-aid measures, speed of transport to a chest surgery centre and comprehensive assessment of injuries are essential to recovery.

Speed in transporting the patient to a chest surgery centre is the essence of success. The only first-aid measures which have priority over transportation are (1) provision of effective airways free from blood and secretions, and (2) application of a piece of cloth or material over a sucking wound connected to the pleural space.

A deeply-penetrating knife should not be extracted.

It should be remembered that visceral damage is often more extensive than the chest wall wound would indicate, particularly in the case of injuries caused by high velocity projectiles.

Because of their size and anatomical position, the lungs are often lacerated. This causes serious bleeding and pulmonary collapse, which in turn causes more extensive haemorrhaging. Dyspnoea, shock and cyanosis are present in all serious injuries. Cardiac tamponade may be produced if the pericardium and the heart are wounded by the penetrating object.

Assessment of injuries is best carried out in the operating theatre while resuscitation measures are still in progress.

Surgery is usually necessary and its extent varies with the severity of injuries.

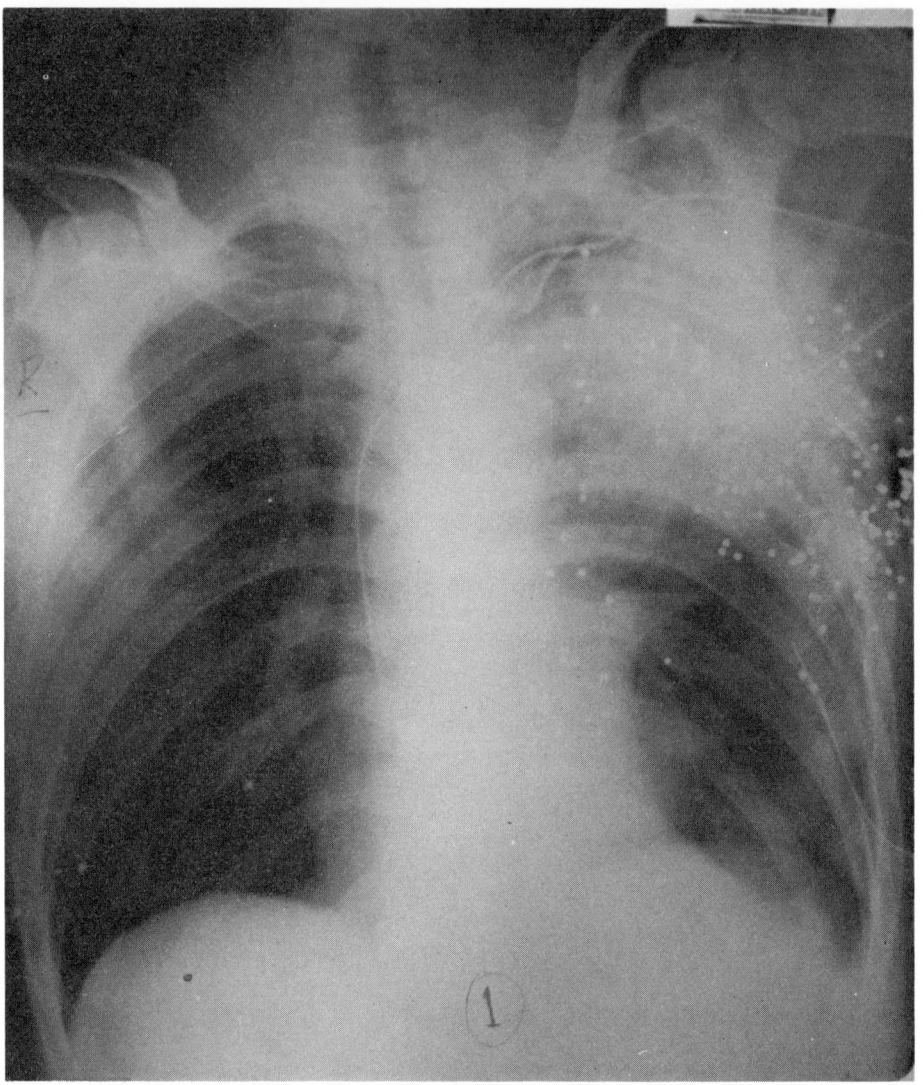

Figure 1.49 Gunshot wound of the chest with extensive laceration of the left lung.
Note *pellets and central venous pressure line* in situ.

9 Pneumothorax

Pneumothorax is the presence of air in the pleural space causing lung collapse (Fig. 1.50). Basically air can enter the pleural space either from within the air ways (i.e. escaping from the lung) or from the outside of the chest through a wound caused by a penetrating injury. There are several types of pneumothorax, all of which can be classified as closed or open pneumothorax.

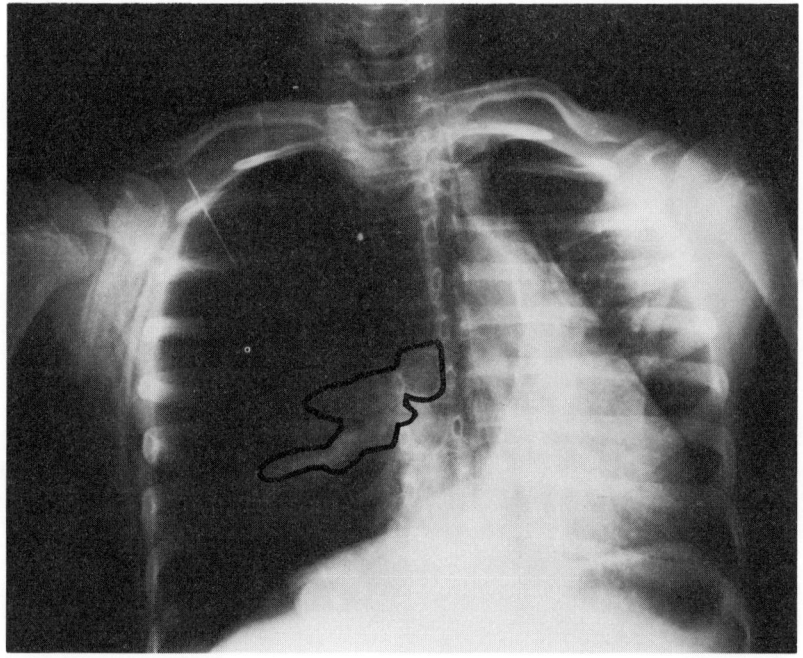

Figure 1.50   Right-sided pneumothorax with shift of the mediastinum to the left (tension pneumothorax).

CLOSED PNEUMOTHORAX

In this type, air is leaking from the lung and enters the pleural space. The opening in the lung acts as a one-way valve admitting air on inspiration only. A great deal of air can be present in the pleura with an increasing pressure (tension pneumothorax). This produces lung collapse with a shift of the mediastinum to the opposite side, and interference with blood circulation.

OPEN PNEUMOTHORAX

Air enters and leaves the pleural space which is continuous with the atmosphere and therefore at the same pressure. The lung collapses and the mediastinum swings from side to side with each breathing movement.

Aetiologically pneumothoraces can be classified as:

1. *Traumatic.* Caused by blunt or penetrating injury to the chest.
2. *Spontaneous.* This type is distinguishable from the others by its spontaneous occurrence as a result of rupture of an emphysematous bleb, bulla or cyst.

CLINICAL FEATURES AND DIAGNOSIS

The majority of pneumothoraces are spontaneous and caused by rupture of an emphysematous bulla; they are usually of the closed type and cause great tension. The patient experiences a sudden pain in the chest followed by acute dyspnoea. Clinical examination shows absence of or reduction in breath sounds in the affected area and shift of the mediastinum (as revealed by tracheal displacement above the supra-sternal notch). A chest radiograph confirms the diagnosis of pneumothorax and collapse of the lung.

TREATMENT

This is based on evacuation of the air and expansion of the lung and maintenance of the expansion.

Treatment must take into account the cause of pneumothorax. Effective air evacuation from the pleural space usually, but not always, results in expansion of the lung.

EVACUATION OF AIR

Air evacuation can be achieved by one or two methods:

1. *Pleural aspiration.* Simple pleural aspiration sometimes deals successfully with a shallow closed pneumothorax.
2. *Continuous drainage of air.* The use of an intercostal catheter connected to an underwater sealed system provides continuous drainage and ensures expansion of the lung.

MAINTENANCE OF EXPANSION

Evacuation of air and lung expansion deal with the immediate situation, but a continuing air leak must be prevented and expansion maintained. This can be effected by either drainage and pleurodesis, or thoracotomy and pleurectomy.

Drainage and pleurodesis

Expansion is maintained by abolishing the space between the visceral and parietal pleura, allowing the lung to adhere firmly to the chest wall. This is achieved in practice by inserting a catheter in the pleural space thus removing the air and expanding the lung. At the same time a chemical irritant is introduced into the pleura, producing an inflammation and the desired adhesion of the pleural surfaces (pleurodesis). The chemical used can be silver nitrate 10 % (1–2 ml), iodised talc (2 g) or camphorated oil.

The technique commonly used by surgical units consists of (1) thoracoscopy and assessment of the underlying pathology of the pneumothorax, (2) spraying the surface of the lung with iodised talc, and (3) inserting an apical pleural catheter connected to the underwater sealed drainage system. Following pleurodesis the main points to be observed are:

1. Care of the drainage tube and the underwater sealed drainage system.
2. Relief of pain as pleurodesis induces chemical pleuritis which is very painful.
3. Physiotherapy which is frequently difficult because of the pain.
4. Active mobilisation.

It should be noted that the patient will have a fever for a day or two following the procedure.

Thoracotomy and pleurectomy

Thoracotomy is carried out to allow exploration of the lung and assessment of the causative pathology. This is frequently found to be the rupture of an emphysematous cyst or a large bulla. They can usually be plicated, but occasionally lobectomy becomes necessary. The parietal pleura is then stripped from the chest wall, the surgical wound is repaired, drains are left in the pleural space. In this procedure pleurodesis is achieved by the adhesion of fibrin and raw surface of the chest wall after pleurectomy. It is generally agreed that chronic and repeated spontaneous pneumothoraces are best treated by this method.

EMPHYSEMATOUS BULLAE OF THE LUNG (AIR CYSTS)

Since Laënnec first described emphysema many attempts have been made to define it in a phrase which incorporates all its characteristics. This has led to many descriptions, all of which contain two of the characteristics of the disease: namely, destruction of the lung tissue and enlargement of air spaces beyond the bronchioles. One could say that emphysema is a condition in which there is distension and over-inflation of the alveoli, the walls of which are destroyed. In addition there is a reduction in the capillary bed of pulmonary circulation. These structural changes cause impairment of pulmonary function and respiratory failure.

Emphysema itself is a medical and not a surgical condition. However in some instances its complications require surgical treatment. It is necessary to define some of the terminology commonly used in connection with emphysema.

Bleb: A collection of air beneath the visceral (pulmonary) pleura, that is, outside the alveoli.

Bulla: A collection of air within the distended alveoli. Bullae can become very large, occupying a whole hemithorax.

The two complications of emphysema in which surgical treatment plays a role are: spontaneous pneumothorax and bullous emphysema and air cyst of the lung.

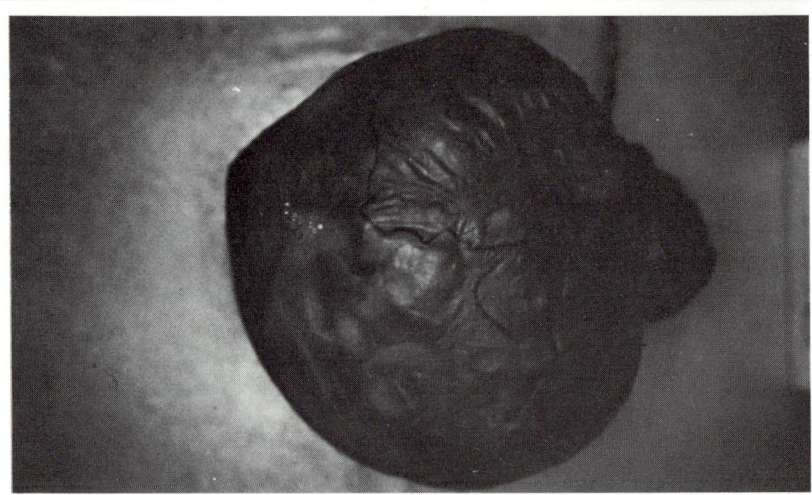

*Figure 1.51   (a) Emphysematous cyst of the left upper lobe with collapse of the left
lower lobe. (b) Specimen of the excised cyst.*

SPONTANEOUS PNEUMOTHORAX
Rupture of a bleb or bulla causes spontaneous pneumothorax (see Pneumo-thorax, p. 79).

AIR CYSTS (emphysematous bullae)
When the size of a bulla is such that it collects a great deal of air, it compresses the healthy or healthier portion of the lung and acts as a space-occupying mass collapsing the underlying part of the lung. The result of this is a further reduction of the respiratory capacity already impaired by emphysema.

Patients can remain asymptomatic, even with a large bulla, as long as the remaining pulmonary tissues are healthy. In the majority of cases, however, respiratory symptoms are present. These can be intermittent episodes of acute exacerbation of dyspnoea and wheeze caused by an increase in the size of the bulla and resulting pressure effects.

Investigations are directed toward assessing the suitability of the case and of the patient for surgery. Surgical treatment is indicated (1) when the bulla is large and exerts pressure over the lung, (2) when it causes symptoms, and (3) when the remaining lung is of good quality.

A chest radiograph shows the size of the bulla and the space it occupies (Fig. 1.51a). Bronchography and arteriography show the degree of compression exerted on the rest of the lung, the broncho-vascular pattern of the bulla and of the unaffected part of the lung. Pulmonary isotopes can demonstrate perfusion and ventilation of the bulla compared with the rest of the pulmonary parenchyma.

Full pulmonary function tests are carried out to assess the patient's suitability for surgery. The degree of benefit to be expected is estimated by careful consideration of the results of anatomopathological and functional investigations.

SURGICAL TREATMENT
A thoracotomy is carried out to allow excision or plication of the bulla (Fig. 1.51b). The underlying lung usually expands when pressure exerted by the cyst is abolished.

10 Pulmonary Suppuration

This chapter deals with a group of diseases of differing aetiopathology, but sharing the common characteristic of being essentially inflammatory conditions with pus formation. Inhalation of foreign bodies has been included here for the sake of convenience and because of the occurrence of pulmonary suppuration when the inhaled object is not extracted or when infection supervenes.

FOREIGN BODIES IN THE AIRWAYS

Accidental inhalation of foreign material is not uncommon particularly among children. Each thoracic surgery unit has a collection of curious objects recovered from the air passages (Fig. 1.52).

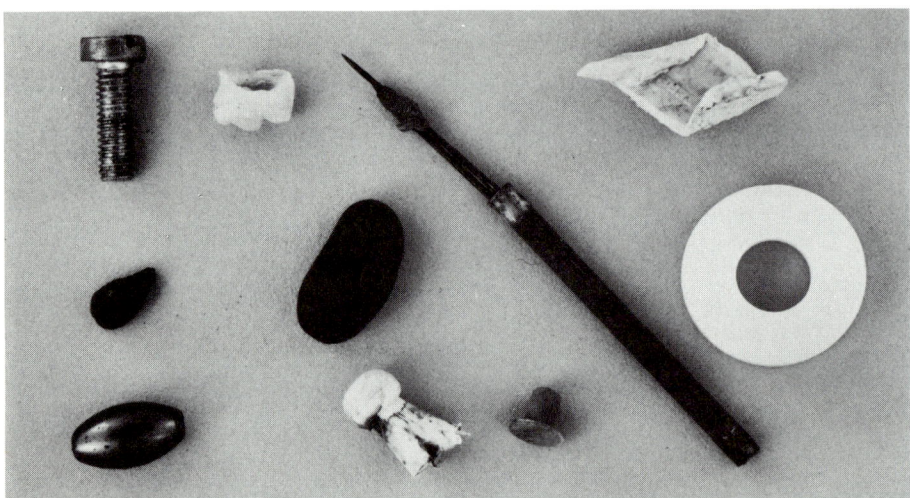

Figure 1.52   Collection of foreign bodies removed from the airways; (screw, tooth, fragments of plastic, grape pip, bead, peanut, sweet, pen cap, cartridge cap, blow pipe and dart).

The effect of a foreign body in the trachea and bronchi is dependent on the age of the patient, the size of the object inhaled, the nature of the object and the site and the duration of impaction.

In an infant a small solid object can be almost fatal, whereas in an adult the same object or even a larger one can remain in a segmental bronchus unnoticed until the obstruction causes collapse of the segment and infection occurs, with subsequent infection and suppuration, (see *Lung Abscess*, p. 86).

84

CLINICAL FEATURES AND DIAGNOSIS

It is important to obtain a full detailed history of events leading to the attack of cough, wheeze and dyspnoea, particularly in children. Sudden dyspnoea and cough in a previously healthy individual, when accompanied by a history of probable inhalation, points to impaction of a foreign body. Auscultation reveals a wheeze or the absence of breath sounds over the area of the lung ventilated by the obstructed bronchus.

Chest and neck radiographs show radio-opaque objects only. As nowadays many objects are plastic compounds, negative radiological findings do not rule out the existence of a foreign body. A chest radiograph can be of assistance even if it fails to outline the inhaled object. Segmental or lobar atelectasis occurring a few hours after the presumed inhalation is good evidence of bronchial obstruction. Occasionally there are no radiological abnormalities except for a relative hyper-clarity of a part or the whole of one lung indicating the entry of air into the alveoli through a partially obstructed bronchus which cannot empty. This results in pulmonary hyperinflation, hence the hyper-clarity on the X-ray picture in the area of the retained foreign body.

Anatomical considerations

Foreign bodies can lodge in the larynx, trachea, lobar or segmental bronchi. In an adult small objects can migrate within the bronchial tree. The right main bronchus is more directly in line with the trachea, and therefore receives incoming objects more readily. So do the lower lobes for obvious reasons.

TYPES OF FOREIGN BODIES

Insoluble solid objects

They can be sharp (nails, pins, screws), or blunt (pen caps, teeth). In recent years most blunt objects have been non-metallic foreign bodies. When an object is

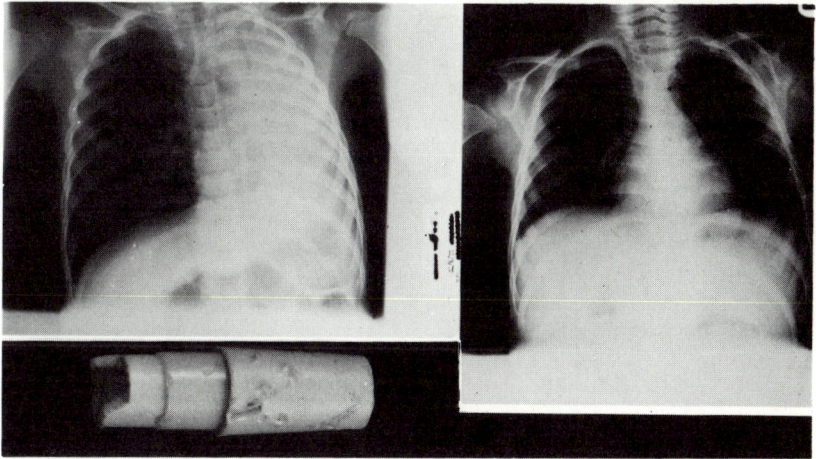

Figure 1.53   Radiograph (left) showing complete collapse of left lung. Radiograph (right) showing re-expansion after removal of pen cap (insert) from the left main bronchus.

lodged in the larynx (usually in an infant), dyspnoea and stridor are intense and the removal of the object demands speed.

The impaction of a blunt foreign body in a bronchus can cause complete obstruction with immediate collapse of the corresponding segment, lobe or even the whole lung (Fig. 1.53). If this is not treated retention of the object is followed by infection leading to pneumonic changes or the formation of a lung abscess. A sharp object causes in addition ulceration of the bronchial wall.

Soluble material

Inhalation of sweets and the like can cause obstructive symptoms initially, but as the material dissolves obstructive symptoms decrease. However, sugar, additives and oil in the sweets can cause severe inflammation. Peanuts are particularly harmful as they swell and fragment causing serious inflammation and infection.

TREATMENT

Removal of foreign bodies

Endoscopy. Laryngoscopy (direct) can show the object which can then be removed. Sometimes a bout of coughing during this procedures dislodges a small object and projects it out of the airway.

Bronchoscopy with a rigid bronchoscope allows visualisation and removal of the object. The bronchial lumen is inspected and washed thoroughly with warm saline solution, especially when sweets and peanuts are inhaled.

Thoracotomy and *bronchotomy* may be necessary when a sharp object has penetrated the bronchial wall. The bronchial wall is incised, then repaired after the object has been removed. When a foreign body has been lodged for some time and has penetrated the lung, causing an abscess with parenchyma destruction, pulmonary, excision is necessary.

Micro-biological studies

During bronchoscopy, a sample of bronchial secretions is taken for bacteriological studies including antibiotic sensitivities.

Antibiotic therapy

This is required for a few days until symptoms disappear. If systemic infection is present or if there is a radiological abnormality the appropriate antibiotics are continued.

Physiotherapy

Breathing and coughing exercises and sometimes postural drainage are used particularly when the foreign body has been within the bronchi for some time.

LUNG ABSCESS

An abscess can be defined as a localised collection of pus within the substance of an organ. Pus consists of a liquid containing proteins, dead and dying leucocytes, micro-organisms and the products of tissue break-down.

A lung abscess is a collection of pus within the pulmonary parenchyma. The incidence of lung abscess has greatly decreased since the advent of anti-microbial agents.

The causes of lung abscess are as follows:

BRONCHOGENIC FACTORS

The most frequent cause of lung abscess formation is inhalation of septic material during and after an operation (usually gastro-intestinal contents). Inhalation is more likely to occur after naso-pharyngeal surgery or in patients with upper gastro-intestinal obstruction.

Inhalation of septic material causing lung abscess need not be connected with operations although it usually is.

The second most frequent factor is the obstruction of the bronchial lumen (by a tumour, a foreign body or a mucous plug). The abscess develops beyond the blocked bronchus.

Complications and extension of an existing pulmonary disease

These complications can lead to abscess formation. This can be the case for patients with bronchiectasis, pneumonia, collapse of a segment or a lobe or pulmonary infarcts.

Haematogenous factors

These factors also play a role. Blood-borne abscesses are due to the migration and deposit of septic material in the lung, secondary to infection in another part of the body or as a result of septicaemia.

Pyogenic infection

Extension of pyogenic infection from neighbouring structures (liver, mediastinum) can also be a contributing factor.

Micro-organisms most commonly responsible for the formation of lung abscesses are *Streptococcus viridans*, *Staphylococcus aureus* and *E. Coli* and, less frequently, anaerobic bacteria.

When the abscess is caused by inhalation, there is a definite relationship between its localisation and broncho-pulmonary segmental arrangement. In a supine position the right main bronchus and the postero-lateral segments of both lungs are in direct postural line for accommodating any inhaled material. It is therefore easy to see that, during sleep or anaesthesia, these areas become the most likely to be invaded.

Once the abscess is formed it can expand to a large suppurating area within the lung. It then usually drains and empties its pus into the bronchus. This is coughed up and accounts for the patient's copious purulent expectoration and the appearance of air in the abscess cavity with the radiological appearance of fluid level. After the abscess has drained into the bronchus, healing occurs with fibrous tissue formation and scarring of the lung, or a pulmonary cyst, may develop.

Various complications can occur:

1. Rupture of the abscess into the pleural space leading to the development of an empyema (pyothorax), or of a pyopneumothorax (air and pus).

2. Chronic abscess formation with recurrent exacerbation of symptoms.
3. Development of bronchiectasis.
4. Metastatic abscesses in other parts of the body.

CLINICAL FEATURES AND DIAGNOSIS

In acute cases fever, malaise and toxaemia are present, in addition to symptoms of respiratory diseases, in particular expectoration of copious purulent material. In chronic cases general ill health, anorexia and respiratory symptoms are predominant.

Diagnosis is established by clinical history and copious expectoration of purulent material, radiological evidence, and bronchoscopic findings.

TREATMENT

Many abscesses can be treated conservatively along the following lines:

1. Administration of antibiotics based on microbiological and sensitivity tests.
2. Physiotherapy and postural drainage.
3. Bronchoscopy and bronchial toilet. This is of great help and can be repeated.
4. Administration of mild analgesic for relief of pain.
5. Scrupulous hygiene and isolation of the patient to prevent secondary and cross infection.
6. High calorie and protein diet to combat protein loss.
7. Aspiration of the abscess (in some cases).

The patient's progress has to be monitored by recording the temperature, doing repeated blood counts, chest radiographs and bacteriological examinations of the sputum.

Surgery is indicated in acute cases not responding to conservative treatment, in chronic cases with repeated acute exacerbation, in cases with associated pleural empyema, and in all cases where neoplasm is suspected.

As the patient's sputum must be reduced to a minimum before operation, appropriate antibiotics are given as part of the pre-operative preparation.

A thoracotomy is carried out for segmental resection or lobectomy. In cases of empyema drainage of the pleural space may be sufficient.

In the light of what is known on the formation of lung abscesses, it is obvious that prophylactic measures should be an essential part of the treatment of most thoracic diseases. The tracheo-bronchial lumen should be cleared by physiotherapy and bronchoscopy if necessary, and antibiotics should be administered when indicated. Prevention of inhalation of food material by weak or elderly patients, and following anaesthesia, must be kept constantly in mind.

STAPHYLOCOCCAL LUNG ABSCESS IN INFANTS AND CHILDREN

This particular type of lung abscess deserves separate mention because of its characteristic behaviour (Fig. 1.54).

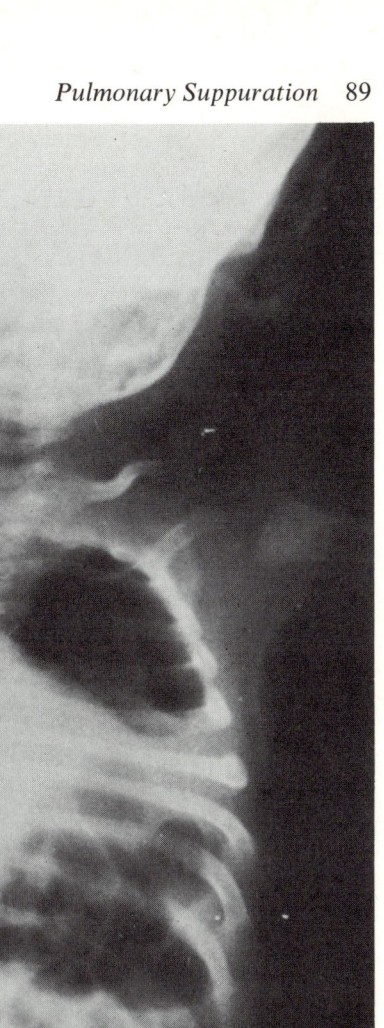

Figure 1.54   Left pyopneumothorax following staphylococcal abscess in an infant.

It usually occurs in infants and children with acute general and respiratory symptoms. There is a sudden attack of dyspnoea, stridor and cyanosis which can lead to cardiac arrest. This is due to the formation of a staphylococcal abscess in the lung, followed by the development of a tension cyst or a tension pneumo-thorax. The latter results from rupture of the abscess into the pleural space.

MANAGEMENT

When diagnosed in the early stages, the abscess is treated conservatively with appropriate antibiotic agents and attention to the general health of the infant.

When a tension cyst is present, or in cases of pyopneumothorax, the chest is drained with an intercostal pleural drain connected to an underwater sealed system. This usually controls both the infection and the pneumothorax.

Infants and children with lung abscess have to be nursed carefully, as the sudden onset of tension cyst or pneumothorax can be fatal if not treated promptly.

BRONCHIECTASIS

The literal meaning of bronchiectasis is 'abnormal dilitation of the bronchi'. But the pathological features of the disease are not limited to bronchial calibre. Mucosal abnormalities and functional changes are also present.

Both the frequency and the severity of the condition have decreased since it was first described by Laënnec in the early nineteenth century.

AETIOLOGY

Several factors can be responsible for the development of bronchiectasis, either individually or collectively; the most important of which are:

1. *Congenital.* The condition or a tendency to develop it is usually discovered in childhood. Kartagener's syndrome associates bronchiectasis, sinusitis and dextracardia.

2. *Obstructive.* Long-standing obstruction of the bronchus by a foreign body or a benign tumour causes distal infection and bronchiectasis.

3. *Respiratory infection* in infancy and childhood. In neonates and children bronchial lumens are narrow and easily obstructed by inflammatory exudates and oedema of the bronchial wall. In addition some infections are accompanied by lymphadenopathy causing extrinsic pressure and obstruction of the lumen.

CLINICAL FEATURES

Clinical examination reveals features such as chronic productive cough, purulent and abundant sputum, repeated haemoptysis, repeated episodes of chest infection with fever and pleuro-pulmonary inflammation often with associated sinusitis and in severe cases partial or complete destruction and collapse of a lung.

Children suffering from this condition miss school frequently because of recurrent 'chest colds'. In adults symptoms can be less pronounced. Marked systemic symptoms such as lack of energy and loss of appetite often draw attention to the condition.

DIAGNOSIS

A sample of sputum is sent for microbiological examination to identify the infecting micro-organism and assess sensitivity. Bronchoscopy reveals obstructive lesions and shows the presence of purulent secretions.

Chest radiograph does not always show abnormal findings although signs of atelectasis and pulmonary infiltration are often visible.

Bronchography (Fig. 1.55a,b) is the most useful diagnostic procedure and the condition cannot be diagnosed without bronchographic confirmation. A bronchogram will indicate the topography, severity and type of bronchiectasis.

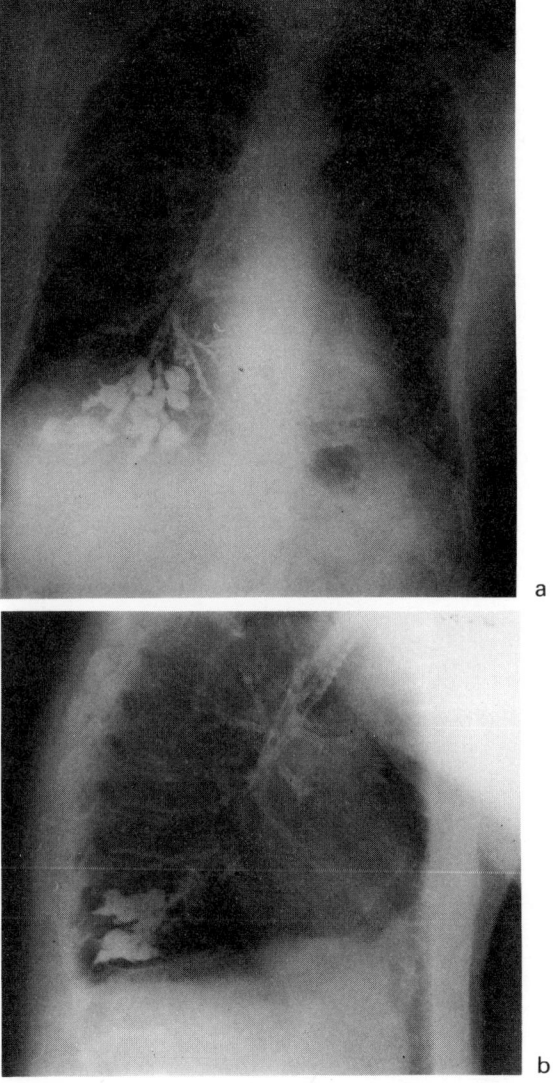

a

b

Figure 1.55   (a) Postero-anterior bronchography showing cystic bronchiectasis of the right lower lobe. (b) Right lateral view of same.

There are two types of bronchiectasis described according to their broncho-graphic appearance:

1. Tubular or cylindrical bronchiectasis in which, as the name implies, dilatation extends over the whole length of the bronchus.

2. Saccular bronchiectasis in which the bronchogram shows the grape-like appearance of the bronchi. It is sometimes called cystic bronchiectasis.

Microscopic examination of a specimen will show inflammed areas, suppuration and changes in the bronchial mucosa and the covering epithelium.

COMPLICATIONS
Complications of bronchiectasis range from:

1. Progressive damage to the lung due to repeated inflammation and infection and gradual destruction of the parenchyma leading to emphysema and respiratory failure.

2. Lung abscess and empyema.

3. Brain abscess. A rare complication nowadays but once not uncommon.

4. Heart failure (cor pulmonale) due to progressive interference with pulmonary circulation caused by lung destruction and the development of pulmonary hypertension.

Treatment
Since aetiological factors, such as infections, stasis of secretions and obstruction of the bronchus, play such an important role then preventive measures should be applied whenever possible. They range from physiotherapy and bronchoscopy to remove a foreign body or an obstruction, to prompt specific treatment of chest infections especially in childhood.

Treatment itself is either medical or surgical.

Medical treatment
Cases with minor symptoms and little sputum, or for cases with widely scattered bronchiectasis in both lungs, indicate the need for medical treatment. Particular attention is paid to expectoration with the help of physiotherapy. The patient is taught how to perform postural drainage once or twice a day. Antibiotics should be reserved for acute episodes and be used according to sensitivity tests. Caution should be exercised over the long-standing use of antibiotics, as bacteria can become resistant to them and be replaced by fungus colonies against which antibiotics are powerless.

In cases of extensive and long-standing bronchiectasis regular bronchoscopy and bronchial lavage prevent colonisation by fungi. It provides bronchial disinfection and obviates repeated use of antibiotics.

Surgical treatment
When medical treatment is ineffective then surgical treatment is considered. Localised bronchiectasis causing severe symptoms and abundant sputum production may require an operation. Segmental resection, lobectomy or, more rarely, pneumonectomy is carried out. Before surgery patients are fully investigated and prepared.

Following operation no effort should be spared to obtain full expansion of the residual lung and to prevent infective complications. Particular attention should be paid to posture, especially in younger patients.

FUNGAL DISEASES OF THE LUNG

Lungs can become infected by a variety of fungal organisms. The frequency with which a particular type of fungus occurs is subject to geographical variations.

Many fungal organisms live in the soil and enter the respiratory tract by inhalation (e.g. Histoplasmosis and Aspergillosis—see *Glossary* for more details). Others live in a symbiotic state on the skin and in the mouth, assuming a pathogenic role when the opportunity arises (e.g. Moniliasis and Actino-mycosis—see *Glossary* for more details).

Such an opportunity arises following prolonged use of antibiotics, immuno-suppressives and cortico-steroids, or in cases of poor general health and chronic suppurations. Pulmonary fungal infection can be sub-clinical and asympto-matic, or it can cause cough, sputum, haemoptysis and other manifestations of respiratory diseases.

Laboratory tests, immunological investigations for detecting antibodies and skin hypersensitivity testing are neither specific nor reliable enough to establish diagnosis. Radiological examinations reveal pulmonary infiltration, cavitation and solitary nodules, none of them specific to fungal infection.

Identification of organisms in the sputum and histological examination of pathological specimens are the only reliable diagnostic procedures.

Treatment of fungal diseases is principally medical. Surgery plays a minor role in the treatment of complications and in establishing diagnosis by exploration. Antibiotics are avoided as their use promotes the propagation of fungal organisms (except in the case of Actinomycosis for which Penicillin is the drug of choice).

Antifungal drugs such as Amphotricin B, Natamycin (Nystatin), Rifampicin and Saramycetin are useful in specific cases.

ASPERGILLOSIS

Among fungal diseases Aspergillosis is the commonest in Britain and has surgical relevance. The disease is caused by Aspergillus Fumigatus which is a secondary invader of the lung. Typically the disease occurs in individuals with debilitating conditions, or those suffering from long-standing pulmonary sup-puration as in bronchiectasis. The organism has a particular affinity for tuberculous cavities where it forms a rounded mass called Mycetoma composed of necrotic tissues, organisms, fibrin and inflammatory cells.

Clinically there are two important forms:

Aspergillus bronchitis which manifests itself by a wheeze, cough, bronchitic and radiological signs of pulmonary infiltration.

2. *Mycetoma-type Aspergillus* with symptoms of pulmonary suppuration and haemoptysis and characteristic radiological features.

Treatment is usually conservative and medical. It is based on anti-fungal chemotherapy and bronchial disinfection, using bronchoscopy and bronchial lavage.

Surgical excision can be necessary for the mycetoma-form, particularly when complicated by haemoptysis.

11 Tuberculosis

Pulmonary tuberculosis results from infection by Mycobacterium Tuberculosis (Koch Bacillus or Tubercle Bacillus).

For generations this disease has caused not only illness and death, but also social disruption and prejudice. The causative agent was not discovered until the nineteenth century and for centuries the treatment of tuberculosis remained speculative and in some respects reminiscent of witch-doctoring.

Though tuberculosis is still with us and still a common condition in some parts of the world, it is no longer a great killer nor an incurable disease. In 1882 Robert Koch discovered the rod-shaped (bacillus) organism, Mycobacterium Tuberculosis (Koch Bacillus, Tubercle Bacillus) and succeeded in reproducing the disease in animals using a culture of the organism. This discovery, together with the later advent of anti-tuberculous chemotherapeutic agents and improvement in hygiene, nutrition and living standards, contributed to the removal of the mysteries and prejudices surrounding tuberculosis.

THE ORGANISM

The Tubercle Bacillus is a slender rod-shaped Gram-positive organism 2 to 3μ long. It consists of lipids, proteins and carbohydrates. The lipid chain constitutes the outstanding feature of the organism forming a waxy sheath round it. The protein fraction is antigenic and is responsible for the immune response of the host. The culture of the bacillus requires a special medium containing egg yolk and glycerol, with provision of air. Six weeks should elapse before the culture is examined.

There are several strains or types of Tubercle Bacilli: human, bovine (affecting cattle), avian (affecting birds), piscine (affecting fish), murine (affecting voles) etc. Man is affected by the human and bovine types.

MODE OF INFECTION AND LESION

The majority, if not in all, of cases human tuberculosis is caused by inhalation of bacilli. The alimentary tract rarely constitutes a route of infection; infection by inoculation or a cutaneous route is extremely rare. In pulmonary tuberculosis Tubercle Bacilli produce a specific inflammatory reaction. The formation and progress of this inflammation depends on the individual's previous contact with tuberculous infection. In individuals with no previous exposure, the infection is referred to as the primary complex (primary infection). When there has been previous exposure to the disease, it is referred to as a secondary infection.

PRIMARY INFECTION

The inhaled bacilli are carried by the lymphatics to form a small sub-pleural focus of infection, the tubercle follicle, which is the tissues' specific inflammatory response to the Tubercle Bacilli. The tubercle follicle is recognisable under the microscope and is differentiated from other non-specific inflammatory reactions.

This sub-pleural tuberculous follicle is accompanied by pulmonary hilar lymphadenitis (inflammation of lymphatic nodes). The tuberculous follicle and its lymphadenitis are known as the primary focus (Gohn's focus) (Fig. 1.56). In the majority of cases the primary focus heals and calcifies; infection is then controlled.

The tuberculous follicle is formed by a mass of cells and a central necrotic acellular material called caseum. The cells are arranged in zones and are of three types:

1. Epitheloid cells (special cells derived from monocytic white cells as well as from tissue macrophages).
2. Some large multi-nucleated cells called Giant Cells (Longhans).
3. Smooth rounded cells surrounding epitheloid cells.

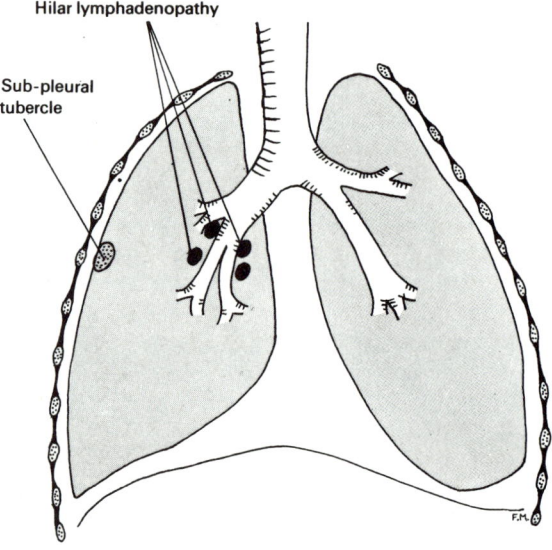

Figure 1.56   Gohn's focus.

In Western communities the primary complex usually occurs in childhood, and is accompanied by minor clinical symptoms which often go unnoticed. Progress of the primary infection depends on several factors, of which the individual's general health is the most important. Poor general health and malnutrition promote the spread of the primary infection, leading to generalised tuberculosis and eventually death. Spread occurs essentially via lymphatics, but also along the bronchial lumen and by way of the bloodstream.

SECONDARY INFECTION

A second exposure to Tubercle Bacilli differs in many ways from the primary infection. It causes symptoms of respiratory disease. Greater local involvement of the lung with tissue destruction and necrosis is usual, but widespread infection is less likely.

The inhaled bacilli cause a large lesion usually at the apex of the lung. The lesion cavitates: its centre becomes hollow as the necrotic contents are expectorated (Fig. 1.57).

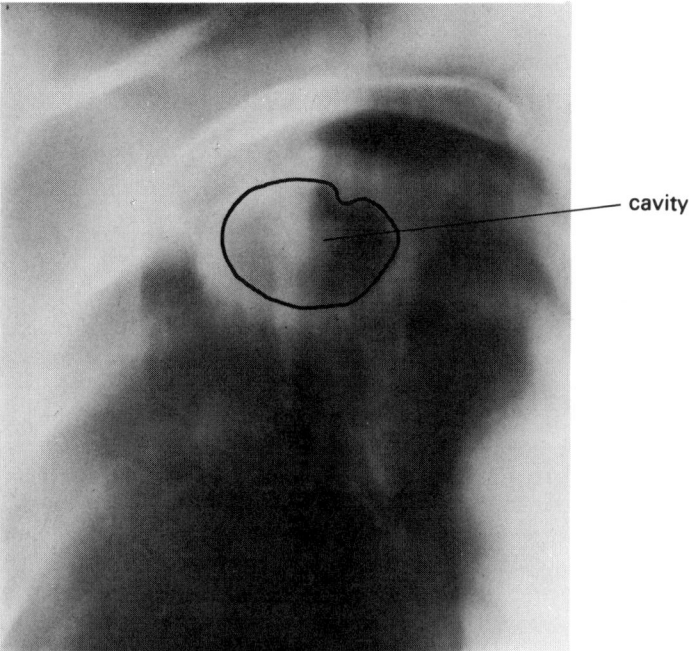

Figure 1.57   *Tuberculous cavity in the apex of the right lung.*

The secondary lesion can progress in different ways: (1) It either heals completely with fibrosis and scarring; or it spreads locally; or it spreads to distant organs and leads to miliary tuberculosis, or (2) The spread occurs via the bronchial channels, the lymphatics and blood circulation.

CLINICAL FEATURES AND DIAGNOSIS

The primary complex can go completely unnoticed or can be accompanied by cough, malaise and mild fever. In generalised tuberculosis, symptoms and signs of severe infection together with manifestations of pulmonary disease are usually present.

In secondary infection, symptoms are varied and related to the extent and severity of the lesion on the one hand, and degree of destruction of the lung on the other. Constitutional symptoms (excessive fatigue, weight loss, fever and night sweats) are present together with respiratory signs and symptoms (cough, sputum, haemoptysis, pain and signs of pleural effusion). Occasionally no definite respiratory symptoms are present.

INVESTIGATIONS

CLINICAL INVESTIGATIONS
The history of contact and exposure to tuberculosis and history of previous respiratory illness are recorded.

LABORATORY EXAMINATIONS
They are essential for diagnosis. A full blood count and ESR are carried out. The latter is repeated and gives an indication of the progress of the disease and its response to treatment.

A fresh specimen of sputum is sent to the laboratory for identification by ZN staining (see p. 58), by culture of the organism and if necessary by inoculation into a guinea pig.

When no sputum can be obtained, gastric lavage is a useful method of obtaining material for laboratory examination.

RADIOLOGICAL EXAMINATION
Chest radiography and tomography are most useful. They reveal infiltrations and cavitation which is a diagnostic feature of tuberculosis.

IMMUNOLOGICAL TESTS
Mantoux and Heaf tuberculin tests are helpful investigations (see *Immunological Investigations*, p. 63). It should however be noted that, whereas a negative reading definitely indicates that the lesion is not tuberculous, a positive reading means that the patient may have or has had tuberculosis.

ADDITIONAL INVESTIGATIONS
They can be required in individual cases and include:

1. Biopsy of the lymph nodes (scalene nodes or mediastinal nodes), of the pleura and pulmonary tissues.
2. Bronchoscopy for the detection of endobronchial disease and to obtain bronchial secretions for the identification of organisms.

MANAGEMENT OF PULMONARY TUBERCULOSIS

The discovery and development of anti-tuberculous drugs in the 1940's can be considered as the greatest single step toward the eradication of tuberculosis. The treatment of pulmonary tuberculosis has pursued a changing course and now the disease is considered a medical condition treated with anti-tuberculous drugs. However in some cases there is still a place for surgery.

When considering the management of patients with pulmonary tuberculosis it is important to ascertain whether the disease is active, inactive or quiescent.

In active tuberculosis Tubercle Bacilli are recoverable, there is radiological evidence of the disease, the patient's health deteriorates and complications such as empyema appear. In inactive tuberculosis the criteria above are absent. In quiescent tuberculosis, although bacilli are not recoverable, activity is radiologically detectable. The patient is generally in reasonable health.

SURGICAL TREATMENT

Surgery is indicated when medical treatment has failed to control the disease. Pulmonary resection and thoracoplasty are the two procedures employed. All patients are operated on under coverage of anti-tuberculous drug therapy. Most often segmental resection of the apical and posterior segments of the upper lobe is carried out for an apical cavity. Lobectomy or pneumonectomy is necessary in cases of complete destruction of a lobe or the whole lung, or when severe tuberculous bronchiectasis is present. Thoracoplasty is performed when the disease is extensive or when the patient does not respond to drugs. Before surgery, patients are fully investigated and prepared (see Chapter 14).

Since the introduction of potent anti-tuberculous drugs, surgery plays a minor role in the treatment of pulmonary tuberculosis. But it still plays a major part in the treatment of its complications.

Complications of pulmonary tuberculosis requiring surgical treatment are:

1. Empyema. It can require thoracotomy and decortication (see p. 37).
2. Resection for bronchiectactic lobe or segment.
3. Dangerous and repeated haemoptysis requiring thoracotomy and resection.

HYPERSENSITIVITY AND IMMUNITY

Hypersensitivity can be defined as an individual's abnormally high sensitivity and excessive reaction to a substance which causes little or no reaction in others. Immunity is the protection conferred to an individual by previous exposure to an infectious disease.

Tuberculosis appears to confer a degree of acquired immunity so that in subsequent exposure there is some protection against the dissemination of the disease. At the same time previous exposure to disease produces a state of hypersensitivity. This can be demonstrated by the skin reaction to intradermal injection of tuberculine (as in Mantoux test).

VACCINATION (BCG)

Based on experimental and clinical experience, it appears that vaccination with Tubercle Bacilli provides some measure of protection against tuberculosis. Immunisation is done with BCG vaccine (Bacille Calmette Guérin) which is a bovine strain of tubercle bacilli attenuated (rendered less virulent without loss of its effectiveness to confer immunity) by articifical culture. BCG inoculation only produces a mild localised reaction.

A Mantoux test is carried out before vaccination. If the reaction is negative, BCG is inoculated.

MEDICAL TREATMENT

The basis of treatment is multiple drug therapy. Traditionally Streptomycin, Isonizid and PAS (ParaAmino Salicyclic Acid) were used for as long as 18 months. With the advent of newer anti-tuberculous drugs, a variety of combination therapies and regimes of differing duration have been developed. Ethambutol, Rifampicin, Viomycin and Cyclocerine are currently available.

The present trend in Britain is to administer a short course (9 months) of Isonizid and Rifampicin, supplemented by Streptomycin or Ethambutol for 2 months (British Thoracic and Tuberculosis Association's Recommendation, 1976).

Studies carried out in various countries indicate that the treatment programme has to be adapted to social and geographical considerations. It is to be noted that all chemotherapeutic agents possess some degree of toxicity.

Isolation, bed rest and hospitalisation

There is no general agreement about the duration of isolation, bed rest and hospitalisation in tuberculous patients. This is partly because of social, economic and geographical differences existing between communities, and because of differences in severity and extent of the disease in individuals. The general consensus is:

1. Only very ill patients with extensive tuberculosis are kept in bed, but progressively mobilised as they improve.

2. Patients with positive sputum and extensive disease are considered infectious and are isolated.

3. The initial course of chemotherapy is usually started at hospital.

4. The length of hospital stay depends on the severity of the disease, the patient's general condition and sputum positivity on direct smear.

The tendency is therefore to limit hospitilisation and to allow, as far as possible, ambulatory treatment.

12 Miscellaneous Lung Diseases

This chapter deals with some primarily medical pulmonary conditions in whose treatment and management, surgery plays a role.

PULMONARY EMBOLISM

Pulmonary embolism is the migration into the pulmonary artery of a solid mass (the embolus) originating in the venous system. The embolus lodges in the pulmonary artery, and/or its branches, causing arterial occlusion leading to pulmonary infarction, major circulatory embarrassment or immediate death. In the great majority of cases the embolus is a thrombus (fibrin clot) formed in a deep vein of the leg or the pelvis.

Three groups of factors are responsible for venous thrombosis which is at the root of embolism:

1. Factors associated with the flow of blood within the vein (e.g. stasis).
2. Factors affecting vessel walls such as inflammation or injuries.
3. Factors derived from changes in blood-clotting factors.

Once thrombosis is formed within a vein it propagates and a portion of it, in the form of the thrombus, can become detached from the main mass and migrate as an embolus.

Consequences of pulmonary embolus depend on several factors of which the size of the embolus, the site of its final impaction and the state of the individual's cardiac and respiratory systems are the deciding ones. A small embolus may cause little more than chest pain, temporary haemoptysis and a limited pulmonary infarct. Large emboli, particularly those affecting both sides, can cause death.

In non-fatal cases large pulmonary emboli can produce pulmonary arterial occlusion severe enough to cause dyspnoea, cyanosis and severe hypoxia. The cardio-respiratory condition of the patient becomes an important factor in determining the outcome.

CLINICAL FEATURES AND DIAGNOSIS

A massive pulmonary embolus can cause immediate death before an attempt at diagnosis can even be made. It is suggested that sudden death could be the result of mechanical obstruction of the pulmonary arteries, with the arrest of circulation. Alternatively death could be caused by a 'reflex'. The precise cause of death at the onset of pulmonary embolus is not clearly understood.

A non-fatal pulmonary embolus causes shock, chest pain, tachypnoea, dyspnoea, cyanosis, haemoptysis and raised central venous pressure. Most of these symptoms and signs are non-specific and may not be of diagnostic value.

101

Further investigations are therefore necessary to establish diagnosis, particularly if surgery is being considered.

A chest radiograph shows signs of pulmonary infarct or pleural effusion. If the embolus is largish the lack of pulmonary vascular marking becomes evident. ECG and CVP recordings are helpful, particularly the latter. Pulmonary scanning shows lack of perfusion in the corresponding area of occlusion. Pulmonary arteriography is the most important investigation in the diagnosis of pulmonary embolism. It demonstrates the filling defect in the blocked artery, the anatomy or the occluded pulmonary artery and the extent of occlusion (Fig. 1.58a,b). Arteriography therefore helps not only to establish diagnosis but also to make a therapeutic decision.

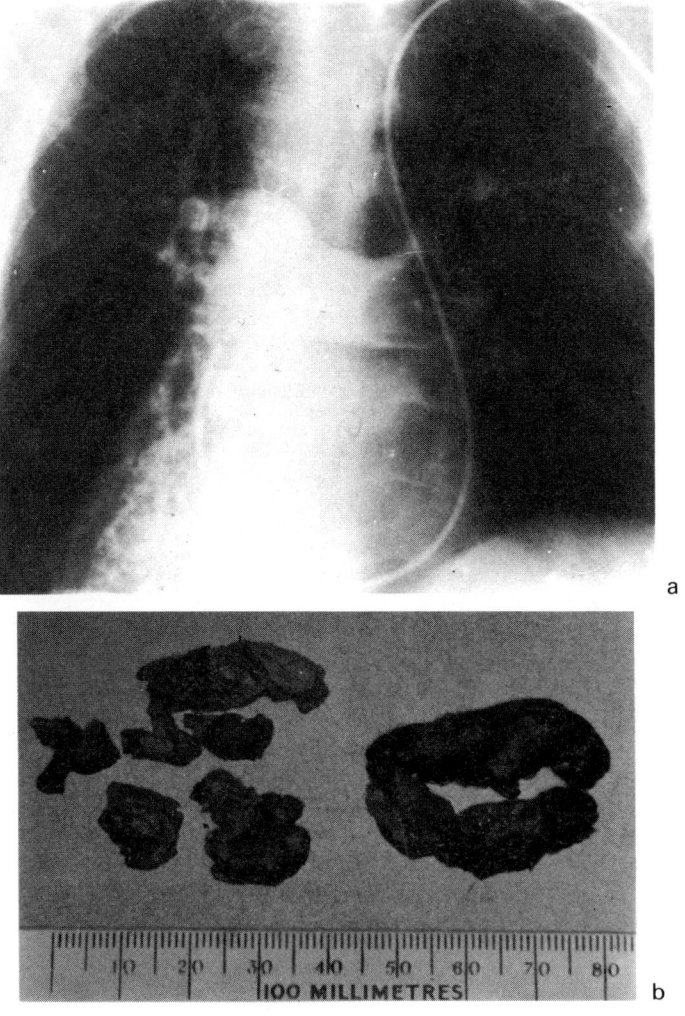

a

b

Figure 1.58   Pulmonary embolism. (a) Pulmonary angiogram showing filling defect. (b) Clots removed from the pulmonary arteries.

TREATMENT

For some years now a great deal of effort has been centred round the pathogenesis of pulmonary embolism and its prevention, particularly after major surgery. Risk factors have been identified. These include prolonged bedrest and major surgery. Patients who are particularly at risk are the elderly and those with cardio-vascular and respiratory diseases.

Preventive measures such as early mobilisation after surgery and prophylactic anticoagulant therapy have been advocated in these high-risk individuals. Recently low dosage subcutaneous Heparin (5000 units 12-hourly starting a day before operation and continuing for a few days) has been recommended in patients undergoing major surgery. This appears to have reduced the incidence of post-operative pulmonary emboli.

When diagnosis is established the choice of treatment, whether conservative or surgical, depends on the extent and severity of the occlusion on the one hand, and the general, cardiac and respiratory performance of the patient on the other. Anticoagulant (Heparin) and fibrinolytic agents have been used successfully in cases of small to moderate-size emboli. Larger pulmonary emboli require surgical embolectomy. This is best carried out under cardio-pulmonary by-pass using a pump oxygenator. The pulmonary artery is opened and thoroughly cleared of emboli. The source of thrombi, that is the site of venous thrombosis, is also defined radiologically and explored. Thrombectomy and venous ligation are carried out.

HYDATID DISEASE (CYST) OF THE LUNG

Hydatid cysts (Synonym Pulmonary Echinococcosis) are caused by the parasitic worm *Taenia Echinococcus*, whose life cycle is shared between dog and sheep. Human infestation occurs through ingestion of food contaminated with the ova contained in the faeces of a diseased dog. The complete life cycle of the parasite is shown in Fig. 1.59.

In man the ingested ova form larvae which pass into the liver through the portal vein. The liver becomes the first station for the development of hydatid cysts. Some of the larvae pass into the lung and form cystic lesions. With the life cycle of the parasite, it is easy to see the prevalence of the disease in countries with a high number of sheep and dogs; New Zealand, Australia, South Africa and some Southern European countries being amongst the high-risk areas.

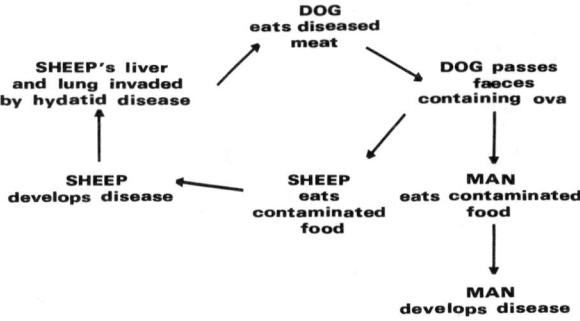

Figure 1.59   Life cycle of the hydatid disease parasite.

In the lung the parasite forms a cyst which expands. The cyst contains a fluid with scoleces, and is surrounded by its own germinal layer and hyaline membrane. In addition, pulmonary tissue around the cyst is compressed and forms a further fibrous membrane round the cyst. Rupture of the cyst will produce daughter cysts. In many cases the disease is discovered in the course of a routine chest radiograph; at other times minor symptoms of respiratory disease can be manifest. Occasionally the cyst is ruptured and the fluid expectorated.

Casoni test is based on skin hypersensitivity reaction, as in Mantoux test (hydatid fluid is injected intradermally). Although it is helpful in diagnosing some cases, it is said to be not entirely reliable.

Treatment

In many cases diagnosis is made at operation. Enucleation of the cyst, or excision of the segment or the lobe containing large cysts (if enucleation is not possible), is carried out. Many surgeons inject formaline solution into the cyst prior to enucleation or excision, in order to minimise the risk of spread, should contamination occur by accidental rupture of the cyst at operation.

SARCOIDOSIS

This is a granulomatous condition of unknown aetiology involving many parts of the body. Lungs, lymph nodes, skin and lymphoid tissues are the sites usually affected. Sarcoidosis was so named by Boek in 1889 because of the flesh-like appearance of the tissues involved by the disease (*sarkos* = flesh).

Pulmonary sarcoidosis can take several forms. Sometimes mediastinal lymph nodes are enlarged by the disease, causing compression of the bronchus resulting in pulmonary collapse. At other times the disease causes direct pulmonary infiltration following by pulmonary fibrosis.

The pulmonary manifestations of sarcoidosis resemble that of tuberculosis. Clinical manifestations of the disease are variable, ranging from no to severe respiratory symptoms. Diagnosis is suspected on radiological findings and confirmed by lymph node biopsy (scalene node or a mediastinal node) and a Kveim test. Sometimes diagnosis is obtained at exploratory thoracotomy. Sarcoidosis is treated medically by cortico-steroids.

COLLAGEN DISEASES OF THE LUNG

As the name implies this is a group of conditions in which there are anatomical changes of connective tissues. The aetiology of these diseases is generally obscure. In some cases altered immune response and auto-immune phenomena are incriminated.

Lungs are affected early and predominantly in some cases with the result that the respiratory manifestations may be the presenting symptoms of collagen diseases.

WEGNER'S GRANULOMATOSIS

The disease is characterised by granulomatous lesions, vasculitis and nephritis. Pulmonary lesions appear as necrotic granulomas with abscess formation.

SYSTEMIC LUPUS ERYTHEMATOSIS

This is a general systemic condition with pleuro-pulmonary involvement. The latter consists of pleural effusion, pulmonary infiltrations and patchy consolidation.

RHEUMATOID DISEASE

Lungs can become involved in this disease. Pulmonary manifestations appear either as general fibrotic changes or rheumatoid nodules. When rheumatoid nodules in the lungs are associated with coalminers' pneumoconiosis, the condition is called Caplan's syndrome.

13 Tumours of the Chest Wall and Lung

CHEST WALL TUMOURS

Soft tissue tumours of the chest are no different from those found in any other part of the body. Exceptions should be made for breasts which can be considered as appendages of the skin. Breast tumours are not considered here even though chest wall involvement can occur in cases of recurrence after mastectomy. Chest wall tumours can be benign or malignant. In the latter category they can be primary tumours arising from various chest wall diseases, or metastatic tumours migrated from other sites of the body and deposited in the chest wall.

RIB AND STERNAL TUMOURS

In most cases these tumours present themselves as a slow growing lump on the chest. Sometimes sternal and rib tumours are diagnosed after investigations of pain in the chest. Occasionally they are discovered accidentally in the course of chest radiography.

Histologically, sternal and rib neoplasms are usually chondromatous benign tumours or slow-growing malignant tumours. Hodgkin's disease, lymphoma and myeloma occasionally involve the sternum and ribs. Not infrequently the sternum and ribs become the seat of secondaries, particularly in cases of cancer of the bronchus, thyroid and kidneys (hypernephroma). Carcinoma of the chest wall following radical mastectomy or as a result of direct invasion by carcinoma of the bronchus through the thoracic cavity is seen from time to time.

Treatment

Whenever possible rib and sternal tumours are excised. Excision of a large portion of the chest wall in addition to the tumour can present some problems. These include extensive loss of chest wall tissue, the replacement of which is necessary purely to provide coverage for the thoracic viscera, and loss of bony chest frame, the integrity of which is mandatory for the proper physiological function of the chest and the mechanics of breathing. Problems arise in cases of extensive resection of the sternum or excision of several ribs and large areas of soft tissues. Extensive bone excision requires the use of prosthesis and sometimes some type of skin grafting or refastening.

PROSTHESIS FOR CHEST WALL RECONSTRUCTION

Several types of prosthesis are used to reconstruct the sternum and body chest wall. They should fulfil the following requirements: (1) rigidity and firmness, (2) ready incorporation into the tissues, (3) chemical and biological acceptability to the host tissues and (4) lack of antigenicity and rejection by the host organism.

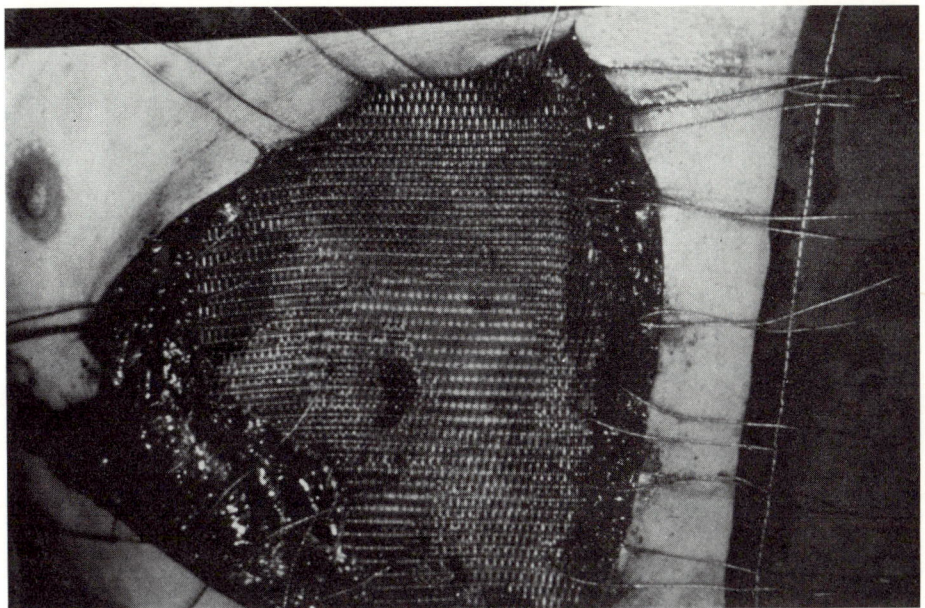

Figure 1.60   Reconstruction of the chest wall using Heavy Marlex Mesh after removal of a malignant tumour.

Heavy Marlex Mesh is used by many surgeons with good results (Fig. 1.60). Marlex is a high-density polyethylene different from low-density polyethylene in many respects. When produced as mesh it is inert but allows ingrowth of the host granulation tissues within the mesh. It is provided as a sheet and has to be tailored to a given defect. A piece of suitable size and shape is cut from the sheet, then the edges are heat-sealed with a live cautery. Once the Marlex Mesh patch is in place it is covered with soft chest tissues.

TUMOURS OF THE LUNG

It is difficult to define a tumour in a sentence which incorporates all its characteristics and features. However the following description provided by Willis* can be quoted:

'A tumour is an abnormal mass of tissue, the growth of which exceeds, and is unco-ordinated with, that of normal tissues and persists in the same excessive manner after the cessation of the stimuli which evoked the change.'

Two important characteristics are outlined: growth beyond the boundaries of normal tissues and autonomous growth of tissues.

According to their behaviour tumours are classified as benign or malignant and their salient features can be described as:

1. *Benign tumours* do not invade, but compress, surrounding tissues as they expand. They do not produce distant satellite lesions (metastases, secondaries) and their constituent cells resemble the parent cells.

*Willis, R. A. 1967. The Pathology of Tumours. 4th edn. London, Butterworth.

2. *Malignant tumours* invade and destroy surrounding tissues. They produce secondary satellite lesions of an equally destructive nature, and their cells vary in the degree of resemblance to the parent cells. The closer the degree of resemblance the more 'differentiated' the tumour is said to be. When there is no resemblance whatsoever between the tumour and the parent cells the tumour is said to be undifferentiated. An anaplastic tumour displays an extreme degree of dissimilarity to its parent cells.

Tumours of the lung generally, and cancer in particular, make up the greatest part of the work of a Thoracic Surgical Unit. Advances in oncology, chemotherapy and radiotherapy have so far failed to achieve decisive changes in the therapeutic approach to lung cancer for which the principal method of treatment is still surgery.

The lungs can be involved by a variety of benign and malignant tumours, but only the most common tumours are discussed here.

BRONCHIAL ADENOMA

This is the most common of the benign tumours (Fig. 1.61). It affects individuals of a younger age group than carcinoma and is more common in females than in males.

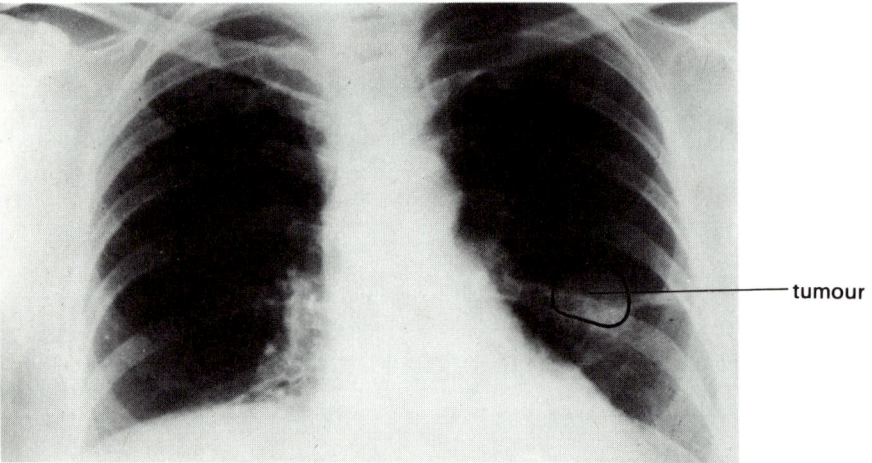

tumour

Figure 1.61   Adenoma of the left lower lobe.

Respiratory symptoms usually draw attention to the condition. These can extend over a long period, sometimes a year or more. Haemoptysis, repeated chest infections, signs of bronchial obstruction and pulmonary collapse are usually present.

Diagnosis

From the above clinical symptoms and signs and radiological investigations, a diagnosis may be reached. A chest radiograph may show no abnormalities when the tumour is small, but larger tumours show as an opacity in the lung fields or as pulmonary collapse, bronchiectasis and inflammatory changes. Diagnosis is confirmed by bronchoscopy and biopsy.

Treatment
Surgical treatment is usually curative. In early cases when the pulmonary tissue has not been altered by repeated infection minimum pulmonary resection is required. Even involvement of the larger bronchi does not exclude economic excision as bronchoplastic procedures are applicable in these cases. More extensive surgery with segmental lobar resection is required when the pulmonary parenchyma is involved.

HAMARTOMA
This benign tumour-like lesion consists of normal lung cells and tissues with an abnormal architectural arrangement. The lesion is asymptomatic and is discovered in the course of routine chest radiograph.

Treatment
As exact diagnosis of hamartoma cannot be established with absolute certainty, and, although the tumour is innocent, it is usually removed by simple enucleation in the course of an exploratory thoracotomy.

OTHER TUMOURS
Other benign tumours such as adenoma and leiomyoma rarely affect the lungs.

Carcinoma (synonym cancer) of the bronchus
Carcinoma is the commonest of the malignant lung tumours, derived from the epithelial elements of the bronchus and the lung. It affects males 4 to 5 times more than females. Practically no age group is spared although most sufferers are in their fifties and sixties.

As with the majority of cancers although no definite causative agent can be found many factors are known to play a prominent role in its development. There is evidence that cigarette smoking leads to the development of lung cancer and that prolonged exposure to asbestos, cobalt, radium, nickel, coal, arsenic and chrome derivatives is responsible for the high incidence of lung cancer among workers in these industries.

Clinical features and diagnosis Essentially bronchial carcinoma presents itself in two ways:

1. *Asymptomatic.* The tumour is discovered in the course of a routine chest radiograph or on investigations for other conditions.
2. *Symptomatic* Because signs of respiratory disease are present the tumour is discovered in the course of planned investigations.

All bronchial carcinomas become symptomatic in time. The type and severity of symptoms vary according to the site and the extension of the disease. Of all the manifestations of respiratory disease, previously described (see *Investigations*, p. 54), cough and haemoptysis are the most frequently observed. These, when accompanied by a wheeze and clubbing of the finger nails in patients over fifty, suggest a strong likelihood of bronchial carcinoma.

INVESTIGATIONS

Clinical
Pulmonary involvement by the primary tumour and secondary involvement of glands in the neck, liver, bones and the central nervous system, which are the commonest sites of metastases can be brought to evidence.

Laboratory
Blood examination may or may not reveal any abnormalities. Sputum examined for cytological studies may reveal the presence of abnormal malignant cells.

Radiological
Postero-anterior and lateral chest radiographs show the tumour as an opacity (Fig. 1.62) or show segmental or lobar collapse caused by bronchial obstruction. Additional radiological investigations such as tomography and bronchography can be required for more accurate diagnosis.

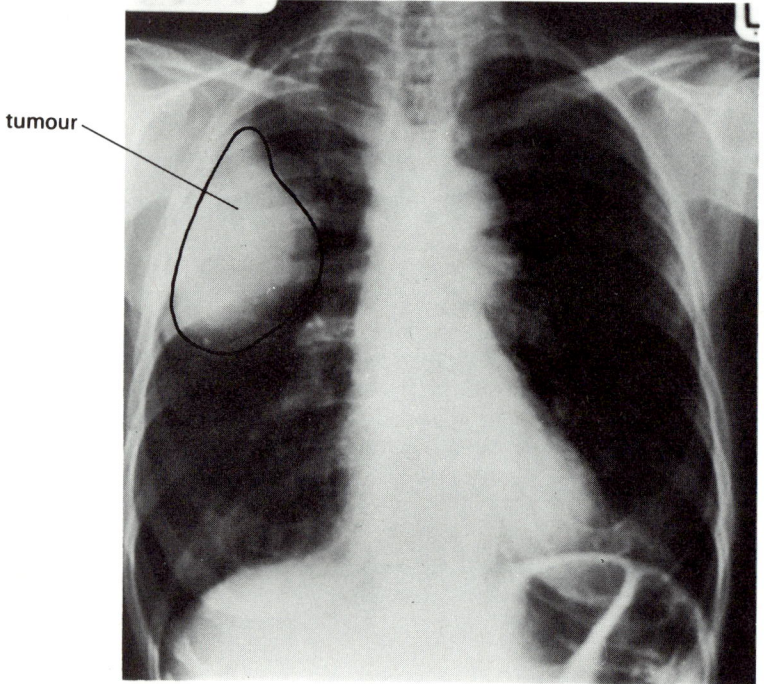

Figure 1.62   Primary malignant tumour of the right upper lobe.

Bronchoscopy
This is the most useful investigation as it can demonstrate intraluminal bronchial pathology and bronchial involvement. It also indicates therapeutic measures to be taken in a given case.

Mediastinoscopy

It is now carried out routinely by some surgeons to assess the involvement of the superior mediastinum and the paratracheal chain of glands. A biopsy of these glands is taken for histological examination.

Scalene node biopsy is carried out in some cases.

TREATMENT

When diagnosis is definitely established, therapeutic possibilities are considered. It must be stressed that sometimes diagnosis is strongly suspected and not definitely established. An exploratory thoracotomy is then advised. Treatment entails either one or a combination of surgery, radiotherapy, chemotherapy, or symptomatic treatment with analgesics and sedatives.

The choice of treatment depends on anatomical site and extent of the growth, histological type of the tumour, presence or absence of secondaries, and general condition and respiratory function of the patient.

Surgery

It is universally agreed that a patient in good general health and with a tumour limited to the lung, should be given the chance of surgical treatment involving either removal of a lobe (lobectomy) for a growth limited to one or two lobes, or removal of a lung (pneumonectomy) and satellite lymph nodes.

Radiotherapy

Radiotherapy is mostly used for:

1. An inoperable growth involving the mediastinum, with impending obstruction of the venous return to the heart in the area of the superior vena cava.

2. Other central tumours, particularly in the young and in cases of rapidly growing and highly malignant anaplastic and oat-cell carcinomas.

3. In cases of localised skeletal secondaries causing pain.

4. In recurrent growth.

5. In symptomatic tumours (i.e. causing pain) haemoptysis and other definite local symptoms.

Chemotherapy

Cytotoxic drugs have a limited use and before they are prescribed their beneficial effects should be carefully weighed against their toxic side-effects. They are usually prescribed in cases of inoperable tumours which have spread to multiple distant sites. Relief and survival of up to one year have been observed in some cases.

Combined therapy

Multi-modal treatment in cancer of the lung has attracted surgeons from time to time. At present it is reasonable to state that the results of combination therapy cannot be judged and that isolated reports of benefit from such therapy have not been sustained by an independent body of workers or well-planned trials.

Symptomatic treatment

This consists of the administration of drugs which have no specific effect on the tumour but simply remove the pain and ease suffering. Analgesics and sedatives should be prescribed for patients with an extensive and painful growth to alleviate symptoms.

PATHOLOGY OF LUNG CANCER

Cancer (synonym carcinoma) is a general term applied to malignant epithelial tumours. In most cases cancer of the lung develops from the bronchial wall and is a true bronchial carcinoma, even though it presents itself like a mass within the pulmonary substance. As it progressively expands the tumour involves pulmonary tissues indiscriminately, spreading locally and to distant sites. Spread along the lymphatic channels and the nodes occurs early with the formation of satellite tumour masses. The rich vascular and lymphatic supply of the lung provides tumour cells with easy circulatory access and the possibility of invading distant organs via the blood stream. The tumour originates in the periphery of the lung at times and at others near the hilum. By definition all malignant tumours metastasise at some stage of their development. Many complex factors operate in determining at which stage and site secondary deposit occurs. Although secondary tumours can be deposited in any part of the body, the most frequent sites for metastases of lung cancer are the vertebrae, the brain, the liver and suprarenals.

Four types of lung cancer have been described and classified according to the predominance of the cell type and their arrangement on microscopic examination:

1. Squamous cell carcinoma.
2. Adenocarcinoma.
3. Undifferentiated oat-cell carcinoma (small or anaplastic).
4. Alveolar cell carcinoma.

EPIDERMOID OR SQUAMOUS CELL CARCINOMA
Between 35–40% of all malignant pulmonary tumours are of the squamous cell variety. These tumours are derived from bronchial epithelial cells. They are more frequently seen in males than females. They commonly spread through lymph nodes.

ADENOCARCINOMA
Some 20% of cases of pulmonary cancer are derived from bronchial glandular or peripheral pulmonary tissues. The spread of these tumours is primarily effected through the blood stream although lymphatic spread can also take place.

UNDIFFERENTIATED SMALL CELL CARCINOMA
Some 30–35% of pulmonary tumours are undifferentiated. This means that their cell of origin cannot be distinguished. One type in this group is characterised by small and undifferentiated cells: it is known as oat-cell carcinoma.

These tumours are particularly malignant and spread rapidly. They are also capable of producing extra pulmonary signs and symptoms (e.g. neurological) without actual metastases in CNS (non-metastatic syndromes).

ALVEOLAR CELL CARCINOMA

This is an uncommon type of pulmonary cancer. The tumour develops beyond the bronchiolar system. It disseminates by way of the blood and lymphatic streams.

SECONDARY TUMOURS OF THE LUNG

By virtue of their rich vascular and lymphatic capillary networks and owing to their high blood flow, the lungs are commonly involved by secondary tumours. Tumour cells of various origins and from almost every part of the body can migrate to the lungs where they form secondary satellite tumours. Common sources of secondary pulmonary tumours are:

1. *Malignant tumours* of the respiratory tract including bronchogenic carcinoma. The latter may at times present itself as multiple cancerous foci in both lungs as shown in Fig. 1.63 and poses difficult diagnostic and therapeutic problems.

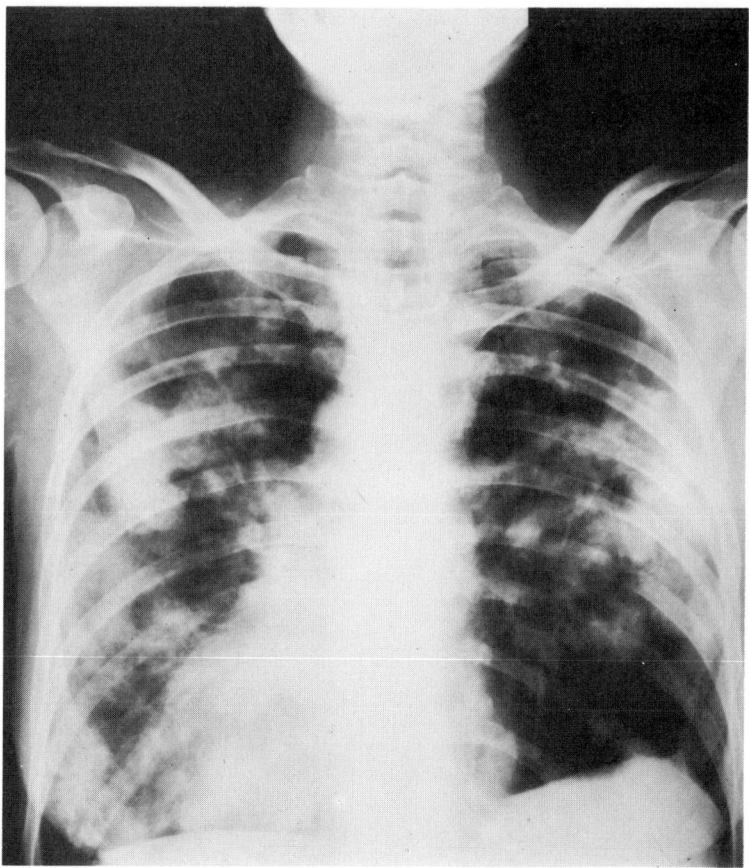

Figure 1.63   Scattered secondary tumours in both lungs.

2. *Gastro-intestinal cancer* frequently spreads to the lungs which then present with multiple secondary tumours.

3. *Cancers of the breast*, kidneys, testicles and the female genital tract can also spread to the lung.

The treatment of multiple secondary tumours of the lungs is that of disseminated cancer.

When the lung presents with a single secondary tumour in the form of a mass shown on a chest radiograph, surgical excision may be carried out. This excision is indicated providing that the primary tumour from which the pulmonary secondary is derived is treatable and that there are no secondary deposits in other tissues of the body.

14 Preparation of Patients Undergoing Lung Surgery

The aim of surgery is to cure the disease or improve the quality of life. The patient should be in the best possible condition, both physically and psychologically, in order to make a successful recovery. Patients are naturally apprehensive when surgery is planned, particularly if it is likely to be extensive. A warm welcome and good atmosphere in the ward, introduction to other patients, and knowledge of the general ward layout and routine, can all help to alleviate some of the patient's fears.

Admission to hospital is arranged a few days prior to operation so the patient may be fully investigated and prepared.

PSYCHOLOGICAL PREPARATION

It is the nurse's duty to ensure that the patient is psychologically prepared for operation. This means establishing a relationship with him so that he will talk about problems which are worrying him. If possible, these should be dealt with either by the nursing staff or a medical social worker. Ensuring adequate rest and sleep both pre- and post-operatively is important to aid healing. Finding time to listen to the patient helps to establish a relationship of trust. Increasingly, research is showing that giving a patient full information pre-operatively speeds recovery, prevents post-operative complications and may reduce the amount of post-operative analgesics required for pain.

Whilst it is the doctor's responsibility to give a patient information about the operation, the nurse can help by talking it over with the patient and ensuring he understands. In addition, the patient should be told about the presence of drainage tubes, intravenous infusion or any other apparatus he will see post-operatively. This gives him a chance to prepare himself mentally for coping during the post-operative period, an important aspect of preventing anxiety which can interfere with recovery.

During the post-operative period, the nurse will need to 'reassure the patient'. This is aimed at helping the patient to come to terms with his condition and develop hope for the future. It comprises many different nursing techniques among which are giving the patient accurate information about what is happening to him, showing calmness and efficiency when giving nursing care, showing faith in the medical staff, taking immediate action in emergencies, demonstrating well coordinated team work, and good relationships among members of staff, encouraging the patient to talk about his anxieties and worries, recognising the patient as an individual, and giving a friendly welcome to his relatives and friends.

A patient who has successfully undergone the same operation can be invaluable in giving information and boosting the morale of another patient prior to operation.

Psychological preparation of patients undergoing lung surgery is particularly important, as they are understandably apprehensive. Neoplasm of the lung is such a common and publicised condition that the majority of patients know of someone who has had the 'same operation' or remember a relative who may have died from lung cancer. Tuberculosis can still cast a dark shadow on people's minds and it is therefore the surgeon's task to explain and reassure the patient about the forthcoming operation. Doctors and especially nurses should discuss with the patient his condition and the state in which he will be returning to the ward. By doing so the patient will not be too alarmed when intravenous fluid or blood are in progress, and/or when he finds himself attached to an intercostal drain. The nurse plays a very important pre- and post-operative part in reassuring and helping the patient through this very difficult period.

CLINICAL PREPARATION

HYGIENE
The patient's general hygiene is important. This applies to the skin, nails and external body orifices which harbour pathogenic organisms. A daily bath will help to cleanse the skin. Dental hygiene has a special place in thoracic nursing, as bacteria in the teeth can cause post-operative infection that will affect recovery.

NUTRITION
Many patients suffer from a lack of appetite and may be in a poor nutritional condition. The presence of a chronic infection and sepsis (e.g. empyema) which withdraw protein from the general body pool can be a major contributing factor to the state of malnutrition. These patients should receive a high protein and calorie diet.

CORRECTION OF ANAEMIA
Patients suffering from lung neoplasms can become severely anaemic because of haemoptysis, sepsis or merely as the result of the malignant tumour preventing valuable proteins and chemicals being utilised for normal cell metabolism. Anaemia should be corrected before surgery.

HEART
A good functioning of the heart is extremely important particularly in older patients and treatment may be necessary to control the heart rate and rhythm.

BLOOD
Before surgery a specimen of blood is taken for grouping and cross-matching so that blood will be readily when required.

ANTIBIOTICS
Antibiotics are prescribed prophylactically by most surgeons.

BOWELS

Care should be taken to ensure regular bowel action. A small enema the day before operation is still favoured by many surgeons.

PHYSIOTHERAPY

All patients undergoing thoracic surgery must be taught how to breathe correctly by using the respiratory muscles effectively and economically, so as to increase their effective ventilation. This is brought about by breathing symmetrically, deeply and slowly. The nurse should know the principles of chest physiotherapy so that in the post-operative period she can help the patient when the physiotherapist is not in the ward area. It cannot be overemphasised that retention of sputum causes collapse or atelectasis of the lung distal to the blocked bronchus.

If sputum is contaminated and contains pathogenic organisms, then infection leading to a lung abscess will result. Patients undergoing thoracic surgery are particularly liable to sputum retention and infection as breathing and coughing are more difficult because of the thoracotomy. It is therefore essential that the patient be taught to breathe correctly *before* his operation. It is a good idea to let the patient try breathing with an oxygen mask if he is likely to be given oxygen post-operatively.

SPECIAL DISINFECTION AND DECONTAMINATION

All sources of infection should be eliminated prior to surgery. Sputum is examined for organisms and for sensitivity to antibiotics. Nasal swabs are taken for microbiological studies as the nose is part of the air-conducting system and can harbour pathogenic micro-organisms.

TEETH

Particular attention should be paid to infected or carious teeth and all patients who are to have thoracic surgery must have a dental check and treatment as required.

SKIN

The skin is widely exposed to an environment containing a variety of micro-organisms; some micro-organisms are permanently present (e.g. staphylococci albus)—these are known as resident flora. Other species are less frequently present and are known as transient flora (e.g. staphylococcus pyogenes, pseudomonas pyocyanae).

The skin has its own disinfecting processes provided by its own mechanical strength and the chemical properties of glandular secretions. In addition it has biological properties conferred by bacteriological agents living on its skin.

The purpose of skin preparation is to eradicate micro-organisms from the surface of the skin in order to prevent their introduction into the body through a combination of surgical incision and suppression of local and general auto-disinfection mechanisms.

Different techniques exist and each department has its own routine for skin preparation, but the following approach seems to be prevalent:

1. The skin over the anterior aspect of the chest from the clavicles down to the umbilicus and over the corresponding posterior area is shaved.

2. The patient has a bath the night or morning before operation.

3. The chest and abdomen are washed with soap and water an hour or so before the operation.

4. The skin over the chest and upper abdomen is painted with a solution of 1–2 % iodine in 70 % alcohol.

5. The iodine solution is wiped off with 70 % alcohol solution.

6. A sterile towel is wrapped over the painted area.

The patient is sent to the operating theatre with this towel over the chest. In the theatre a further disinfection of the skin is carried out by the surgeon before towelling the patient for operation.

BEFORE THEATRE

OPERATION CONSENT FORM
The nature of the operation would have been explained to the patient by a member of the surgical team the day before the operation, or at least prior to premedication. The patient should sign the form in the presence of the doctor.

FASTING
The patient should have been fasted for the four hours immediately before the operation.

EMPTYING THE BLADDER
The patient should be sent to the theatre with an empty bladder.

IDENTITY BAND
Before the patient goes to the operating theatre an identity band is fastened onto his wrist so that he can be identified if unable to respond verbally (in many hospitals such an identity band is fastened on admission).

PREMEDICATION
It is administered as per prescription. Its effect should be explained to the patient.

RECORDS
Radiographs, case-notes, treatment cards and operation consent form should be readily available, to be taken to theatre by the nurse who accompanies the patient.

15 Bronchoscopy

This visual examination, through a bronchoscope of the larynx, trachea and the bronchial trees, is carried out for the following purposes:

1. Diagnosis of broncho-pulmonary lesions.
2. Removal of inhaled foreign bodies.
3. Clearing the bronchial tress of excessive normal and abnormal secretions (suction bronchoscopy).
4. Obtaining a sample of secretions for laboratory investigations, in particular cytology and microbiological studies.
5. Obtaining biopsy material for histological examination.

Bronchoscopy can be performed under either local or general anaesthesia, but all diagnostic bronchoscopies and bronchoscopies for the removal of foreign bodies are carried out under general anaesthesia. Suction bronchoscopy is best carried out in the ward or in an intensive care unit with the patient in his own bed.

For whatever reason bronchoscopy is performed, the patients should be told about the procedure and reassured. They should be warned of possible blood stains in the sputum afterwards as a bronchial biopsy may be taken.

Patients for local anaesthesia should be specially reassured. The procedure should be explained clearly so that all necessary cooperation is obtained. A sedative should be provided.

BRONCHOSCOPY IN THE OPERATING THEATRE

The patient lies on the table and is anaesthetised. The operator stands behind. A towel is wrapped around the patient's head covering and protecting the eyes from accidental injuries. The nose is left free. Many operators protect the teeth and gums with two gauze swabs. The nurse hands the bronchoscope over to the operator and has ready (in the other hand) a suction catheter connected to a powerful suction machine. At all times the nurse should support the suction tubing and the bronchoscope cable, preventing them from pulling on the instrument when *in situ* in the patient's respiratory tract.

BRONCHOSCOPY IN THE WARD

The patient sits in an upright position in bed, with his head slightly extended. In post-operative cases in particular, it is distressing to the patient to lie flat. Furthermore, the supine position is no more advantageous to the operator. The patient's eyes are covered with a towel after a general or local anaesthetic has

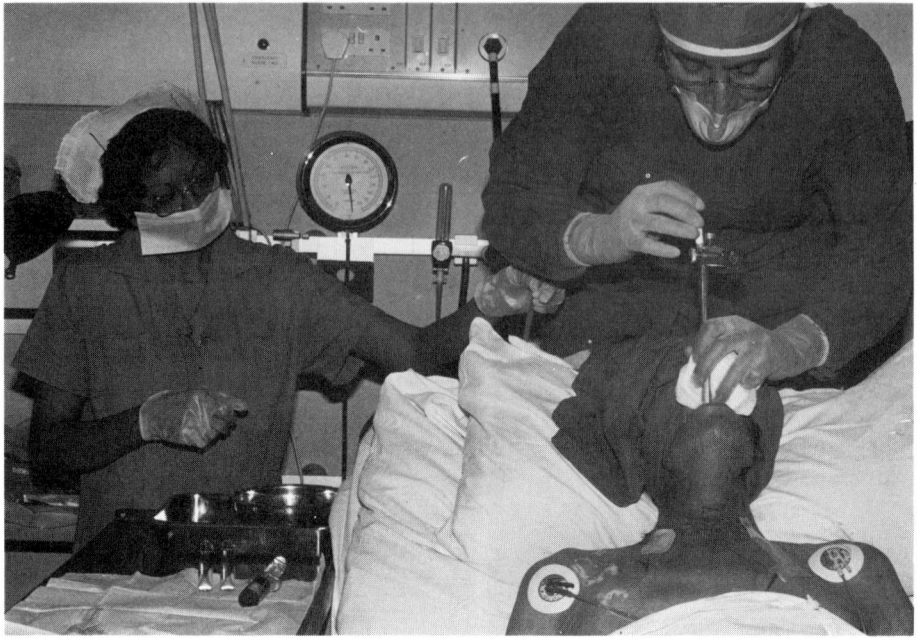

Figure 1.64　Suction bronchoscopy in the ward.

been given. The operator stands on a suitable stool behind the patient (Fig. 1.64). A step by step explanation of the procedure should be given to the patient, in terms of what he will feel.

PROCEDURE FOR SURFACE ANAESTHESIA
The patient sits upright with the neck extended. The operator, standing in front, injects 2 ml of 4% Lignocaine through the crico-thyroid membrane into the tracheal lumen. It is emphasised that this injection is made into the actual lumen. It trickles over the mucosal surface of the trachea and produces a bout of coughing, which splashes the local anaesthetic onto the surface of the larynx. Additional local anaesthesia of the oro-pharynx and the laryngo-pharynx is carried out by spraying the mouth and the pharynx with Lignocaine (or using laryngeal swabs soaked in local anaesthetic and held with laryngeal forceps).

EQUIPMENT
Equipment for bronchoscopy can best be described under (1) local anaesthetic requirement, (2) diagnostic bronchoscopy requirements, and (3) emergency (post-operative) suction bronchoscopy.

Local anaesthetic requirements
These consist of swabs; skin disinfectant solution (e.g. Hibitane in spirit); 5 ml syringe and matching needle; lignocaine 4% (for surface anaesthesia); gallipot for disinfectant solution; laryngeal spray; *Krause laryngeal forceps; *small

swabs suitable for laryngeal forceps; *additional gallipot for local anaesthetic (for soaking the swabs held in the Krause forceps).

* Items required only when the operator wishes to apply local anaesthetic to the pharynx and pyriform fossa.

Diagnostic bronchoscopy apparatus
The apparatus, as illustrated in Figure 1.65, is as follows:

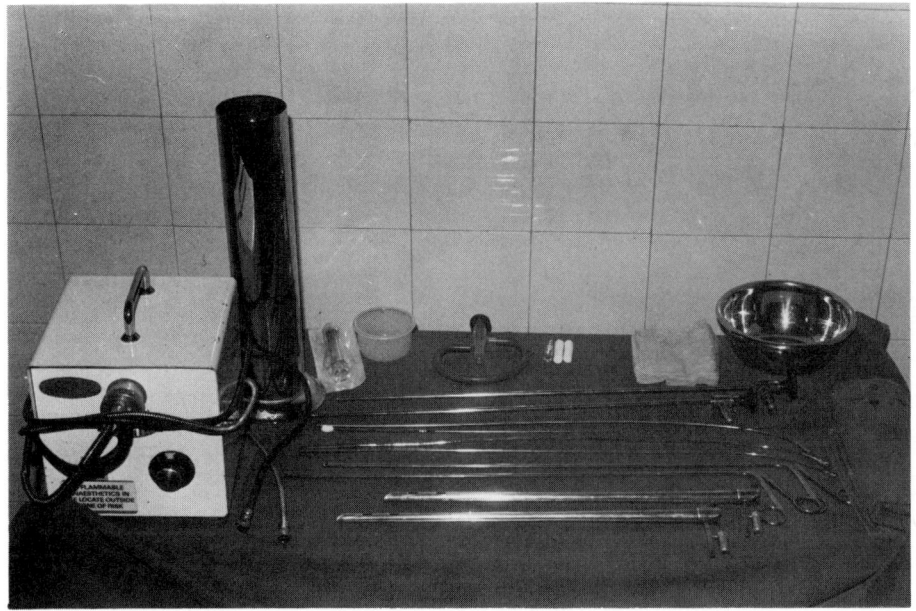

Figure 1.65   Diagnostic bronchoscopy trolley. (See text for details.)

Bronchoscope   There are principally two types of instrument:

1. A rigid direct bronchoscope (see Fig. 1.36, p. 60) available in different diameters and lengths adapted to the size of the patient (adult, adolescent, child and infant).

2. A flexible fibroptic indirect vision instrument (see Fig. 1.37, p. 60).

Most surgeons prefer the rigid bronchoscope and use the flexible one only occasionally for some specific diagnostic purpose. For both types it is necessary to have a light carried (fibroptic), a cable and its connector, a light source, and a lubricant (sterile glycerine or lignocaine lubricant).

Suction apparatus   This consists of one suction catheter (metal with attached plastic tip or disposable catheter); a suction tube; a powerful suction machine; a secretion sample container: Luken's tube or a disposable type; a warm (body temperature) sterile, normal saline solution; a gallipot; a 10 ml disposable syringe; a bowl of sterile water to clear suction tubes.

The solution, gallipot and syringe are used when a sample of bronchial secretions is required for laboratory investigations and in cases where secretions are slight or non-existent. A small quantity of saline can be injected and collected to provide a sample specimen.

Telescopes   One direct and one right angle telescope is usually sufficient, along with a cable and connector and a jar containing warm sterile water with a large protective pad at the bottom. Telescopes are kept in this jar ready for use. Warm water facilitates vision by preventing the distal (objective) side of the telescope from becoming misty. A light source is also required.

Biopsy apparatus requirements consist of one straight and one right-angled pair of biopsy forceps (e.g. Brock's or Patterson's); a biopsy specimen container with 'fixative', specially supplied by the pathology laboratory; a gallipot containing normal saline (for rinsing forceps if it is necessary to use them a second time on the same patient); an intra-bronchial swab holder; small size swabs to fit swab holder; ampoules of 1/1000 Adrenaline solution.

The swab holder, swabs and solution are useful for surface application in case of bleeding after a bronchial biopsy.

Swabs

Head towel for patient

Emergency ward bronchoscopy
As this is not for diagnostic purposes, and as a sizeable tray cannot be made available at short notice, minimum apparatus only is required (see Fig. 1.66).

Bronchoscope   Apparatus consists of an appropriate sized or portable bronchoscope, with attached batteries (check working order frequently), and a lubricant (sterile).

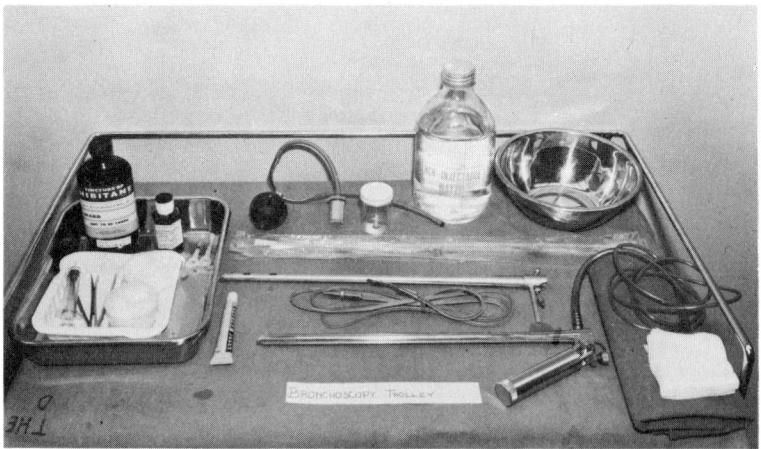

Figure 1.66   Simple suction ward bronchoscopy trolley. (See text for details.)

Suction apparatus consists of suction catheters (disposable); suction tubing and connector; a suction machine or wall suction; a sample container to receive secretion for microbiological studies; a bowl of sterile water, to clear the suction catheter; swabs; one towel; oxygen and connecting tube to fit the side of the bronchoscope.

BRONCHOSCOPY AFTER-CARE

When bronchoscopy is carried out under general anaesthesia in the operating theatre, the patient remains in the recovery room (or area) until full consciousness is regained. During the patient's journey back to the ward the accompanying nurse carries a kidney dish, disposable sputum container and gauze swab (or disposable tissues). In most cases the patient is sent back to the ward from the recovery room after the return of full cough reflex. If this practice is not adhered to then the nurse should also carry an airway tongue forceps and mouth gag. Oxygen should also be available on the carrying trolley.

If the patient is fully conscious and coughing, an upright sitting position is satisfactory. When the patient is not fully conscious a semi-prone position should be adopted. When a biopsy is taken from the right bronchial tree, the left semi-prone position is adopted (i.e. right side down). The right semi-prone position is adopted after a biopsy of the left bronchial tree.

The duty of the nurse is to look after the patient and not play the role of porter. She should not take her eyes off the patient. Her duties are:

1. To ensure that the upper airways are clear from secretions and blood at all times.
2. To ensure that respiration is unobstructed.
3. To check the pulse during the journey.

If these are not satisfactory, then she must deal with the problem as a matter of first priority and must get assistance.

Before the patient's return to the ward, the duty of nurses is to have the necessary equipment available near the bed, i.e. oxygen supply and equipment for its administration, a suction machine, with suction head and tubing, a kidney dish and gauze swab, or disposable tissues, and a sputum container.

An unconscious or semi-conscious patient must not be left alone, not even 'for a minute'. On arrival in the ward the following observations are made and recorded:

1. State of consciousness.
2. Arterial pressure, pulse rate and volume.
3. State of respiration.
4. The patient's colour (i.e. whether cyanosis is present or not).
5. Any other abnormalities, such as nausea, vomiting, bronchospasm or haemoptysis.

If there is any doubt about the patient's breathing a senior member of the nursing staff or medical officer should be requested to see the patient.

If observations are satisfactory and the patient is conscious, with a good cough reflex, he may be left to rest. Observations are then made only two or three times on that day. Otherwise, the above observations are repeated according to instructions and requirements. Patients are usually given food and drink four hours later.

COMPLICATIONS OF BRONCHOSCOPY

Bronchoscopy in itself has no complications when carried out by an expert. However, there are definite complications related to general anaesthesia and bronchial biopsy, which are part of the overall procedure.

ANAESTHETIC COMPLICATIONS

Respiratory complications
These complications are connected with airway obstruction and are due to (1) secretions, saliva and vomitus, (2) the tongue falling back, (3) laryngeal and bronchial spasm, and (4) signs and symptoms of airway obstruction are essentially those related to hypoxia and carbon dioxide retention (see p. 150).

Gastro-intestinal complications
Nausea and vomiting are not common complications, but it is absolutely essential that the respiratory tract remains clear at all times, and that respiration is unobstructed.

BIOPSY COMPLICATIONS

Bleeding
Haemorrhage from the site of the biopsy is checked by the operator in the operating theatre. Any additional blood-stained secretion is dealt with in the recovery room (or area), before the patient is returned to the ward. In the ward there will be some expectoration of blood-stained secretion, but frank haemoptysis is not common. In the case of haemorrhage the following procedure should be undertaken:

1. The patient should be reassured.
2. Clear the mouth and respiratory tract.
3. Incline the patient towards the side from which the biopsy was taken (i.e. biopsy side down).
4. Monitor the pulse rate and volume arterial BP, and breathing rate.
5. Monitor the progress by observing:
    (a) If the bleeding is fresh.
    (b) If there are blood clots.
    (c) The volume lost.

If haemoptysis continues, and particularly if there is the slightest doubt about the patient's breathing, the medical officer should be informed.

Pneumothorax
This is a rare complication. It can cause dyspnoea and mediastinal shift, or be discovered by a subsequent chest radiograph. If this is suspected, the position of the mediastinum should be checked by palpating the trachea above the supra-

clavicular notch, oxygen supplied and the medical officer informed. He will have to deal with the pneumothorax and therefore an aspiration set and/or intercostal pleural drainage apparatus should be prepared and made available.

Surgical emphysema
This too is a rare complication, usually occuring with a pneumothorax, but sometimes on its own. If surgical emphysema is present on return to the ward, the medical officer should be informed.

16 Surgical Access to the Chest

THORACOTOMY

Thoracotomy is the surgical opening of the chest; it is carried out for operative access to all intrathoracic structures.

Anterior, antero-lateral, posterior and postero-lateral thoracotomies are carried out on the right or the left side of the chest, depending on the type of operation and the structure upon which surgery is to be carried out. The chest, or more precisely the mediastinum, can also be opened in the mid-line by splitting the sternum.

POSTERO-LATERAL THORACOTOMY

The standard thoracotomy for pulmonary surgery is the postero-lateral one. The position of patient on the table is either lateral or prone.

Lateral position

The patient is placed on the table with the side of the chest to be opened upwards, and the spine near the edge of the table (see Fig. 1.67). The patient's position must be firmly secured. This can be achieved by placing a pillow between the legs then using a groin support, an anterior chest support and the belt, all of which are among the accessory fitments of the operating table. Care must be taken to safely apply the diathermy pad (electrode) and to protect the patient from hard and metallic parts.

The surgeon stands by the patient's back, the assistant by the patient's front. The skin incision is made below the angle of the scapula along the line of the rib. Posteriorly the incision runs upwards along the vertebral border of scapula. Two muscular layers have to be divided. The superficial layer consists of the trapezius posteriorly, and the latissimus dorsi more anteriorly. The deeper layer consists of

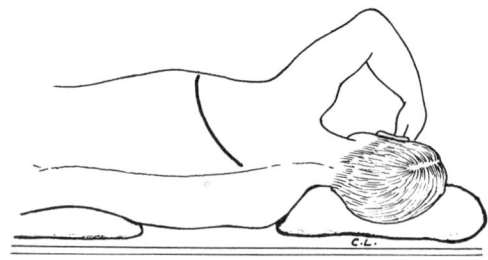

Figure 1.67   Postero-lateral thoracotomy—lateral position.

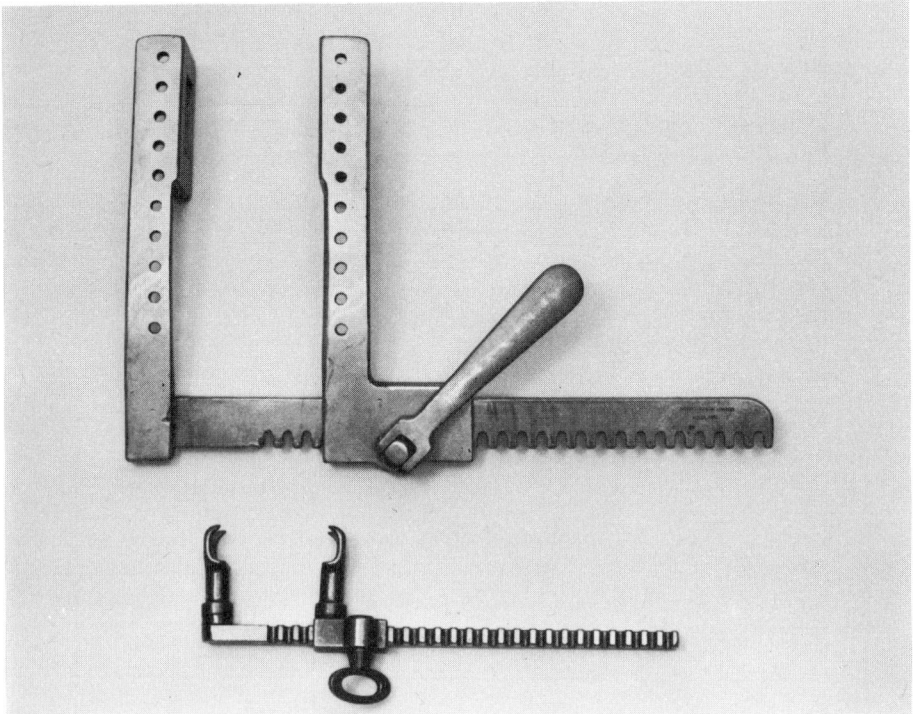

Figure 1.68   Chest spreader (top); Sellor's combined rib approximator and spreader (bottom).

rhomboid muscles posteriorly and the serratus anterior anteriorly. The deepest layer of the chest wall consists of the ribs and the intercostal muscles between them. Entry into the chest is made by peeling off the periosteum from the upper border of the rib, then incising this and the parietal pleura—some surgeons prefer to resect a rib in its greater extent and enter the chest through the bed of the rib.

The next step is to provide a wide opening by using a chest spreader (Fig. 1.68).

Prone position
This position (see Fig. 1.69) used to be a favourite before the advent of one lung anaesthesia with the use of a 'double lumen' tube, particularly when dealing with

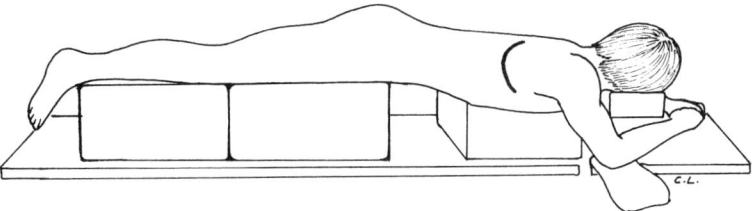

Figure 1.69   Postero-lateral thoracotomy—prone position.

bronchiectatic patients and those with bronchopleural fistulae. The surgeon usually sits on a stool on the operative side. The incision and entry into the chest are made in the same manner as for lateral thoracotomy.

Repair of thoracotomy wound
The closure of the thoracotomy wound is carried out in five layers:

1. Intercostal layer, suturing the periosteum and the intercostal muscles. For this it is necessary to use an approximator (see Fig. 1.68) which facilitates the reduction of the intercostal space which has been widely opened by the spreader.
2. Deep muscular layer suture (rhomboids and serratus anterior).
3. Superficial muscle layer (trapezius and latissimus dorsi).
4. Subcutaneous tissue layer.
5. Skin sutures.

ANTERO-LATERAL THORACOTOMY
The patient is positioned obliquely on the table—by placing and fixing the pelvis as for the lateral position and rotating the shoulder backwards (Fig. 1.70). The skin incision is made in the submammary groove along the line of a rib. The pectoralis major, latissimus dorsi and serratus anterior are divided and the chest entered by raising the periosteum and the perichondrium and incising the pleura.

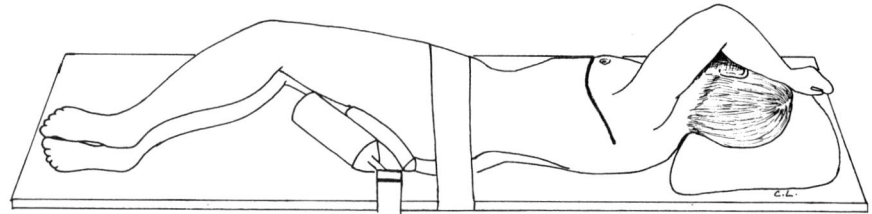

Figure 1.70   Antero-lateral thoracotomy.

ANTERIOR THORACOTOMY
The patient is positioned lying on his back (Fig. 1.71). An incision is made over the desired interspace from the lateral border of the sternum to near the mid-axillary line. Except for high thoracotomies the incision is done below the breast (submammary incision) and the breast can be reflected upwards with the skin if necessary. The muscle layers and parietal pleural are divided to enter the thorax.

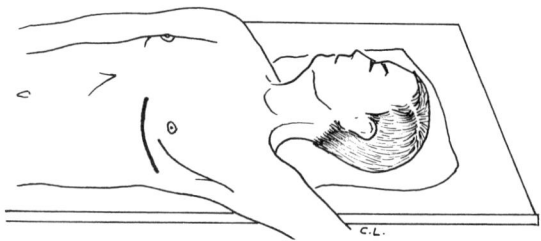

Figure 1.71   Anterior thoracotomy.

MEDIAN STERNOTOMY

This is used for access to the anterior and superior mediastinum (e.g. for thymectomy), and in particular for intra-cardiac operations under cardio-pulmonary by-pass (Fig. 1.72).

A vertical incision is made over the sternum which in turn is divided through its centre vertically using Gigli's or Striker Saw. At the end of the operation the two edges of the sternum are approximated and held firmly together by interrupted wire sutures. Soft tissues are then repaired in layers.

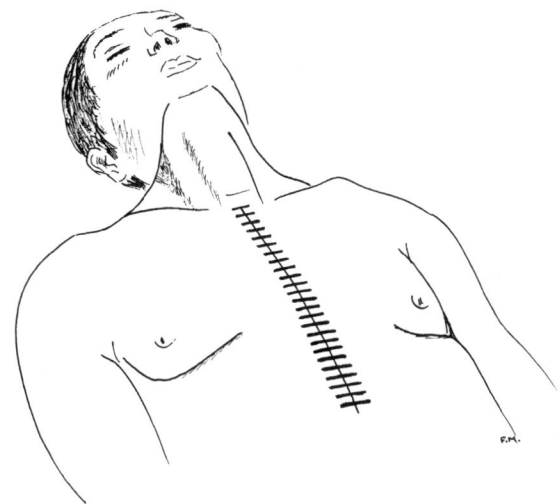

Figure 1.72   Median sternotomy.

PULMONARY RESECTION

Pulmonary resection requires exposure of the lung through a thoracotomy with dissection and identification of the vascular and bronchial branches in order to ligate and divide the former, and incise and suture the latter.

Pulmonary resection can be limited to the smallest pulmonary unit, i.e. a broncho-pulmonary segment, or can extend to the whole of the lung as a pneumonectomy.

PNEUMONECTOMY

This is the resection of the entire lung. With the patient in the prone or lateral position, a postero-lateral thoracotomy is carried out to expose the lung hilum. The vascular pedicle of the lung consists of a pulmonary artery (before it divides into lobar and segmental arteries), and two pulmonary veins. These are ligated and divided outside the pericardium, though at times it is necessary to ligate and divide these structures inside the pericardium. The main bronchus is then divided and the bronchial stump sutured with interrupted stitches. The thoracotomy wound is then repaired.

After a pneumonectomy, some surgeons prefer to drain the chest, others do not drain the pleural space (see Chapters 4 and 5).

LOBECTOMY

This is the resection of a lobe of the lung. As already seen the right lung is divided into three lobes and the left into two. Individual lobes can be excised when pathologically affected. On the right side upper, middle and lower lobectomies are carried out, and upper and lower lobectomies only on the left side.

The operation entails thoracotomy and exposure of the lung hilum. The lobar arteries and veins, which are as many or more than the number of segments in the lobe, are dissected, ligated and divided. The lobar bronchus is divided and sutured. Following a lobectomy the pleural cavity is usually drained by two drains, namely an apical and a basal drain, connected to underwater sealed drainage system (see Chapter 5).

SEGMENTAL RESECTION (Segmentectomy)

This is resection of one or more pulmonary segments. The broncho-pulmonary segments and their arrangement are described in Chapter 2 and further illustrated in Figure 1.14, p. 17). It has been pointed out that each pulmonary segment is an independent part supplied by an identifiable segmental artery and vein (at times more than one) and a segmental bronchus.

In segmental resection, the segmental vessels are ligated, divided and sutured proximally. Although pulmonary lobes are delineated by fissures lined by visceral pleura, segments are attached to one another but can be stripped away when bronchovascular pedicles are divided. This leaves a rather raw surface with multiple, fine air-leaks.

Segmental resection is particularly suitable for diseases such as tuberculosis and bronchiectasis. Following segmentectomy, the chest is closed leaving an apical and a basal drain (see Chapter 5).

SPECIAL TYPES OF PULMONARY RESECTION AND BRONCHOPLASTIC PROCEDURES

In this type of operation the aim is to achieve economic pulmonary resection. That is to excise the whole of the diseased structures with as little pulmonary parenchyma as possible. This is done when the airways are diseased and the parenchyma intact, or when the airways are more extensively affected than the parenchyma.

Surgical excision in these cases should include removal of the diseased parenchyma together with the involved bronchus. As the latter provides bronchial branches not only to the pulmonary tissue which is to be excised but also to the areas of the lung which are free from the disease and are to be retained, some type of airway reconstruction becomes necessary. A typical example of this is the resection of the right upper lobe of the lung containing a neoplasm which not only involves the right upper lobe bronchial branches, but also the right main bronchial branch which subdivides into bronchial branches in the right lower lobe of the lung. A standard right upper lobectomy is insufficient and would mean leaving behind some of the involved tissue in the right main bronchus. On the other hand removal of the right upper lobe, together with excision of a 'sleeve' of the right main bronchus clears the tumours up (Fig. 1.73), but leaves a gap necessitating airway reconstruction. This is achieved by attaching the lower lobe bronchus to the right main bronchus below the carina and above the upper limits of the line bronchial excision. This

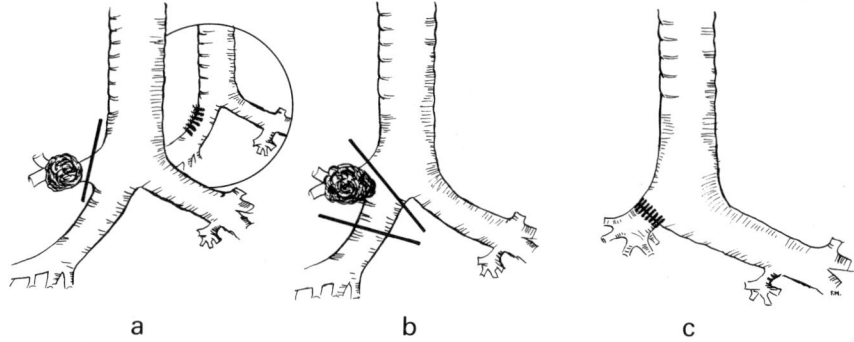

Figure 1.73   (a) Standard right upper lobectomy (inset shows closure of the bronchus). (b) Right upper lobectomy with sleeve resection of the right main bronchus. (c) Reconstruction following sleeve resection.

procedure is referred to as right upper lobectomy sleeve resection. Bronchial reconstruction (broncho-plastic procedures) plays an important role in pulmonary surgery for benign tumours and in some malignant tumours.

THORACOPLASTY

Thoracoplasty consists of resecting a number of ribs, dividing the intervening intercostal bundles (that is intercostal muscles, nerves and vessels), and mobilising the apex of the lung. The aim is to collapse the apex and a variable portion of the lung and to maintain it permanently in that state. This is achieved by the collapse of the chest wall which follows the removal of the ribs.

Nowadays the operation is only carried out in rare cases of apical tuberculous lesions not responding to chemotherapy and unsuitable for excisional surgery. Occasionally the operation is undertaken when, for various reasons, the extent of the chest cavity is to be reduced.

17 Post-operative Management of Patients Undergoing Lung Surgery

Surgical procedures constitute only one phase of the total management of the patient. The post-operative care which follows plays a major part in the overall result. Post-operative nursing care is particularly important in lung surgery because of the anatomical and physiological peculiarities of the lungs and the thoracic cavity.

Post-operative care aims are:

1. Restitution of the vital activities of the body temporarily disturbed by anaesthesia and surgical trauma.

2. Restoration of the lung function which in turn is dependent on full expansion of the residual lung tissues.

3. Assisting local and general effort of the body to repair surgical wounds.

4. Prevention of complications.

5. Preparing the patient physically and psychologically for return to his own environment, that is home, then occupation and work.

These aims can only be fulfilled if medical, nursing and other ancillary staff participate fully in team work. Nurses are the most closely involved. They spend most of their time with patients on the ward, make observations and monitor the patient's progress. They also carry out most of the routine post-operative care. They are responsible for ensuring a continuing high level of care.

It is convenient and logical to describe post-operative care in two stages: *early* (i.e. in the first 24 to 48 hours) and, *late* (from 48 hours to discharge).

EARLY POST-OPERATIVE CARE

Patients are transferred from the operating theatre to the recovery room which should be an integral part of the theatre suite. They should remain there until re-establishment of full consciousness, spontaneous breathing and satisfactory cardiac output is obtained. Their return to the ward or to an intensive care unit should be authorised by the anaesthetist.

The continuation of unconsciousness, lack of effective breathing and an unsatisfactory state of the cardio-vascular system should be reported to the anaesthetist by the recovery room staff.

For descriptive purposes, the early post-operative care can be described as (1) transfer of the patient to the ward, (2) recording of the base-line observations, (3) monitoring of patient's progress by periodic recording of the vital functions, and (4) early post-operative management of patient.

TRANSFER TO THE WARD

In the ward early post-operative care starts before the patient's return. A warm bed is prepared; oxygen and an adjustable suction machine with connecting catheters and tubes (for clearing the airways) are made available near the bed. A pleural suction pump and appropriate tubing should also be ready at hand as suction may have to be applied on the drainage system (Fig. 1.74).

Transfer of the patient from the trolley to the bed must be effected with the minimum of discomfort. During this procedure care must be taken to see that various attachments, such as oxygen tubes and masks, intravenous drips, nasogastric tubes (if *in situ*), are not pulled out or displaced by carelessness, and pleural drains attached to the underwater sealed system are not pulled, displaced or disconnected at the junctions with additional tubes and the underwater glass (or plastic) rod.

In order to transfer the patient from the trolley to his bed without disturbing the drainage system, the bottle and drains have to be lifted—but before this the tube leading from the pleural drain to the underwater rod must be clamped, otherwise fluid and air would enter the chest because of the negative interpleural pressure. Once the patient is in bed the bottles are placed on the floor and the clamp removed.

The site of the surgical wound is inspected (without disturbing the dressing) for local seepage of blood through the dressing, haematoma, and surgical subcutaneous emphysema.

A report on the type of operation, number and position of pleural drains and other attachments to the patient (such as 'airways', oxygen, sites and number of

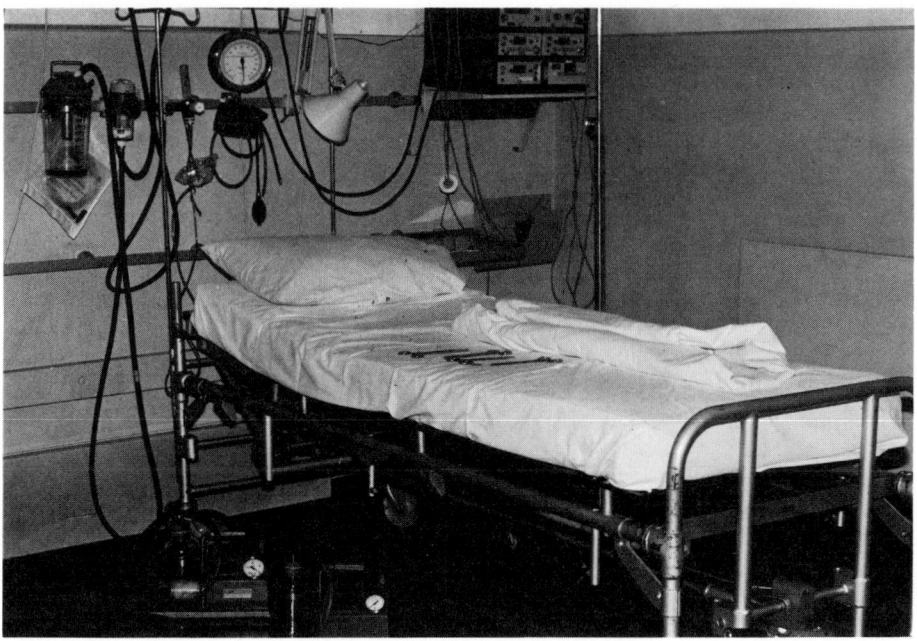

Figure 1.74   Bed and equipment awaiting patient's return to the ward.

intravenous drips, central venous pressure catheters, urinary catheters and ECG) must be received and clearly noted. Instructions with regard to blood and fluid transfusions, supply and rate of oxygen, type and frequency of administration of analgesics should be provided in writing by the medical staff. Further clear instructions about pleural drains should accompany the patient on returning to the ward.

BASE-LINE OBSERVATIONS AND THEIR RECORDING
Base-line observations of vital function are made and recorded. These include (1) state of consciousness, (2) respiratory state, (3) circulatory systems, and (4) pleural drains.

State of consciousness
Consciousness can be defined as a state of awareness of the environment by the individual, and purposeful response to various stimuli. This definition implies various degrees of consciousness. A fully conscious person is aware of the surroundings and responds to simple stimuli such as hearing his name or obeying simple commands (by moving limbs).

An unconscious person is neither aware of the surrounding nor responsive to stimuli. In between, there are several stages which can best be noted in descriptive terms rather than recorded in numerical stages which can be confusing. When consciousness is fully regained the patient should be comforted and told of the completion of the operation.

Respiratory state
The patient's mode of breathing, frequency, depth and the state of oxygenation as judged by the presence or absence of cyanosis, are noted and recorded.

It must be noted that on recovery from anaesthesia the patient goes through stages of unco-ordinated shallow breathing to full rhythmic, deep and co-ordinated respiration.

Careful observation on the nurse's part is necessary to assess the trend of breathing. It is particularly important to have clear airways. A laboured and obstructed breathing at this stage may be due to:

1. The tongue falling back in a patient who is still partially under general anaesthesia.
2. Excessive secretions produced during the recovery from muscle-relaxing agents.
3. Blood and gastric contents.
4. Laryngeal and bronchospasm.

The cause must be investigated and obstruction relieved. If this cannot be achieved readily the medical officer must be summoned.

Circulatory system
On the patient's return to the ward preliminary recordings of the circulatory system must be made. It has been a tradition to judge the cardio-vascular performance by the level of arterial pressure and the pulse rate. It is however more relevant to assess the circulatory state not only by these methods but also by the temperature and venous filling in the extremities as well as central venous

pressure recordings (when a cather is in position). The following recordings are therefore made of the rate, rhythm and volume of the pulse, colour and temperature of the skin in the extremities, degree of venous filling, arterial blood pressure, and central venous pressure.

Pleural drains
In lung and thoracic surgery the pleural drain is of vital importance and a base-line recording of the state of the drain should have priority over other nursing care. Its working cannot be separated from respiratory functions and indeed its malfunction may be the very cause of post-operative cardio-respiratory problems. Therefore, as soon as the patient has returned to the ward, pleural drains should be attended to according to the type of operation and instructions received for their immediate management (see Chapter 5).

The quantity and type of drainage is recorded so that progress can be gauged. While base-line observations on drainage are made, instructions regarding further management of drains are carefully studied and applied by the nursing staff.

Once the base-line observations and information have been recorded proper post-operative care starts. It consists of monitoring at frequent intervals over the next 24 to 48 hours a series of parameters reflecting various bodily activities.

PERIODIC MONITORING OF PATIENT'S PROGRESS
Clinical observations of vital functions are periodically carried out and charted. This is to bring to notice the persistence of disorders in the body's vital activities as a direct consequence of general anaesthesia and surgery, the early trend of the patient's post-operative progress, and early signs and symptoms of complications.

The state of the patient's consciousness is assessed particularly if he was unconscious on arrival in the ward from the operating theatre.

Cardio-vascular and circulatory state
This is monitored by recording pulse rate and volume, arterial blood pressure, and skin colour and temperature. These parameters are recorded and charted as frequently as requested by the medical personnel.

In a satisfactory case the pulse remains regular, steady in rate (only slightly raised compared with pre-operative findings), with a good volume.

Arterial and central venous pressures remain steady over a period of hours; only slight reduction in arterial blood pressure can be considered as normal only if slight. Extremities become warm soon after return to the ward.

Alteration in pulse and blood pressure or change in the circulatory state must be investigated and reported to the medical team.

It is important to be particularly aware of early circulatory complications, the most important of which are shock and haemorrhage (see pp. 144–146). The presenting signs are usually increase in pulse rate, decrease in pulse volume, fall in arterial and central venous blood pressure, and cold and cyanosed extremities. All of these symptoms need not be present during the early development of hypovolumic shock. In particular arterial blood pressure can be maintained over several readings. Changes in pulse rate and central venous pressure are more significant.

Respiratory system

Rate, depth and mode of breathing are recorded as frequently as instructed. Note that early in the post-operative phase the following should be observed:

1. Upper respiratory obstruction and respiratory embarrassment by secretions should be carefully watched and prevented.

2. The patient should be sat up in the bed as soon as possible to improve movements of the diaphragm.

3. Most patients in the early post-operative phase are given oxygen by mask. Some mechanism to humidify the oxygen should always be provided.

4. Duration of oxygen therapy varies according to the patient's needs. Instructions on this point should be received from the medical staff.

Many patients with pulmonary resection are bronchitic, some suffer from some degree of emphysema. In the early post-operative hours it may be difficult or even impossible to get rid of tenacious secretions and sputum. Airway obstruction by secretions and carbon-dioxide retention should be constantly in mind.

The nurse should encourage the patient to take deep breaths and ask him to cough from time to time.

Manifestations of hypoxia and hypocapnia (CO_2 retention) are described on pp. 149–150, and should be known to all staff nursing post-operative lung cases.

Pleural drains

The amount of fluid and its nature should be recorded and the rate of air leak noted.

The management of pleural drains is described in detail in Chapter 5. The commonest cause of post-operative shock in the case of lung surgery is bleeding and the commonest site is in the pleural space. It is therefore important to monitor the drains and evaluate any circulatory disturbance in connection with the amount of drainage.

Some of the early respiratory complications can be related to the malfunction of drains or their mismanagement. For instance, pneumothorax and collapse of the residual lung can be caused by lack of air drainage from the pleural space, itself due to a faulty underwater sealed system, its connections or suction pumps, or obstruction of the air exit. Also, when blood fails to drain, its collection within the pleural space causes a concealed haemo-pneumothorax as well as pulmonary collapse. It is therefore mandatory to relate the recordings of clinical observations in terms of possible early manifestations of a complication. *The pleural drains must always be examined and their functional state re-evaluated when other vital function observations are showing important alterations.*

Monitoring general functions of other organs

After any major operation, it is important to check (1) urinary output and prevent bladder distension, which produces restlessness and irritation in the patient, and (2) nausea, vomiting and abdominal distension.

EARLY POST-OPERATIVE MANAGEMENT

After base-line observations are recorded and found to be satisfactory, and while periodic early post-operative monitoring of various parameters related to vital functions is going on, a comprehensive therapeutic plan should be established. This plan consists of (1) checking any deviation from normal post-operative progress, indicated by abnormal findings in observations of vital functions, (2) taking early measures against any complications arising during periodic observations, and (3) attending to routine post-operative requirements in the absence of abnormal findings and complications.

Measures against deterioration in vital functions, as observed and recorded, are discussed on pp. 146–151, and therapy against complications is discussed on pp. 143–154.

Routine post-operative requirement and management of patients is as follows: when the patient is settled in his bed and base-line observations found to be satisfactory, the backrest and pillows are arranged to allow the sitting-up position. This provides much better respiratory excursion and movements of the diaphragm. Drains must be secured in this position.

An early post-operative chest radiograph is taken as part of the base-line observations. A chest radiograph is usually taken every day while drainage tubes are *in situ*. When drains are removed lung expansion is checked a few hours later by a further radiograph and, following this, regular chest radiographs until the patient's discharge assure radiological monitoring of lung expansion.

Relief of pain and anxiety
It is a good practice to reassure the patient soon after recovery from anaesthesia and tell him that the operation is completed and that he is back in his bed. It is also important to relieve anxiety and pain with drugs.

Pain after thoracotomy has several causes. Apart from the surgical wound, the stretch of the intercostal space and costo-vertebral ligaments, added to reaction in the parietal pleura, can be responsible for pain. The deeper the patient breathes the more pain he experiences. He therefore tends to breathe shallowly. This in turn will reduce the effective tidal volume (see *Physiology*, p. 19). resulting in even more rapid breathing and more pain. If no analgesic is given, quite apart from the patient's discomfort, respiration is affected. On the other hand too much analgesic can upset respiration by adversely affecting the respiratory centre as well as suppressing the cough reflex. Therefore analgesics should be used with caution, in appropriate doses, at the correct frequency.

It is worthwhile mentioning that the patient who becomes restless, excited and even aggressive may be suffering from anoxia. Further doses of sedatives and analgesics only make him more anoxic. The practice of the nursing staff to repeat the dose of analgesic in these circumstances must be actively discouraged. Medical advice should be sought and a doctor requested to see the patient.

The cause of restlessness, excessive pain and excitement must be investigated and remedied. The following case illustrates the point:

A bronchitic man of 59 had a left lower lobectomy in the morning for a carcinoma of bronchus. The operation had been carried out without any particular difficulties, and the immediate post-operative observations were satisfactory. During the afternoon a slight increase in the respiratory rate was noted. In the night the patient was unduly restless and in spite of a repeated dose of analgesic (which had satisfied him during the day) he was manifestly in pain. The matter was reported to the medical officer who, without seeing the patient, made some enquiries about his condition and prescribed a further dose of analgesic (Pethidine) and in addition advised administration of Largactil. An hour later there was no improvement and the dose was repeated on medical instructions. Half an hour later the patient was almost unconscious and had rapid and shallow breathing. He was then seen by a more senior doctor who found collapse of the residual lung and sputum retention. Bronchoscopy and suction were carried out under local anaesthetic in order to expand the residual lung. A bronchodilator and a diuretic were then administered. He improved immediately and his recovery was subsequently uneventful.

This case is presented to point out that in thoracic surgery analgesics and sedatives have to be given with the proviso that irrational behaviour, excessive pain, restlessness and excitability are investigated.

Replacement of blood loss — blood transfusion
Most patients undergoing lung surgery have a blood transfusion during the operation. Many continue to lose some blood in the first 24 post-operative hours.

A survey carried out in 20 consecutive cases at the Cardio-Thoracic Surgical Centre, Castle Hill Hospital showed blood losses (in the first 24 hours after lung surgery) to be 530–535 ml on average. It is advisable to replace this volume following instructions received from medical staff.

Fluid
The patient's fluid requirements are calculated by the medical staff. It is however the nurse's duty to collect precise information about the quantity, the type and the route of administration. It is dangerous to give too much intravenous fluid to patients following pulmonary surgery. The principle of 'keeping the vein open' should be discouraged and a definite volume prescribed.

In most cases only water and a bland fluid are taken, commencing 6 to 8 hours after operation. After the first 24 hours intravenous infusion is discontinued when light diet and fluid by alimentary tract can be given (unless there is a particular contra-indication such as dilatation of stomach and paralytic ileus, nausea and vomiting).

A chart of fluid intake and output must be kept; at least during the early post-operative phase. Urinary output which normally constitutes the major part of output should be measured. If after a reasonable time (12 to 18 hours) no urine has been passed the matter should be reported and the bladder emptied.

Early physiotherapy
Nurses should be acquainted with the principles of breathing exercises, effective coughing and expectoration. In the early stages, and at regular intervals, nurses should encourage deep breathing and coughing. This helps to expand the area of the lungs which may be inactive because of shallow breathing caused by pain.

Humidification of the air, and particularly the oxygen, prevents mucosal dryness and sputum stickiness.

Formal physiotherapy is carried out by professional therapists as soon as possible and no later than 24 hours after surgery. The physiotherapist must be considered as part of the team and should be given sufficient time to carry out this essential treatment.

Medication
Instructions are given by the medical staff with regard to medication, including antibiotics, and should be carried out as prescribed. Analgesics should be administered with the proviso mentioned on p. 137.

Laboratory investigations
These investigations are arranged by the nursing staff during the early post-operative phase and should include (1) blood count: haemoglobin and haematocrit, (2) serum electrolytes and blood urea, and (3) sputum for organism culture and sensitivity to antibiotics.

Routine nursing
Nursing is an integral part of the post-operative care and should be meticulously carried out. This includes early mobilisation of the patient, skin and mouth hygiene, relief of pressure and attention to leg exercises.

It is the practice of many surgeons to move the patient out of bed to sit in a chair after the first 24 hours unless there are definite contra-indications. The drains and other fixtures should not be disturbed.

LATE POST-OPERATIVE CARE

This period of post-operative care extends from 24 to 48 hours after the operation to the patient's discharge from the hospital. On discharge the patient should be fully recovered from the operation, fully mobile and independent. Ideally the surgical wound should be completely healed, requiring no dressings. There should be no symptoms and no signs of infection; the residual lung should be clinically and radiologically healthy and well expanded.

It must be re-emphasised that this division of the post-operative care into an early and a later phase is entirely empirical and that following the base-line recordings of vital functions, all periodic monitoring and other post-operative management should be looked upon as one continuous process. It is nevertheless helpful to the student, and easier for descriptive purposes, to make this distinction.

PATIENT MONITORING AND OBSERVATIONS
Monitoring is less frequent and less elaborate especially in uncomplicated cases.

Temperature, pulse, arterial blood pressure, rate and depth of breathing are recorded twice daily unless otherwise indicated by the medical staff. A check is made on abdominal distension, volume of urinary output, state of alimentation and bowel action.

Intravenous infusion and CVP are discontinued at this stage.

A chest radiograph is taken 2 or 3 days after operation and at weekly intervals until the patient's discharge to monitor lung expansion.

Finally any abnormal symptoms and signs should be investigated and brought to the attention of the medical officers.

MANAGEMENT

Mobilisation
Following any thoracic surgical procedure, mobilisation should be encouraged. While the drainage tubes are still *in situ* the patient should be sat out of bed. If one drainage tube is *in situ* and when the suction pump is not required, a mobile or a 'walking bottle' drainage system (see Fig. 1.28, p. 44) is arranged.

When no drainage tube remains in the pleural space a full mobilisation programme is applied so that by the time the patient is ready for discharge he is capable of returning gradually to normal activities at home and later at work.

Pleural drains
Daily recording of the volume and the type of drainage is made. Constant attention is required until the lung is fully expanded and the drains removed (see Chapter 5).

Surgical wound
In many Thoracic Surgical Units the wound is not touched and the dressing not disturbed or changed until the removal of stitches on the 10th or 11th post-operative day, unless there are complications. Our practice is to take down the original dressing applied in the operating theatre on the 8th or 9th day, clean the wound with an antiseptic lotion and redress it. On the 10th or 11th day the stitches are removed, the area cleaned with antiseptic solution and covered with a layer of gauze held in position by 3 or 4 short pieces of strapping (sleek). This is finally removed after a day or two by the patient at home.

Patient's hygiene
Hygiene must be considered at all times. When the patient is fully mobile and drains removed, he can sit in the bath and when stitches are removed a full bath can be taken.

Physiotherapy
At this stage full chest physiotherapy including deep breathing, coughing and postural drainage should be carried out by professional physiotherapists at least once a day. The more mobile patients can be helped by the nursing staff and physiotherapists. Though chest physiotherapy is obviously most important, movement of the limbs and muscular passive and active exercises should not be ignored. Particular attention should be paid to the movements of the shoulders especially on the thoracotomy side. There is a tendency for patients to limit the arm's movements (because of fear of pain). A 'frozen shoulder', with pain and limitation of movement, is such a common finding that care should be taken to prevent it by early physiotherapy and exercises.

Medication
It is difficult to give a comprehensive list of all possible medication and therefore only the more commonly used are indicated below:

Antibiotics are administered as prescribed. The choice of antibiotic is dependent on the surgeon's preference, based on personal experience, sensitivity of bacteria (particularly that of sputum) and possible infective complications.

Analgesics and sedatives   Night sedation and hypnotics are usually required. The potency, dose and frequency of these are dependent on the individual patient, and although the medical staff prescribe them nurses should exercise discretion as to timing and frequency of administration.

At the time of discharge some patients still have scar pain and a mild analgesic may be required particularly at night for a few weeks.

Aperients After operation constipation is frequent and, when necessary, an aperient should be administered.

Bronchodilators Some patients are specifically prone to frank asthmatic attacks or repeated bronchospasm extending over the post-operative phase. They require special handling and bronchodilator drugs. Since such attacks are frightening patients should be assured that a member of staff is always at hand to give drugs to relieve the spasm.

Mucolytic drugs In many patients bronchial secretions are thick and 'sticky' following operation. This is even more so in bronchitic patients and heavy smokers. Mucolytic agents are used with some benefit. Such drugs as Bisolvon (8 mg tds), Alupent Expectorant and Mucodyn make sputum more liquid and help expectoration by physiotherapy.

Other drugs At times cardiotonic and anti-arrhythmic drugs such as a digitalis preparation are prescribed. An appetite stimulant and a tonic may have to be introduced. In this respect it is important to report lack of appetite and continuous weight loss to medical staff.

Laboratory tests

Blood tests A full blood count including serum electrolytes, blood urea, haemoglobin, haematocrit and white cell count is carried out and repeated at least once a week.

Urine Tests for protein and sugar are carried out once or twice in the ward after operation. More elaborate tests conducted by the laboratory are carried out if necessary and in the case of abnormalities.

Sputum It has already been pointed out that the volume and type should be noted every day. At least once a week a sample should be sent to the bacteriology laboratory for microbiological analysis. In the presence of infected sputum this may have to be repeated, and a therapeutic policy with regard to antibiotics, different from the one already in progress, may have to be adopted.

SPECIAL NURSING CARE OF PATIENTS WITH PNEUMOTHORAX AND EMPHYSEMATOUS CYSTS

Nursing care of these cases differs from the nursing care of post-operative pulmonary resection cases because many of these patients are generally in some degree of respiratory failure with chronic obstructive airway disease. Also, in chronic cases of emphysema, there is a clinical or subclinical element of heart failure, and some patients with chronic bronchitis and emphysema produce a considerable amount of viscous bronchial secretions and have difficulty in expectorating.

Particular attention should be paid to the pleural drainage system. When the underwater sealed drains and bottle are connected to a suction machine the working of the pump should be checked with respect to three specific points:

1. See that the suction pump is working; this should be done frequently.

2. Ensure that the pump is coping with the volume of air which is lost through the drain, and that the air leak is not in excess of the air removed by the pump. When this happens pneumothorax, surgical emphysema and collapse of the lung can follow, leading to hypoxia and death.

3. In some cases the air leak is of such a volume that, when the drainage system is connected to a powerful suction machine (which is also capable of removing a great volume of air), an important fraction of the patient's tidal air volume is sucked out and not used for the purpose of ventilation. The result is complete hypoxia.

Understanding by the nurse of pleural drainage is mandatory for successful outcome.

Physiotherapy and expectoration should be specifically monitored as expansion of the lung is a matter of survival.

Prevention of chest infection is also particularly important. In this respect nurses must be particularly aware of accidental inhalation of food particles by emphysematous patients with severe tachypnoea and dyspnoea.

18 Complications of Lung Surgery

One of the most important aspects of surgery is the realisation by all involved in the patients' care that advanced and skilful surgical techniques can be only partly responsible for the overall success. Pre-operative preparation and post-operative care play major roles in the final results. It has been pointed out that one of the aims of post-operative care is to prevent complications. In fact the basis of many post-operative monitoring and nursing procedures is the prevention or at least the early diagnosis of any complications which may occur. Recognition and treatment of complications are an integral part of every branch of surgery. In thoracic surgery where anaesthetic and surgical techniques are advanced the patient can easily come through the operation but die after post-operative complications.

For the sake of clarity and order, complications of the pulmonary surgery are shown in Table 4 and further discussed under the various headings set out below. For each complication, mention is made as to whether it occurs *early* (i.e. first 48 hours after operation), or *late* (i.e. from 48 hours until the discharge of the patient).

Table 4   Complications of lung surgery

Post-operative Shock
Cardio-vascular Complications
    Haemorrhage
    Thrombo-embolic complications
    Cardiac complications
Respiratory Complications
    Pulmonary insufficiency
    Sputum retention
    Infective pneumonitis and lung abscess
    Pulmonary atelectasis
    Haemoptysis
    Broncho-pleural fistula
    Empyema
Alimentary Tract Complications
    Nausea and vomiting
    Anorexia
    Constipation
Genito-urinary Complications
    Urinary retention
    Urinary infection
    Renal failure
Neurological Complications
Wound Complications

POST-OPERATIVE SHOCK

An important complication to all surgery, and one that is prominent in thoracic surgery, is *shock*.

Shock can be defined as a *state* of severe circulatory and metabolic disorder, characterised clinically by an anxious and apprehensive look and a grey and cyanosed colour. The skin is cold and clammy. The pulse is rapid, thready (small volume). The arterial blood pressure is low. Breathing is rapid, urinary output is nil or very small in volume.

These signs denote signals of serious disorganisation in the body's homeostatic activity culminating in death if urgent and effective measures are not applied.

The outcome of shock depends greatly on the correct management of the patient. This involves early recognition and application of first-aid anti-shock measures by nursing staff, correct aetiological diagnosis and energetic active treatment by the surgical and nursing team.

FIRST AID ANTI-SHOCK MEASURES

The following procedure should be followed:

1. Raise the foot of the bed to allow better distribution of blood and improved perfusion to the brain. The patient lies flat on his back.

2. Apply mask and supply oxygen.

3. Sedate and reassure the patient.

4. Monitor and record arterial blood pressure, central venous pressure (if a central venous line is in position), cardiac apex beat and pulse every 10–15 minutes. Note that the best artery for pulse recording in these cases is the femoral which is reliable and accessible.

5. Record respiratory rate and temperature.

6. Monitor volume of urine if urethral catheter is *in situ* (or insert a catheter, then check).

7. Check chest drains and tubing for patency, correct functioning and monitor the volume of blood loss.

8. Check the proper functioning of drips and enquire about availability of blood left over from the operation, and therefore already matched. Alternatively have plasma or plasma expanders handy.

9. Have the emergency resuscitation trolley near the patient. The medical staff should be immediately contacted while the above first-aid measures are being carried out. If intravenous infusion is not already in progress, the medical officer will have to establish one. Monitoring central venous pressure is an essential part of the management of shock following operation. A central venous line should be established as soon as possible. To detect the cause of shock an ECG may be necessary and this should be carried out with a standard ECG machine or with a cardioscope and attached writer.

AETIOLOGY OF SHOCK

The main causes of post-operative shock can be haemorrhage, neurogenic, or cardiogenic.

Haemorrhage

Cardiac output equals approximately the total circulating blood volume, i.e.

about 5 litre/minute in adults. Any reduction in the circulatory volume by haemorrhage affects the cardiac output unless compensatory mechanisms intervene effectively. These compensatory mechanisms are dependent mainly on increase in the heart rate and redistribution of the blood (i.e. supplying less blood to non-vital parts such as skin, and channelling more towards the essential organs, such as the brain, heart and kidneys). Increase in pulse rate and peripheral vaso-constriction in haemorrhage are the two manifestations of these compensatory mechanisms. These two mechanisms are capable (for a while) of maintaining the arterial blood pressure and securing an acceptable cardiac output and perfusion to essential organs. In severe and rapid haemorrhage however, the compensatory mechanisms are not capable of maintaining sufficient perfusion to essential organs and it is this state of affairs which induces shock.

Neurogenic shock
Shock can be caused by the dilatation of minute vessels, which are normally constricted or closed to circulation, and therefore capable of accommodating only a small volume of blood. The sudden dilatation of these vessels produces pooling and re-channelling of the blood into the corresponding area with consequent deprivation of the essential organs. The autonomic nervous system is responsible for this sudden dilatation.

The signs and symptoms of shock are present because of reduction in the circulating volume. Additionally the adrenal glands release nor-adrenaline and adrenaline which cause changes resulting in the maintenance, or an increase, of arterial blood pressure.

Cardiogenic shock
Shock can appear as the result of severe reduction in the cardiac output by failure of the heart as a pump to eject the blood. It can develop in cases of myocardial infarction and serious abnormality of the heart rhythm and rate. Signs and symptoms of shock are present. There is no haemorrhage. Recording of cardiac beat, pulse and ECG lead to diagnosis.

THERAPEUTIC MEASURES
In pulmonary surgery the commonest cause of post-operative shock is bleeding, and almost invariably this can be diagnosed by observing and monitoring the volume of blood collected in the drainage bottles. The measures to be adopted in haemorrhagic shock are:

1. Replacement blood transfusion guided by monitoring arterial and central venous pressure.

2. Arrangement of an emergency chest radiograph to evaluate the presence of blood in the pleural space.

3. Arrest of haemorrhage, which in these cases means emergency preparation for returning the patient to the operating theatre for a thoracotomy.

In all cases of shock, attention should be paid to oxygenation. This can be monitored by estimating arterial blood gases. A sedative to relieve anxiety is essential. In cardiogenic shock it is important to check cardiac dysrhythmia which can impose a serious barrier to the patient's recovery.

CARDIO-VASCULAR COMPLICATIONS

HAEMORRHAGE

The role of haemorrhage in producing shock has already been discussed (p. 144). Less severe and slower bleeding can be present without producing shock. Post-operative bleeding can be of two varieties; reactionary or secondary haemorrhage.

Reactionary haemorrhage occurs *early* following the operation. Drainage from the chest drains is constant. The volume and rate can be estimated by measurement (providing the underwater sealed system is functioning). It can be demonstrated on a chest radiograph.

Secondary haemorrhage occurs *late* in the post-operative phase (5 to 12 days). Infection and sloughing of a blood vessel is usually the cause. It occurs either (1) by bleeding in the thoracic cavity, not externally apparent but presenting the usual signs and symptoms and visible on a chest radiograph (as by this time the drains are usually removed), or (2) profuse haemoptysis due to infection at the site of the bronchial stump, with erosion of pulmonary vessels. The vessels erode and communicate with the bronchial tree. Sometimes the bleeding is really the manifestation of broncho-pleural fistula, in which case blood-stained pleural effusion is drained into the bronchus and is expectorated.

The symptoms and signs of haemorrhage, viz. increasing pallor, rapid pulse rate, air hunger or deep sighing respiration, and restlessness are present in these cases. If bleeding continues and becomes severe, the extremities become cold, the veins empty, and signs of shock become apparent.

Management of haemorrhage

The general principles of the nursing management of bleeding are common to all types of post-operative haemorrhage and consist of: monitoring the volume and the rate of bleeding; monitoring the circulatory effects of bleeding by frequent (every 10–15 minutes) recording of observations of vital functions in particular the pulse rate, arterial blood pressure and respiratory rate; informing the medical officer; applying the first-aid measures as follows:

1. Reassure the patient.
2. Raise the foot of the bed.
3. Supply oxygen through a mask.
4. Administer a sedative.
5. Replace the blood loss by transfusion of blood, plasma and/or plasma expanders.
6. Have the emergency resuscitation equipment handy.
7. Arrange a chest radiograph.

In the case of a reactionary haemorrhage, as the pleural drains are still in place, the volume and rate of drainage disclose bleeding. At this stage it is essential to check the functioning of the drains. It is important to realise that a faulty drainage system has at least three deleterious effects:

1. It conceals bleeding culminating in oligaemic shock.
2. It causes collapse of the lung through haemothorax.

3. The undrained blood clot displaces the mediastinum away from the operated side towards the normal side. Mediastinal displacement can interfere with circulation and the respiratory function.

When reactionary bleeding is severe and affects arterial blood pressure in spite of replacement transfusion, central venous pressure should be monitored. Often the only effective measure is to return the patient to the operating theatre for thoracotomy and arrest of haemorrhage.

In the case of secondary haemorrhage concealed in the chest, diagnosis may be difficult. Signs of bleeding and evidence of respiratory embarrassment are present. First-aid measures, as indicated above, are applied. Chest aspiration or drainage may be required in the first instance to confirm diagnosis of intrathoracic bleeding.

When the haemorrhage is in the form of haemoptysis the danger of asphyxiation by drowning or airway obstruction is added to the deleterious effects of bleeding. Clearing the airways takes precedence over all other first-aid measures in these cases. The following routine should be adopted:

1. Keep the airways clear by suction.
2. Lie the patient on the side of the operation, that is the operated side down so that the healthy bronchi are drained of any blood which might have spilt from the bleeding side. This also stops the bleeding side from draining into the major airways and causing obstruction.
3. Sedate the patient.
4. Have the emergency suction and bronchoscopy set near the patient.
5. Send for help and summon the medical officer.
6. Apply first-aid measures and monitoring as indicated under general management of haemorrhage.

Arrest of haemorrhage in these cases depends on the cause and can involve a minor procedure or major operation.

THROMBO-EMBOLIC COMPLICATIONS

Thrombo-phlebitis (inflammation of venous walls)
Venous thrombosis of the superficial veins of the arm and the leg can occur following intravenous administration of drugs, infusion of hypertonic solutions and extravasation of irritant substances. Superficial thrombo-phlebitis though unpleasant and painful is unlikely to endanger life.

Management consists of preventing the leak of drugs and infusions out of the vessels, and discontinuing and resiting the drips when there is peri-venous and subcutaneous leakage of infusion. The oedematous area is bandaged (with an elastic bandage) and elevated. At times the site is painful and mild analgesics are required.

It cannot be emphasised strongly enough that intravenous drips must be watched and cared for, as inflammation and oedema due to extravasation of infusions can cause more discomfort than the surgical wound.

Phlebothrombosis (intravenous clotting)
Compression of calf veins at the time of operation (on the table) and during the early post-operative phase can lead to phlebothrombosis. Subsequent extension

of clotting (consecutive clot) can lead to complete occlusion of the vessels. Deep vein thrombosis (DVT) manifests itself on the 8th to 12th day after operation, either by pain in the calf and possible oedema, or by migration of the clot to the right heart and pulmonary artery—in the form of pulmonary embolus.

Prevention In many units patients are given subcutaneous injections of Heparin (in the order of 5000 units b.d.) commencing the day of operation and continuing for a few days. This appears to reduce the incidence of post-operative thrombo-embolic complications. At operation the position of the patient on the operating table is checked, and calves protected from compression.

Following operation, early mobilisation, regular active and passive leg movements are encouraged.

Treatment The general principles consist of an anticoagulant regime, crepe bandaging from the toes to the groin, bed rest with elevation of the leg(s).

The anticoagulant regime in many cases involves an initial dose of 15,000 units of Heparin followed by 6-hourly 5000–10,000 units of intravenous infusion. At the same time an oral anticoagulant (Warfarin 5–10 mg) is given. This regime is continued for 24 hours, following which the oral anticoagulant only is given. In the first 24 hours anticoagulation is monitored by clotting time estimation. From the second day onwards prothrombin time is estimated and the Warfarin dosage adjusted to achieve 1.5 to 2 times the control value.

It is to be remembered that the antidote to Heparin is Prothamine Sulphate, 1 mg of 1% of which neutralises 100 International Units of Heparin. The antidote to Warfarin is Vitamin K (injected) and fresh blood transfusion (if bleeding occurs).

Pulmonary embolus

This is a complication of DVT. A fragment of clot is detached and migrates to the right atrium then to the right ventricle and eventually lodges in the pulmonary artery. This complication occurs some 8 to 12 days after operation. The symptoms and signs vary according to the size of the embolus (clot) and the patient's cardio-pulmonary state. Types of emboli and management have been previously described (see Chapter 12: *Pulmonary embolism*, p. 101).

Surgical treatment may be necessary. Embolectomy is best carried out under cardio-pulmonary by-pass.

CARDIAC COMPLICATIONS

Many patients undergoing lung surgery are elderly and a number of them suffer concomitantly from cardio-vascular disorders. Ischaemic and valvular heart diseases can be present. When diagnosed prior to operation they are sometimes judged to be of relatively low importance, particularly when considering treating a patient with neoplasm.

Following operation, signs and symptoms can increase in severity and result in a definite and specific cardiac condition.

Dysrhythmic complications

The commonest cardiac complication following lung surgery is atrial fibrillation (AF). It is to be expected in patients over the age of 60 who have had a pneumonectomy, and particularly in those whose pericardium had to be opened (for intra-pericardial ligation and division of pulmonary vessels) or partially resected. Typically, AF is noticed 48 to 72 hours after operation. The patient, usually when out of bed or during the physiotherapy, feels unwell, dyspnoeic and sweaty. Pulse and apex beat, then ECG, confirm the diagnosis.

Myocardial infarction
When a patient suffers a massive myocardial infarction he experiences a sudden pain in the chest and can develop cardiac arrest not always responding to resuscitation measures. Smaller myocardial infarctions can produce pain and a variety of dysrhythmic problems. The patient should be put to bed, given a sedative and an analgesic and supplied with oxygen. An ECG is taken and the medical officer is informed.

Heart failure
In some patients heart failure in varying degrees with added pulmonary or peripheral oedema complicates the early post-operative course. Anti-failure drugs relieve symptoms.

RESPIRATORY COMPLICATIONS FOLLOWING PULMONARY SURGERY

Respiratory system complications play by far the most essential role in determining the final results of thoracic and in particular pulmonary surgery. Their importance is such that many of the aftercare procedures are designed to allow their early recognition and prevention.

COMMON RESPIRATORY DIFFICULTIES
Complications affecting the respiratory system following pulmonary surgery, irrespective of type, have a similar presentation and require similar management, with minor variations according to the extent of resection.

Other complications, which present with dissimilar clinical manifestations according to the type and extent of resection, are described individually as they require specific aftercare. However they are mentioned here to provide an overall view of the respiratory system complications following pulmonary surgery.

Immediately after operation, respiratory problems are usually those related to the general anaesthesia with upper airway obstruction resulting from excess salivary and bronchial secretions, vomitus and blood in the tracheo-bronchial trees. These are removed at once by suction. The mouth and pharyngo-larynx are cleared in the recovery room or the operating theatre before the patient is transferred to the ward.

PULMONARY INSUFFICIENCY
Early in the post-operative phase, respiratory problems produce some degree of respiratory insufficiency, that is interference with the process of gas exchanges. In practical terms this means varying degrees of lack of oxygen and excess of carbon dioxide in the blood and the body as a whole. It is helpful, therefore, to discuss briefly the effects of anoxia and carbon dioxide accumulation.

Hypoxia and anoxia

These terms denote relative or total lack of oxygen (O_2) in the body and in the blood (hypoxaemia and anoxaemia). It should be noted that, strictly speaking, anoxia is rarely (if ever) present but that hypoxia and anoxia are used synonymously by clinicians to mean low oxygen pressure (below 70–75 mm Hg in arterial blood). When hypoxia reaches a certain level central cyanosis develops (see p. 55). Lack of oxygen leads to functional and structural changes in cells, tissues and organs of the body. The magnitude of these changes is proportional to the *severity* and the *duration* of lack of oxygen, and is partly dependent on the susceptibility of a particular type of tissue.

Of all the cells of the body the neurones are the most sensitive to anoxia, and amongst them the cells concerned with consciousness are outstandingly so. It is therefore not surprising that very temporary anoxia has a definite effect on patients' consciousness and behaviour.

The respiratory neurones are directly depressed by anoxia. However, the centre responds by increasing its discharges to the respiratory muscles, thus raising the respiratory rate. This reflex is stimulated by the chemoreceptors of the carotid and aortic bodies. If anoxia is prolonged then permanent damage of these cells occurs with depression of breathing.

The effects of anoxia can be summarised as follows:

Central Nervous System   Drowsiness, depression and confusion, or excitement and aggression followed by loss of consciousness.

Respiratory System   Rapid and shallow breathing, then shallow and periodic breathing, with final arrest of respiration.

Cardio-vascular System   Increase in heart rate, slight increase in blood pressure followed by reduction. Final slowing of heart rate and cardiac arrest.

Carbon dioxide accumulation

It has been pointed out that respiration is regulated in such a way as to maintain in the arterial blood an acceptable level of oxygen and carbon dioxide reaching the tissues, particularly the brain. In turn, it is also true to say that arterial blood gases regulate the level of respiration. It is important to realise that while lack of oxygen stimulates respiration, the respiratory centre is more susceptible to stimulation by excess carbon dioxide in the arterial blood than by relative lack of oxygen because of the directly suppressive effect of lack of oxygen on the respiratory centre neurones.

Symptoms of increased carbon dioxide in arterial blood can be summarised as follows:

Central Nervous System   Anxiety, disorientation, convulsions and coma followed by CO_2 narcosis.

Circulatory System   Tachycardia followed by slow rate culminating in arrest, hypertension, bounding (full) pulse, and warm and sweaty skin.

Respiratory System   At first deep and rapid then shallow and rapid breathing.

In practice it is important to recognise the signs and symptoms of respiratory insufficiency and confirm diagnosis by arterial blood gas analysis.

AETIOLOGY OF POST-OPERATIVE RESPIRATORY INSUFFICIENCY
Respiratory insufficiency, with symptoms and signs of hypoxia and excess of carbon dioxide, confirmed by arterial gas estimation indicating low partial pressure of oxygen and high partial pressure of carbon dioxide, is a definite complication of thoracic surgery.

Aetiological factors can be classified as: ventilatory deficiencies and inadequacy of lung parenchyma and perfusion.

Ventilatory deficiencies
These include airway obstruction of any kind (e.g. secretions), neuropathological conditions affecting the respiratory centre or the more peripheral nerves (e.g. phrenic nerve damage), and direct interference with respiratory muscle action and/or the harmonious mechanism of breathing—by disruption of the chest wall integrity (e.g. trauma and flail chest).

Inadequacy of lung parenchyma
These factors include inadequacy of parenchyma through lack of sufficient lung volume (e.g. extensive pulmonary resection), diseased lung, disturbing ventilation and diffusion (e.g. emphysema, pulmonary fibrosis and post-operative pneumonitis), or pulmonary atelectasis following operation.

Inadequacy of perfusion
These are heart failure, or post-operative pulmonary embolus.

Most cases of post-operative respiratory insufficiency are due to ventilatory deficiencies caused by airway obstruction or to the inadequacy of lung parenchyma.

Management
The management of respiratory insufficiency should be carefully designed and occupy an important place in the aftercare of pulmonary surgery. It can be described as follows:

Recognition of symptoms and signs through careful and precise monitoring of the vital functions following surgery, and prompt notification to the medical staff in order to investigate and prevent deterioration.

First-aid measures, consisting of checking clearance of the airways and assisting removal of tenacious expectoration or abnormal secretions by oronaso-pharyngeal suction, checking all drainage tube systems, for proper functioning, and providing oxygen *either* by mask—this can help by providing an increased percentage of oxygen in the inspired air (say 40–50% instead of 20–21% which is the normal percentage), consequently increasing partial oxygen pressure in the inspired and alveolar air—*or* by intermittent positive pressure of oxygen-enriched air using an Ambu bag and a face mask connected to an oxygen supply and placed over the patient's mouth and nose. The bag is pressed in synchronisation with the patient's inspiratory phase. This method is particularly useful for patients who are weak, drowsy and, in spite of clear airways, cannot reach an acceptable blood gas level without assistance. It is necessary to have absolutely clear airways for this method. Secretions causing obstruction have to be cleared by active physiotherapy or suction bronchoscopy.

Treatment of the cause
Treatment is carried out by the medical staff, but nursing staff should have a clear idea of the procedure involved in order to provide suitable equipment such as bronchoscopy sets, aspiration and intercostal drainage equipment.

Prevention of recurrence
Once the cause of respiratory insufficiency is recognised and immediate treatment applied, it is necessary to ensure the maintenance of satisfactory ventilation and an acceptable level of arterial blood gases. The patient is monitored frequently, for a few hours at least, until it is clear that there is no deterioration.

Monitoring should cover (1) state of consciousness, (2) patient's colour, (3) arterial BP, pulse rate, cardiac rhythm and volume, (4) rate and depth of breathing, (5) clearance of upper airway, and (6) pulmonary ventilation judged by the extent of air entry into the lungs.

If the patient deteriorates the medical officer should be informed. It may then become necessary to carry out one of the following procedures: either endo-tracheal intubation or tracheostomy.

Endo-tracheal intubation and positive pressure ventilation using a ventilator.

Tracheostomy with or without positive pressure ventilation. This type of patient should be nursed in an intensive care unit, or a high dependency unit with all the necessary facilities and equipment (see Chapter 24: *Tracheostomy*, p. 247).

SPUTUM RETENTION
Early in the post-operative phase, patients (particularly bronchitic and heavy smokers) can find expectoration difficult. Thoracotomy pain, repeated injection of sedatives and analgesics and general fatigue, all play a part. Some patients become very distressed with definite symptoms and signs of airway obstruction. Others develop in addition pulmonary oedema due to relative anoxia increasing the permeability of the pulmonary capillaries, or due to some degree of heart failure. Respiration in such patients becomes noisy and 'bubbly'. Symptoms and signs of respiratory insufficiency are present in advanced cases.

The severity of symptoms and signs depends on the extent of pulmonary resection and the state of the residual lung.

Management
Sputum retention must be treated actively and energetically before respiratory failure develops. The following measures should be adopted:

1. Monitor and observe the patient's progress.
2. Help expectoration by active and passive physiotherapy and humidification of inspired air.

3. Provide oxygen.

4. Report the matter to the medical officer at an early stage.

5. Do not forget to send sputum specimens for microbiological studies (culture and sensitivity).

Medication

Medication containing mucolytic agents (e.g. Bisolvon) should be administered so as to reduce the viscosity and the stickiness of secretions. An expectorant should also be given in either a humidifier, or systemically (e.g. Alupent Expectorant, Benylin Expectorant); antibiotic based on sputum bacteriology.

More active measures

If there is no improvement then *bronchoscopic aspiration* of tenaceous secretions, or *tracheostomy*, if respiratory insufficiency develops, should be undertaken.

BRONCHOSPASM

Immediately after the operation, that is during the recovery from anaesthesia, bronchospasm can occur. It can at times be so severe as to require a broncho-dilator intravenously.

Early in the post-operative phase and during the first week after operation, spasm can be a manifestation of a small broncho-pleural fistula. *At other times* spasms of various severity can complicate the post-operative course particularly in chronic bronchitis. A broncho-dilator, such as Choledyl (100 mg t.d.s.) can alleviate a mild spasm. In some instances Hydrocortisone has to be administered (100 mg IV).

INFECTIVE PNEUMONITIS AND LUNG ABSCESS

Infection of the residual lung following pulmonary surgery is, on several counts, particularly serious. One of the most serious effects is a further reduction of the functioning parenchyma. When infection occurs in the form of patchy consolidation, then the term pneumonitis is used. When infection is confluent and when there is additional bronchial obstruction, a collection of pus (i.e. an abscess) forms in the residual lung.

The general symptoms and signs of infection, together with dyspnoea and a variable amount of purulent expectoration are present (see *Lung abscess*, p. 86). The outcome depends on the extent and severity of infection, the patient's general condition, the extent of lung resection and the volume of the remaining lung, and the type of organism involved and its sensitivity to antibiotics.

Management

In pulmonary surgery it is far easier to prevent infective complications than it is to treat them.

Prevention consists of early mobilisation and physiotherapy to get rid of post-operative collection of secretion; careful observation and monitoring of post-operative progress to discover imminent infection; attention to the patient's general condition such as anaemia and nutritional state; routine collection of sputum after operation for bacteriological studies.

When infection is present ensure that regular collection of sputum specimens for bacteriological monitoring is carried out, as well as the appropriate antibiotic therapy and repeated chest radiograph.

When the abscess progresses and expands to the pleural space, an empyema follows.

PULMONARY ATELECTASIS
Segmental or lobar collapse following partial pulmonary resection can complicate lung surgery. Following pneumonectomy the onset is more dramatic and the outcome more problematic. This is further described on p. 157.

HAEMOPTYSIS
Post-operatively this complication is usually associated with a broncho-pleural fistula. The latter will be described later in cases of pneumonectomy and partial pulmonary resection.

Haemoptysis can occasionally complicate pulmonary surgery for other reasons (e.g. pulmonary embolus) and its management is described on p. 101.

BRONCHO-PLEURAL FISTULA
This is the most serious of all the complications following pulmonary surgery. Its seriousness, mode of presentation and management are different for each type of resection, and these are considered in detail on p. 155 and p. 158.

EMPYEMA
This complication is usually associated with a broncho-pleural fistula. In the case of pneumonectomy (see p. 156) the outcome is more problematic than in the case of lobectomy or segmental resection (see p. 159).

RESPIRATORY COMPLICATIONS: SPECIAL CASES

AFTER PNEUMONECTOMY
Specific complications usually occur associated with the pneumonectomy space. It is therefore helpful to understand the normal changes taking place in the empty hemi-thorax following pneumonectomy.

During the first 24 to 48 hours residual air in the pleural space is drained (if drains have been inserted) or evacuated by aspiration (if there are no drains). Once the drain is removed residual air is partially absorbed but minor bleeding and fluid exudation from the chest walls continue. A chest radiograph taken after 48 hours shows an 'empty' hemi-thorax, its lower part occupied by fluid, with the level visible just above the diaphragm (Fig. 1.75). During the next few days accumulation of inflammatory exudates, the presence of a protein-rich fluid and the negative intrapleural pressure cause the level of the fluid to rise in the space. After 10 to 12 days the fluid rises to the level of the 3rd and 4th ribs posteriorly. Excessive fluid showing on the radiograph above this level calls for pleural aspiration and evacuation of some of it.

Apart from this accumulation of fluid, the size of the pneumonectomy space reduces and continues to do so in the months and years that follow. This is brought about by several factors. For instance:

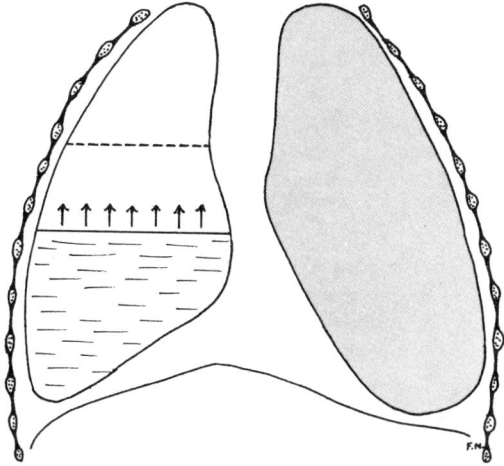

Figure 1.75   Thorax after pneumonectomy.

1. Fibrin deposit and formation of an increasing amount of fibrous tissue over the inside walls of the space.
2. Rising of the diaphragm.
3. Atrophy of the intercostal muscles and approximation of the ribs.
4. Movement of the mediastinum towards the space.
5. Descent of the apex of the thorax.

Examination of the pneumonectomy space many years after operation shows a restricted space with thick walls and fixed mediastinal displacement towards the space, and almost complete disappearance of the fluid.

Complications associated with the pneumonectomy space are as follows:

Broncho-pleural fistula
Early in the post-operative phase this complication is rare, and is usually associated with complete or partial disruption of the bronchial stump stitches. The signs are dyspnoea; haemoptysis; surgical subcutaneous emphysema; large volume of air leak from the pleural drain (if the pleura is drained); great tracheal displacement (if there is no drain); hypotension.

Management of post-operative fistulae   The patient should be reassured and encouraged to sit upright leaning towards the thoracotomy side (i.e. fistula down). He should be given oxygen and his progress monitored (recording of pulse, arterial BP and respiration). The medical officer should be informed. Early disruption of the bronchial stump requires return to the operating theatre, amputation of the stump and reclosure. Broncho-pleural fistulae usually occur *later* in the post-operative phase. Fortunately this complication is now infrequent; a few patients die within hours or days of its development. Some do survive, but have a permanent empyema and broncho-pleural fistula necessitating a drainage tube. Only a small number of patients fully recover. The greatest immediate dangers are spill-over from the pneumonectomy space contents into the airway, and interference with ventilation of the other lung. The signs are:

1. *Haemoptysis:* This, in effect, is the expectoration of old blood and fluid contained in the pneumonectomy space.

2. *Moist sounds:* These are heard in the trachea and the good lung at auscultation or even without a stethoscope. The breathing becomes bubbly and noisy.

3. *Bronchospasm.*

4. *Tachycardia* or other cardiac dysrhythmia especially atrial fibrillation.

5. *Signs of infection:* Fever, general malaise and leucocytosis.

6. *Chest radiograph:* Shows a fall in the fluid level in the pneumonectomy space (in comparison with previous pictures).

Management of late broncho-pleural fistulae   Immediate management is the same as for early fistulae, but with the following additional procedures:

1. Bring the emergency resuscitation trolley near the patient.

2. Prepare a chest aspiration set which, in most cases, will probably be required.

3. Have an intercostal drainage set handy as the chest may have to be drained urgently in the ward to relieve acute symptoms.

Ultimate management depends on the surgeon's decision as to whether the fistula should be closed surgically or treated more conservatively by drainage alone, at the price of a chronic empyema, broncho-pleural fistula and a permanent drain.

Empyema

This is an infection of the pneumonectomy space, with a collection of pus within it. It is usually associated with a broncho-pleural fistula, although an empyema can develop occasionally without a fistula. This complication is revealed by signs of infection (malaise, swinging temperature, leucocytosis, anaemia). There are few or no symptoms referable to the respiratory system and the residual lung. Management does not differ from that of other empyemas (see p. 34).

Excess air or effusion in the pneumonectomy space

When there is no drain in the chest, or after its removal (24 hours after operation), excess collection of air and fluid causes respiratory embarrassment through displacing the trachea and the mediastinum towards the hemi-thorax containing the remaining lung. In addition, the heart and the venous return are adversely affected. Fluid level in the space should be checked clinically and radiologically and tracheal displacement should be evaluated every day in the immediate post-operative phase. Signs of excess fluid and/or air are dyspnoea; tachycardia; displacement of the mediastinum, away from the space (as judged by trachea displacement when palpated above the supra-sternal notch); excess air or effusion is aspirated and pleural pressure adjusted using a Maxwell box.

RESPIRATORY COMPLICATIONS AFTER
PARTIAL PULMONARY RESECTION

It is relevant to describe what changes take place in the pleural space following pulmonary resections, other than pneumonectomy.

Immediately after the operation, a partially vacant space is left within the hemithorax, the size of which corresponds to the extent of the pulmonary tissue removed. Within a few days (if the post-operative course is uneventful), the space disappears and the residual lung fits the hemithorax. This is brought about by the expansion (hyperexpansion) of the remaining pulmonary tissue, the size of the thorax being reduced by the inward displacement of the chest walls (the diaphragm rises, the mediastinum shifts to the operated side, and the lateral walls slightly collapse inwards).

In post-operative care, the expansion of the residual lung and the abolition of the space must receive the greatest attention. The role of the medical and the nursing staff is to ensure effectively functioning pleural drains (to expel all air and to re-establish negative intra-pleural pressure), early expansion of the residual lung (encouraged by chest physiotherapy) and prevention of infection.

Many of the respiratory complications in partial pulmonary resections can be avoided if the residual space is properly attended to.

ATELECTASIS OF THE RESIDUAL LOBES OR SEGMENTS
When the residual lung does not expand or collapses after early expansion, respiratory difficulties occur. The most important causes of pulmonary collapse can be summarised as follows:

Bronchial obstruction
This is due to the retention of excessive and abnormal secretions, caused by something as little as a plug of mucus. Bronchial obstruction produces collapse of the corresponding pulmonary area. This complication usually occurs *early* in the post-operative phase, particularly in bronchitic patients. The patient expectorates with difficulty. Examination shows reduced movements on the side of atelectasis (which is usually the operated side). A chest radiograph confirms diagnosis.

Management   If atelectasis is not extensive, expansion is achieved by physio-therapy, humidification of air and a mucolytic agent and expectorant. Broncho-scopic suction is required if the lung fails to re-expand. This is usually carried out in the ward with the patient in his own bed, under local surface anaesthetic (see Chapter 15).

Collapse due to pneumothorax
Early in the post-operative phase, air leaks from the interfunction of the pulmonary segments and lobes are drained. Drains are left in the pleural space until all leaks stop, and full expansion of the lung is obtained. The malfunction of drains, due to a faulty system, poor connections, blockage due to blood clot, or the patient lying on tubes, is the most frequent cause of early pneumothorax. The cushion of air with atmospheric or higher pressure not only collapses a corresponding volume of residual lung tissues, but reduces the effectiveness of physiotherapy.

Treatment is aimed at re-establishing proper air drainage with subsequent lung expansion. A pneumothorax can occur *late* in the post-operative phase after drains have been removed and the patient is well and progressing satisfactorily.

Sudden or gradual dyspnoea draws attention to lung collapse. A chest radiograph shows a pneumothorax, which can be due to either a small slow leak from the original junctional area of the resected and residual lobes or segments, or a spontaneous pneumothorax from an area of overexpanded and emphysematous lung tissue. Diagnosis is made or confirmed by a chest radiograph and the *treatment* consists of drainage of the pleura usually via a small intercostal tube, inserted in the apex of the chest (see Chapter 9).

Pleural effusion

Accumulation of fluid in the pleural space causes pulmonary collapse. Expansion of the lung depends on prompt evacuation of the fluid. The presence of fluid not only prevents lung expansion but also provides a suitable medium for growth of organisms (promoting the development of empyema).

Early in the post-operative phase, pleural effusion consists of blood and blood-stained fluid which is drained by the drainage tubes when they are functioning properly. After the drains have been removed, fluid can collect.

Increasing dyspnoea, lack of air entry on auscultation, and fullness on percussion in the corresponding area of the chest occupied by the fluid lead to diagnosis. A chest radiograph confirms diagnosis.

Management   Prevention is the best management and this can be done by paying attention to the drainage tubes (as for pneumothorax, see p. 48). When there is evidence of fluid collection chest aspiration is necessary.

Persistent air leak

In the *early* post-operative phase, following lobectomy or segmental resection air leaks are always present, due to intersegmental or interlobar lines of dissection. These lines usually heal within 48 to 72 hours. During this time the residual lung tissue expands and fills the space, and by doing so helps the sealing of these leaks. Air leaks can persist due to slow lung expansion and/or the inability of the lung tissue to expand beyond a certain point.

Management   Nursing staff and physiotherapists should encourage the expansion of the lung by regular effective removal of secretions and prevention of sputum retention, and by checking and rechecking the whole pleural drainage system. If the lung fails to expand and the air leak persists, the matter should be reported to the medical staff.

Broncho-pleural fistula

This complication has become rare since the advent of antibiotics and the infrequency of surgery for pulmonary suppuration. It usually appears late, a week or so after operation when the pleural drains have been removed. A slight infection of the stump is usually the causative agent. Occasionally this complication occurs *early* due to necrosis and dehiscence of the bronchial stump, with the presence and persistence of a large volume of air.

Management   Every effort should be made to prevent this complication. Postoperative occurrence of haemoptysis and swinging temperature should be closely observed and taken seriously.

Treatment   Aspiration or drainage of the pleural space and appropriate antibiotic therapy are effective in some cases. In others a revision operation becomes necessary.

Empyema

This usually occurs *late* in the post-operative phase. It can be associated with a broncho-pleural fistula or can complicate residual air or fluid collection in the pleural space. Patients present symptoms and signs of infection (malaise, pains and aches in the chest, fever, anaemia and leucocytosis). Clinical examination indicates the presence of fluid in the chest and lung collapse. A chest radiograph confirms this.

Management   Prevention should concentrate on encouraging full expansion of the lung by physiotherapy.

Treatment consists of chest aspiration to remove the purulent collection. A sample of pleural aspirate should be sent for bacteriological studies. Appropriate antibiotics are injected into the pleural space after aspiration. Occasionally it may be necessary to carry out further surgery to drain the empyema.

Surgical subcutaneous emphysema

This is air in the tissues, particularly loose subcutaneous tissues. It makes a peculiar crackling sound under the palpating fingers. This post-operative complication arises as a result of an air leak from the bronchial stump or the lung surface (because of inadequate drainage), or an air leak caused by the incomplete closure of the inner layer of the thoracotomy wound, or its early disruption.

Surgical emphysema usually occurs *early* in the post-operative phase.

Management   The entire drainage system must be checked. Other parameters (e.g. breathing) should be monitored, a chest radiograph arranged, and medical officer informed. When drains are *in situ* their patency should be checked. When there is no drain in the chest, it is usually necessary to have one inserted. Sometimes the insertion in the subcutaneous tissue of an underwater drainage tube (with several holes) speeds up relief. Patients do worry about their inflated looks and in severe cases are afraid because they cannot open their eyes. It is very important to reassure them.

ALIMENTARY TRACT COMPLICATIONS

NAUSEA AND VOMITING

Early following operation, patients often feel nauseated and vomit. This usually subsides by the end of the first 24 hours. When this persists the cause must be investigated as this not only interferes with the patient's hydration and alimentary tract feeding but also with respiratory functions. Persistent vomiting is usually due to post-operative ileus and occasionally acute dilatation of the stomach.

Management

Prevention   Ensure that the patient has fasted before being sent to the operating theatre. Attention should be paid pre-operatively to bowels by administering an enema (usually) the day before operation.

Treatment   Decompress stomach by inserting a naso-gastric tube and evacuating the contents (measure fluid removed) and replace the volume of aspirated fluid. Intravenously administered fluid containing appropriate electrolytes (checked against blood electrolyte estimation), for as long as the ileus last. Progress must be monitored by measuring abdominal distension and check for the presence of bowel sounds. Record pulse rate and volume (repeated as requested by the medical staff) and blood pressure twice a day. Antiemetic drugs, such as Maxolon, should be given. If the condition persists beyond 72 hours, associated intra-abdominal causes should be considered and subsequently investigated.

ANOREXIA

This complication usually occurs *late* in the post-operative phase and can be troublesome as anorexia affects smooth recovery and interferes with wound healing. In a number of cases appetite returns after a week or so, and is helped by nurses paying attention to the patient's individual likes and dislikes for particular foods. Appetite-stimulating agents are sometimes required.

CONSTIPATION

Constipation is another complication that occurs in the *late* post-operative phase. Insufficient attention is paid to this common complication, which makes many patients very unhappy. It can easily be prevented by a careful diet and aperients. In severe cases, bowel action stops, faecal impaction occurs; an enema and manual disimpaction are needed before any relief is obtained.

GENITO-URINARY COMPLICATIONS

URINARY RETENTION

This condition is not unusual in the *early* post-operative phase. Contributing factors are:

1. In male patients, some degree of prostatic enlargement.
2. Post-operative pain inhibiting the start of micturition.
3. Analgesics given repeatedly.
4. The inability to start micturition when in bed in a reclining or semi-reclining position.

If no urine is passed within 12 to 18 hours after operation, patients should be put out of bed or sat at the edge of the bed, and encouraged to micturate. In case of failure a urinary catheter should be passed into the bladder (observing antiseptic techniques).

Late in the post-operative phase, retention or presence of residual volume in male or female patients is usually caused by urinary tract pathology.

URINARY INFECTION
Any urinary symptoms (dysuria, haematuria, frequency of micturition) should be reported to the medical staff for investigation.

RENAL FAILURE
This complication occasionally occurs in patients with extensive surgery complicated by haemorrhage, hypotension and/or shock. The manifestations are anuria and oliguria, rise in blood urea and metabolic acidosis. It should be remembered that anuria should not be confused with urinary retention. In the latter no urine is passed, but the bladder does contain urine.

MENSTRUAL DISTURBANCES
Early in the post-operative phase many young women start a rather heavy menstrual period, irrespective of the expected date. This is not really a complication, but it is worth mentioning as it can cause anxiety. Nurses should reassure the patient.

NEUROLOGICAL COMPLICATIONS OF PULMONARY SURGERY

Neurological complications are rare after a pulmonary operation and only a few can be directly attributed to surgery. For instance:

Hemiplegia, hemiparesis or other neurological deficit can occur as a result of the migration and cerebral embolisation of tumour or clot particles from the affected pulmonary vein. This complication is usually noticed soon after operation or *early* in the post-operative phase. Occasionally neurological complications occur *later* in the post-operative phase. A cerebral embolus or haemorrhage can be the cause. Early secondaries in the vertebral column cause spinal injuries and consequent neurological disturbances.

Mental confusion and temporary personality changes are occasionally encountered following pulmonary surgery in older patients, particularly those who may have suffered some degree of post-operative hypoxia.

Psychological complications It is not rare to have patients who recover well from an operation and physically show all the signs of satisfactory progress but develop changes of personality. Some of them later on show evidence of cerebral metastases, others do not. The underlying cause should be investigated and every attempt made to discover the reason. Occasionally it may be necessary to seek advice from a psychiatrist.

THORACOTOMY WOUND COMPLICATIONS

The care of the thoracotomy wound constitutes an important part of the post-operative management. Wound complications prolong hospitalisation and have a demoralising effect on the patient, who has already had a long stay in hospital.
Certain features of the thoracotomy wound need consideration. For instance:

1. The wound is usually extensive and, when repaired, it should be air-tight in order to keep separate the outside atmospheric pressure from the intra-pleural sub-atmospheric pressure.

2. Repair of the wound involves several layers of suturing (see Chapter 16: *Thoracotomy*, p. 128).

3. On the anterior aspect of the chest, intercostal spaces are wider and the ribs and their cartilages are covered by a thinner layer of soft tissues. In addition the anterior end of the wound is the lowest part, when the patient is sitting or standing, and is the area most dependent on drainage. Therefore, any collection of fluid or pus appears and discharges anteriorly.

4. The wound is constantly subjected to the trauma of respiratory and other movements (i.e. coughing). Pain can therefore be very severe. Analgesics have to be repeated frequently early in the post-operative phase. This can divert attention from abnormalities of the wound.

EARLY COMPLICATIONS
Early in the post-operative phase complications of the wound are:

1. *Wound disruption.* In this the skin sutures remain intact. Dehiscence of the intercostal layer with presence of surgical emphysema, and a definite sensation of bulging on coughing can be easily felt on palpating the wound even without removing the dressing.

2. *Haematoma* associated with, or without, disruption of the muscular layers.

3. *Superficial bleeding* and oozing from the skin suture line.

Management
Management of early post-operative wound complications consists of examining the wound on the patient's return from the operating theatre (without disturbing the dressing) and if any abnormality is noticed the examination is repeated at intervals so as to assess progress. The medical staff's attention should be drawn to any abnormality. In some cases the patient may have to be returned to the theatre for exploration and resuturing.

LATE COMPLICATIONS
Late complications of the thoracotomy wounds are:

1. *Disruption,* usually of the muscular layers, becoming obvious when skin stitches are removed. This can require a few deep sutures (taking skin and muscular layers together). At other times resuturing in the operating theatre is necessary.

2. *Sepsis and wound discharge.* Discharge occurs usually through the anterior lower part of the wound.

Management
Management consists of providing proper drainage, by removing a few stitches, or opening up with a pair of sinus forceps a small area of the wound (taking care not to enter the pleura). The medical officer should be informed of cases where the discharge tunnels between the muscular layers. The wound must be kept clean with an antiseptic solution, and the sloughing tissues removed. A dressing, and appropriate packing to prevent leakage, must be applied. The dressing is kept in position by stretch net material. Swabbing is done repeatedly for bacteriological studies and antibiotic sensitivity and antibiotics, the choice of which is guided by sensitivity tests, are administered. Attention to the patient's

general condition and state of nutrition should be observed.

In some cases the wound has to be treated surgically.

Discharging sinus

Discharge can come from a source in the subcutaneous or muscular layers or even the pleura. The source and the size of the collection can be assessed by gentle probing or a sinography. *Management* depends on the source and usually requires surgical exploration and drainage. Nursing care is the same as for wound discharge.

Scar pain

Of all the wound complications this is the most difficult to treat. It is brought to attention by the patient after the wound has completely healed, usually without complications. Thorough examination of the scar usually reveals no abnormality. Occasionally there is a history of pleural effusion, sometimes the chest wall is involved by recurring neoplasm. All efforts must be made to find the possible causes to reassure and to help the patient who should not be simply dismissed as 'neurotic'.

Part 2
The Oesophagus

This section deals with surgery of the oesophagus. A description of surgical pathological conditions is also included.

19 The Oesophagus and Investigations of Oesophageal Diseases

The oesophagus, or gullet, is the part of the alimentary tract extending from the pharynx to the stomach. It is a 25 cm (10 inch) long muscular tube whose wall consists of three layers (Fig. 2.1):

1. An inner layer of mucous membrane with squamous stratified epithelium, under which mucous glands lie.
2. A middle layer of longitudinal and circular muscle.
3. An outer layer of loose fibrous connective tissue.

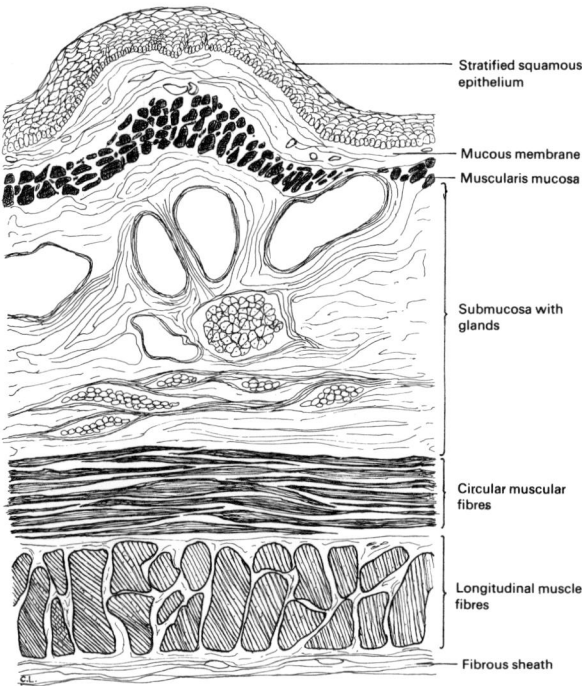

Figure 2.1 Histology of the oesophagus.

166

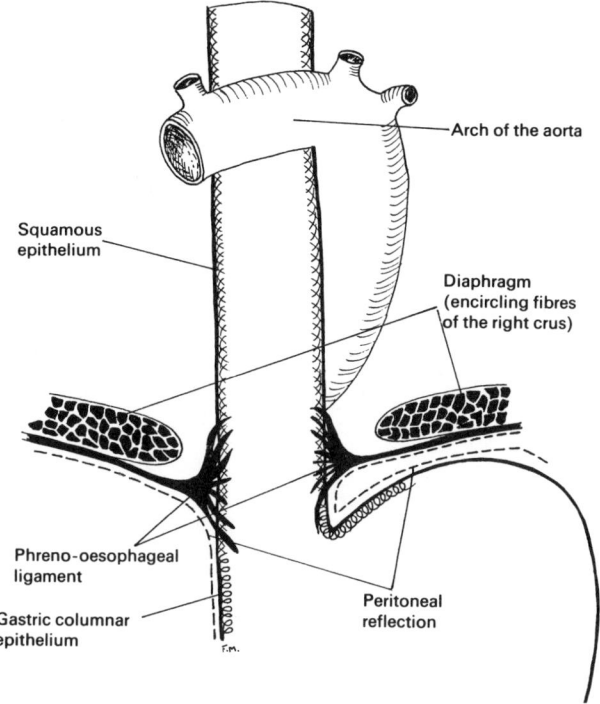

Figure 2.2   Arrangement of the oesophageal hiatus and entry of the oesophagus into the abdomen.

The entrance to the oesophagus is guarded by the muscular ring of the inferior constrictor muscle of the pharynx. This is the crico-pharyngeal muscle. The lower end of the oesophagus, the cardia, has a valvular sphincteric action at its junction with the stomach. It has an important function in preventing gastro-oesophageal reflux.

The oesophagus is divided into a cervical, a thoracic and a short abdominal portion. The greatest part of its length is situated in the thorax. In its course from the chest to the abdomen the oesophagus passes through the oesophageal hiatus, an opening in the muscular part of the diaphragm formed by the encircling fibres of the right crus (Fig. 3.1, p. 226). At the hiatus the oesophagus is attached to the diaphragm by peritoneal reflexion and a fascia. This is referred to as the phreno-oesophageal ligament (or membrane). The phreno-oesophageal ligament indicates the external landmark of the thoracic and abdominal oesophagus although the gastro-oesophageal mucosal junction lies some 2–2.5 cm below it (Fig. 2.2).

It is important to notice that in its passage from the neck to the abdomen the oesophagus is posteriorly in close contact with the body of the cervical and thoracic vertebrae (from the 6th cervical to the 12th thoracic vertebra). In the chest it is situated in the superior and posterior mediastinum. In the neck and the upper part of the chest the trachea is directly situated in front of the oesophagus.

FUNCTION OF THE OESOPHAGUS

The essential function of the oesophagus is to provide a passage for the bolus from the pharynx to the stomach. The transit of food from the mouth to the stomach involves swallowing and lubrication.

MECHANISM OF SWALLOWING

Following mastication and mixing with saliva in the mouth the bolus passes into the pharynx. The initial stage of swallowing is voluntary and is achieved by the elevation of the floor of the mouth and the projection of the tongue against the hard palate, forcing the bolus backwards into the pharynx.

The next stage of swallowing, that is the entry of the bolus into the oesophagus proper, is an involuntary action (reflex). The larynx is shut off from the pharynx by the epiglottis and by the approximation of the vocal cords. Contraction of the palatine and pharyngeal muscles causes the bolus to enter the oesophagus. Once in the oesophagus the co-ordinated peristaltic contractions propel it downwards towards the stomach. Swallowing is achieved by orderly co-ordinated action involving many muscles, is dependent on the integrity of the glosso-pharyngeal and the vagus nerves, and governed by the medullary centre. At the oesophago-gastric junction the cardia acts like a one-way valve, permitting the entry of bolus in the stomach but preventing reflux of stomach contents back into the oesophagus.

MANIFESTATIONS OF OESOPHAGEAL DISEASE

When investigating pathological conditions affecting the oesophagus careful consideration should be given to manifestations, that is symptoms and signs of the disease. These are dysphagia, heartburn, anaemia, haematemesis, flatulence and loss of weight.

DYSPHAGIA

Difficulty in swallowing can define as dysphagia. The passage of food, which is usually unnoticed, becomes noticeable to the patient. When dysphagia is severe food cannot go down the oesophagus and has to be ejected. A distinction must be made between dysphagia and vomiting. In the former the swallowed bolus is ejected up the oesophagus. In the latter, food reaches the stomach but is then brought up with some of the gastric contents. Dysphagia can be caused by a variety of neurological, muscular or obstructive lesions affecting the oeso-phagus. It is convenient to record severity of dysphagia in Grades (I to IV) according to the consistency of the food that cannot be swallowed.

Grade 0   — No dysphagia.
Grade I   — Dysphagia to solids.
Grade II   — Dysphagia to semi-solids.
Grade III   — Dysphagia to purees.
Grade IV   — Total dysphagia including liquids.

HEARTBURN

A sensation of burning pain and discomfort in the epigastrum and behind the lower part of the sternum indicates heartburn. It is often accompanied by regurgitation of gastric contents into the oesophagus and 'throat'.

This symptom is not specific to oesophageal diseases and can be present in some pathological conditions of the stomach or duodenum. Heartburn is often associated with inflammatory changes of the lower oesophagus (oesophagitis) due to incompetence of the cardia and gastro-oesophageal reflux, as seen in cases of hiatal hernia.

PAIN

It is difficult to localise pain originating in the oesophagus. Upper abdominal, retrosternal and chest pain radiating upwards towards the neck may be caused by oesophageal conditions.

Oesophageal pain can however be difficult to differentiate from angina pectoris or coronary arterial insufficiency.

ANAEMIA

In some oesophageal conditions there is frank or occult bleeding resulting in hypochromic and iron deficiency anaemia. When bleeding is severe and sudden, the patient has haematemesis and presents signs and symptoms of shock.

HAEMATEMESIS

This is vomiting either fresh or altered blood. A penetrating ulcer, oesophageal varices or a mucosal tear can cause an acute emergency situation with obvious vomiting of blood, hypotension and shock.

FLATULENCE

This is the presence of excessive gas in the gastro-intestinal tract with associated abdominal discomfort. It is present in some oesophageal conditions, but it is not specific to oesophageal diseases.

LOSS OF WEIGHT

In many of the long-standing oesophageal obstructive lesions, particularly malignant tumours, loss of weight is present at the time of the patient's admission to hospital.

INVESTIGATIONS OF OESOPHAGEAL DISEASES

Investigations can be classified as clinical and non-specific or specific.

CLINICAL AND NON-SPECIFIC INVESTIGATIONS

A systemic examination is usually carried out on admission by a doctor. Clinical history is taken with particular reference to clinical manifestations of the oesophageal disease. It is important to weigh the patient and, when dysphagia is present, to ascertain its severity and duration.

Non-specific, routine investigations include blood count, blood biochemical profile, and ward urine examination for protein, sugar and acetone.

SPECIFIC INVESTIGATIONS

Radiological studies

Chest radiograph may indicate the nature of the condition (e.g. perforation of the oesophagus). At other times it can help diagnosis (e.g. by demonstrating extrinsic pressure on the oesophagus from an intrathoracic tumour).

Barium contrast examination   A thin or thick solution of barium preparation is used to outline the lumen of the oesophagus. A series of X-ray films taken at short intervals show the precise location and the extent of the pathology (Fig. 4.3, p. 258).

Cine-barium swallow using an image intensifier and a special camera. A motion picture of the barium transit is taken. This technique is useful when studying the swallowing pattern and the downward progress of the bolus from the mouth to the stomach. A cassette video recording of a barium swallow simplifies the viewing of the film.

Manometric studies

The pattern of peristaltic activity, particularly the relaxation of the cardia distal to the oncoming bolus, can be recorded and studied. This is done by placing a catheter in the oesophageal lumen and connecting it to a transducer and an electronic manometer. The resulting series of pressure waves recorded from various parts of the oesophagus indicates functional peristaltic activity.

pH studies

The secretion of gastric acid and its reflux into the oesophagus may be gauged by intra-luminal oesophageal pH measurements. Oesophageal pH studies are particularly relevant in cases of gastro-oesophageal reflux associated with a hiatus hernia or a malfunctioning of the cardiac sphincter.

The pH is the negative logarithm of the hydrogen ion concentration (H^+), or $pH = -\log_{10}(H^+)$.

H^+ concentration of pure water at $25°C = 10^{-7}$ g ions/l.

$\log_{10}$ of $10^{-7} = -7$

As $pH = -\log_{10}(H^+) = (-7)$.
Therefore pH of water $= 7$.

The pH of a neutral solution will always be given by the figure 7. The pH of an acid solution by a figure less than 7, and an alkali solution by a figure greater than 7.

Endoscopy

Oesophagoscopy is a visual examination of the oesophageal lumen with an instrument called an oesophagoscope (see Chapter 21: *Oesophagoscopy*, p. 206). Alterations of the mucosa such as inflammation and ulceration can be observed. The nature and the level of an obstructive lesion can be determined macroscopically. It is customary to refer to the level of the lesion in cm from the upper incisors (or the upper alveolus of the maxilla). A biopsy can be taken in the course of the procedure for histological examination.

Bronchoscopy   The trachea and main bronchi have a close anatomical relationship with the oesophagus and therefore this examination is carried out for some oesophageal conditions, e.g. neoplasms (see Chapter 15).

Mediastinoscopy is performed when the oesophageal condition is due to or accompanies involvement of the mediastinal structures (see Chapter 23).

20 Diseases of the Oesophagus

A description of all the pathological conditions affecting the oesophagus is both unrealistic and unnecessary and therefore only the more common diseases and conditions are discussed here.

CONGENITAL OESOPHAGEAL ATRESIA AND TRACHEO-OESOPHAGEAL FISTULA

The word 'atresia' means absence of natural opening due to abnormal canalisation in a tubular organ. In the case of oesophageal atresia the continuity of the upper alimentary tract is interrupted by the abnormal oesophagus. There are several variants of this condition the commonest being where the upper oesophagus has a blind end, and the lower portion opens into the trachea, therefore establishing a tracheo-oesophageal fistula (more than 70 % of cases). The other variants are illustrated in Fig. 2.3.

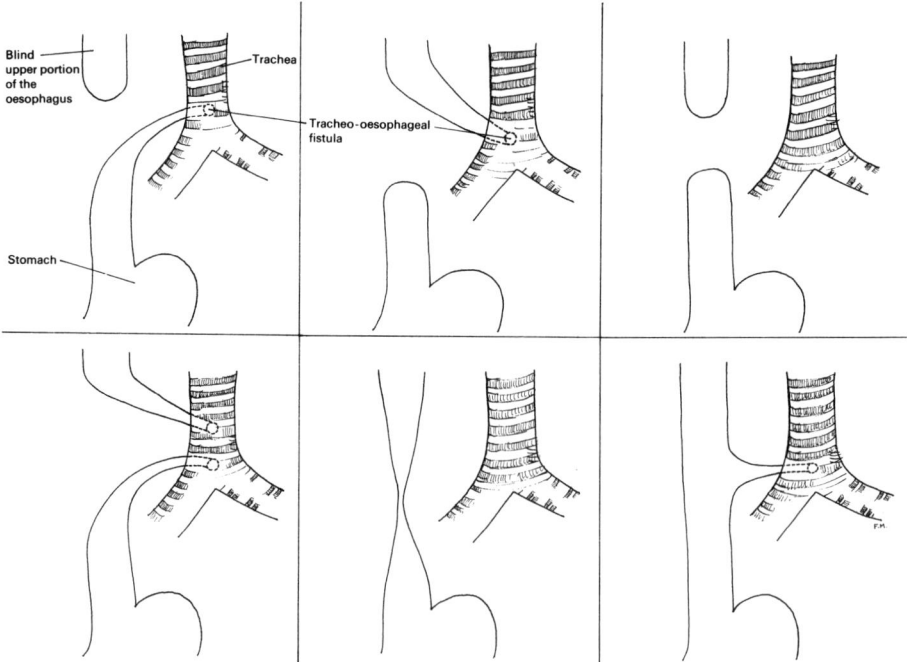

Figure 2.3   Types of oesophageal atresia with or without fistula (commonest type is shown in upper left diagram).

The existence of the condition is frequently suspected before birth because of the presence of maternal hydramnios. At birth the baby cannot swallow saliva which collects in the mouth and appears as frothy liquid. Any attempt at feeding produces an accumulation of fluid which spills into the lungs and causes choking and cyanosis. In addition there is also distension of the stomach when a tracheo-oesophageal fistula is present. If untreated the baby suffers from respiratory embarrassment (respiratory distress syndrome) resulting in death.

DIAGNOSIS

At birth, diagnosis is based on the above clinical findings and confirmed by the impossibility to pass a naso-gastric catheter into the stomach. Further confirmation is provided by an X-ray film showing the tip of the firm radio-opaque catheter in the upper oesophagus and a gas-filled stomach. A drop or two of Dianosil in the naso-gastric catheter will outline the blind pouch (Fig. 2.4). Care should be taken not to spill the opaque medium into the trachea.

Neonates with oesophageal atresia may have other congenital anomalies that should be looked for (e.g. congenital heart disorder).

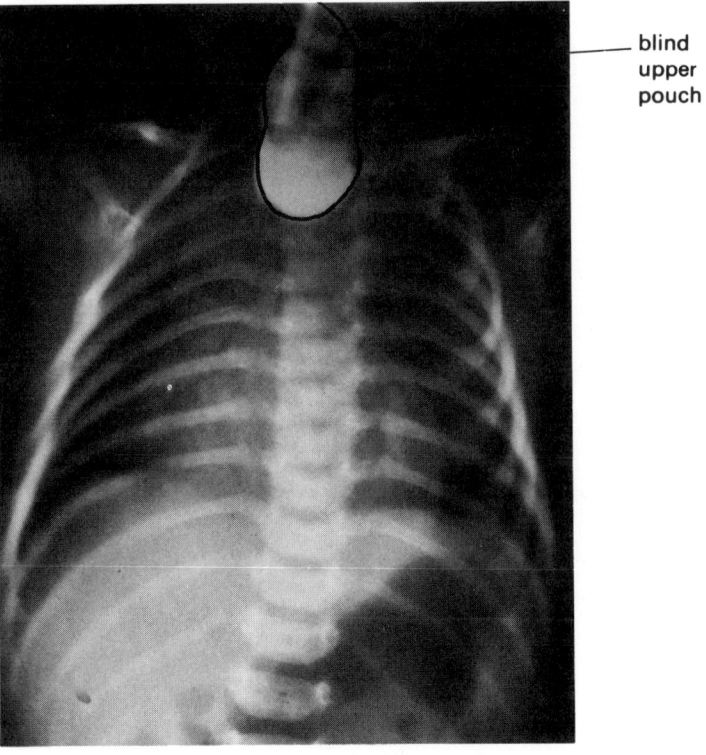

blind
upper
pouch

Figure 2.4   Barium examination of oesophageal atresia showing the blind upper pouch.

Pre-operative care

Pre-operatively, nursing care is directed towards clearing the baby's airways and assisting respiration. Feeding is stopped and the infant is nursed in an incubator. During diagnostic procedures, especially during radiological examination, the nurse should ensure the availability of oxygen, suction machine and catheters. An intravenous infusion is established before surgery.

Surgery

This is the only treatment and consists of closure of the tracheal fistula and establishment of oesophageal continuity. A right thoracotomy is carried out and a one-stage operation can be performed in the majority of cases. Occasionally, this is not possible because of the unsuitable anatomy of the oesophagus. The oesophago-tracheal fistula is repaired (if there is one), a cervical oesophagostomy and a feeding gastrotomy are established (Fig. 2.5).

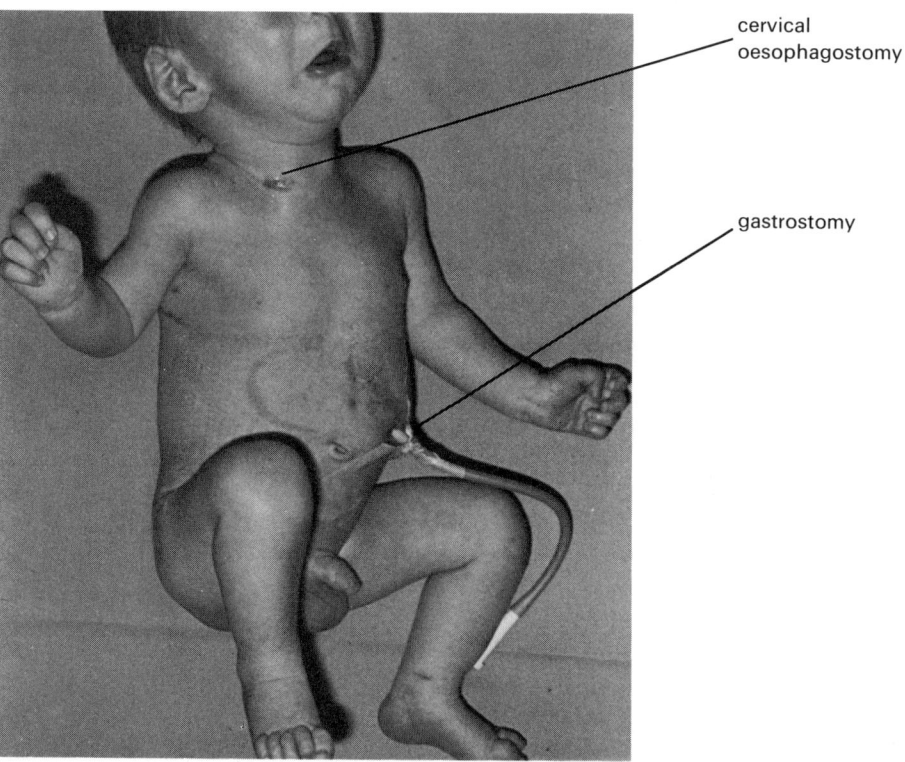

cervical oesophagostomy

gastrostomy

Figure 2.5   Infant on whom the first stage of oesophageal reconstruction for atresia has been carried out.

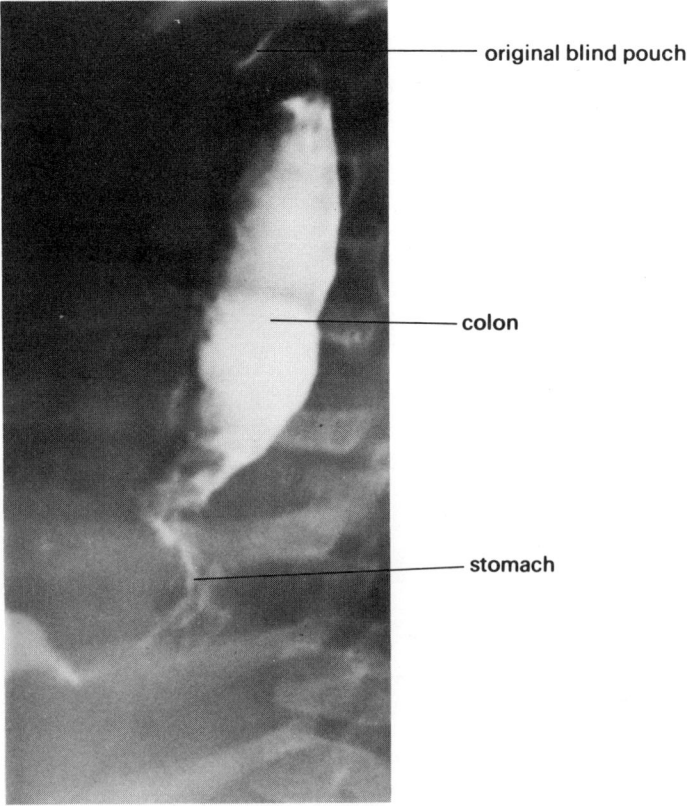

original blind pouch

colon

stomach

Figure 2.6   Colon interposition in a case of oesophageal atresia treated by two-stage oesophageal reconstruction. X-ray shows the colon filled with barium and functioning as thoracic oesophagus.

Oesophageal reconstruction is undertaken at a later date (12 to 18 months) when a loop of colon with its blood supply is implanted in the neck and chest, re-establishing the continuity of the cervical thoracic and abdominal oesophagus with the stomach (Fig. 2.6) (see *Reconstructive surgery of the oesophagus*, p. 209).

Post-operative care
Post-operatively the baby is nursed in an incubator for a few days. Particular attention should be paid to fluid and nutritional requirements, prevention of stomach distension and lung collapse, and the intercostal catheter.

The intercostal catheter is usually discarded 24 to 48 hours after surgery. Naso-gastric tube feeding is started 24 hours after the operation and the intravenous drip discontinued 24 hours later.

At all times, particularly during the first 4 or 5 days, expansion of the lungs is checked especially on the thoracotomy (right) side.

FOREIGN BODIES IN THE OESOPHAGUS

Various blunt or sharp objects can lodge in the oesophagus. A blunt object has to be relatively large to remain in the oesophagus, unless there is a pre-existing obstructive lesion. Impaction of a foreign body in the oesophagus causes obstruction of the lumen and generally total dysphagia. A sharp object can penetrate the mucosa and cause an ulcer. Or it can perforate the oesophagus producing severe mediastinitis and a peri-oesophageal abscess.

The patient is usually aware of having swallowed an object. When this is not the case, the onset of acute dysphagia is the only guide to diagnosis. Radio-opaque objects are visible on an X-ray film (Fig. 2.7), but objects made of plastic, for instance, are not radiologically detectable. In such cases barium swallow shows an obstruction and the foreign body is seen at endoscopy.

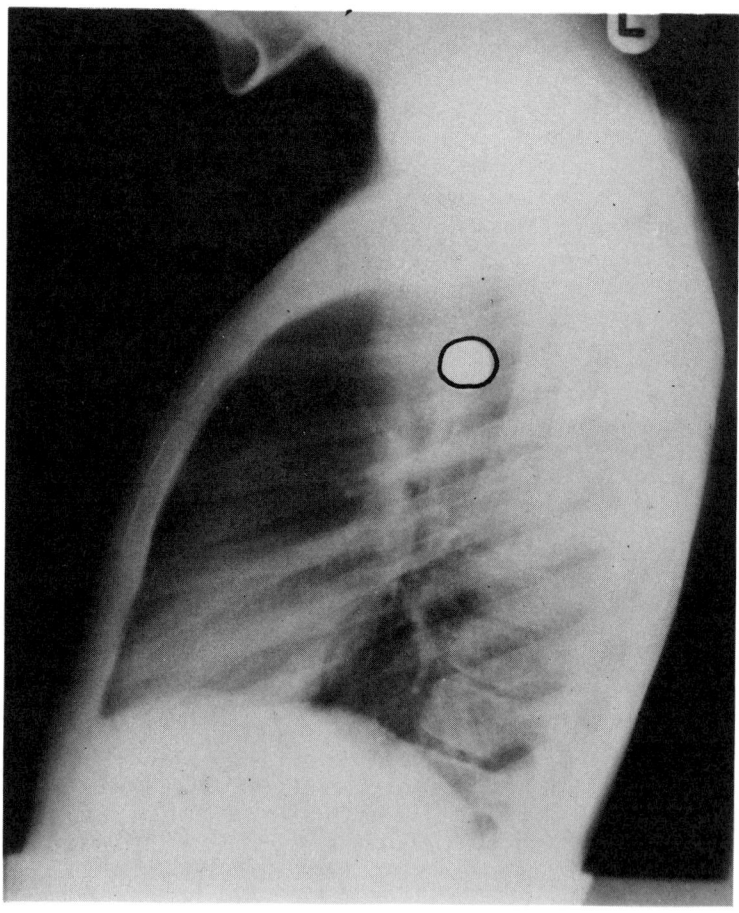

Figure 2.7   Foreign body (coin) lodged in the oesophagus.

MANAGEMENT

When the X-ray film has shown the location of the foreign body oesophagoscopy is carried out and the object removed. Following endoscopic removal, patients should not be given fluids or food before a perforation has been excluded on radiological and clinical evidence.

In rare cases when the foreign body cannot be removed by oesophagoscopy, surgical removal becomes necessary. When sharp objects have caused perforation of the oesophagus, the neck or the posterior mediastinum, or both, are usually surgically drained following the removal of the object and the repair of the tear.

HIATAL HERNIA

A hiatal hernia is the protrusion (herniation) of the stomach into the chest through the oesophageal hiatus of the diaphragm. Hiatus herniae fall into three types:

1. *Sliding:* The cardiac end of the stomach is drawn upwards into the chest some distance above the hiatus.

2. *Para-oesophageal:* Part of the stomach, usually the fundus and the body, enters the chest through the oesophageal hiatus and lies along the oesophagus.

3. *Mixed:* The features of the sliding and para-oesophageal herniae are combined.

SLIDING HIATUS HERNIA

Regurgitation of gastric juice into the oesophagus is mainly prevented by the sphincter action of the cardia assisted by the arrangement of the diaphragmatic muscles around the lower oesophagus. In patients with sliding hiatal hernia (Fig. 2.8) severe gastro-oesophageal reflux is often present. It is caused by weakness in

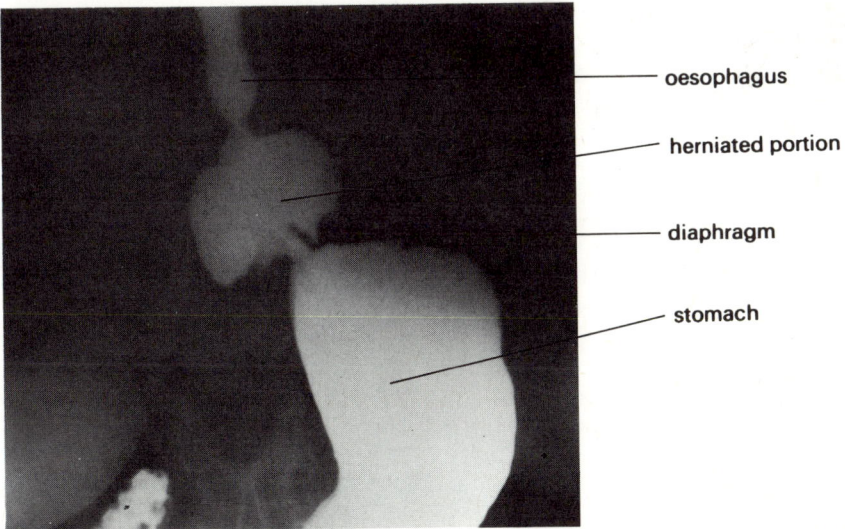

oesophagus

herniated portion

diaphragm

stomach

Figure 2.8   Sliding hiatal hernia.

the diaphragmatic muscles, upward displacement of the gastro-oesophageal junction and malfunctioning of the cardiac sphincter. Refluxed gastric contents eventually create inflammation (oesophagitis) and ulceration of the mucosa leading to scarring and stricture formation. It is because of associated gastro-oesophageal reflux and oesophagitis that hiatal hernia can be a serious condition.

Clinical features
Hiatal hernia is a common condition found more frequently in women. The majority of sufferers are overweight. The patient usually seeks medical advice because of dyspepsia, heartburn, retrosternal pain, flatulence, vomiting after meals and dysphagia. Symptoms are exacerbated by bending and lying down. Existence of the hernia is sometimes suspected because of chronic or acute anaemia due to frank or occult bleeding related to the complications of the condition. Dysphagia occurs with the development of spasm in cases of severe oesophagitis, ulceration and scarring. At first it is intermittent and only mild (Grade I), later becoming permanent and severe (Grade II, III, IV) (see Chapter 19: *Manifestations of oesophageal diseases*, p. 168).

Diagnosis
A barium swallow demonstrates the presence of the hernia with free reflux. Oesophagoscopy and biopsy of the mucous membrane show the presence of oesophagitis. Lower oesophageal pH studies indicate the degree of severity of the reflux. Manometric studies reveal a reduction in pressure in the lower (sphincter) oesophageal segment.

Management
It is usually advisable to treat the patient medically for at least 4 to 6 months. The patient should sleep in a propped-up position, with the end of the bed raised on wooden blocks or bricks, and an anti-acid anti-spasmodic medication prescribed. Obese patients should lose weight.

Symptoms that persist in spite of medical treatment, i.e. dysphagia associated with severe oesophagitis and ulceration, are indications for surgery. Surgical treatment consists of repairing the hernia and providing an anti-reflux mechanism.

PARA-OESOPHAGEAL HERNIA
The stomach is herniated through the oesophageal hiatus with its cardiac end remaining in position below the diaphragm (Fig. 2.9). There is no gastro-oesophageal reflux, therefore no oesophagitis.

Although a considerable portion of the stomach can be herniated patients are often asymptomatic and only diagnosed on routine chest X-rays showing a fluid and gas-filled stomach in the chest. Those who do develop symptoms complain of fullness, pain in the chest and occasional vomiting after meals. Patients are frequently anaemic for the same reason as in sliding hiatal hernia.

Sometimes the sufferer is admitted as an emergency suffering from shock with severe pain in the chest. This is due to gastric volvulus (distortion of the stomach) and obstruction of the hernial sac at the hiatus, with consequent distension of the fluid- and gas-filled stomach.

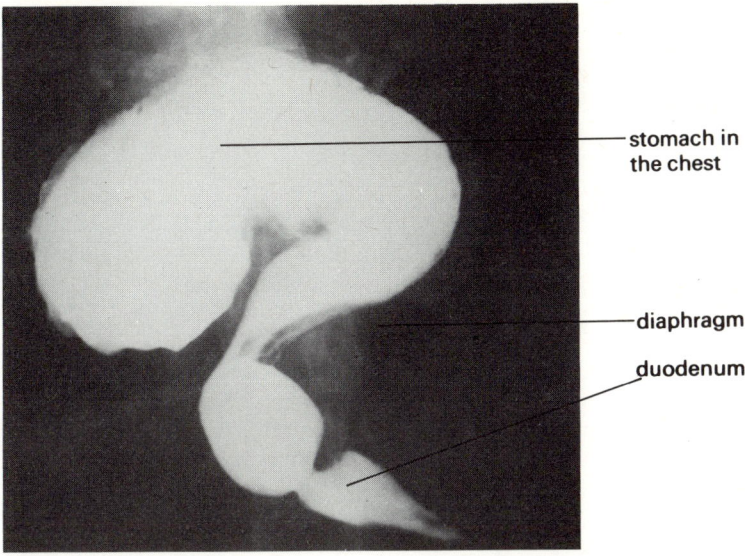

stomach in
the chest

diaphragm

duodenum

Figure 2.9   Para-oesophageal hernia. The whole of the stomach is in the chest and has rotated on a horizontal axis.

Diagnosis

A chest radiograph shows the stomach in the chest behind the heart. Barium swallow examination confirms the diagnosis.

Management

Although these herniae may be asymptomatic the possibility of volvulus, obstruction, severe anaemia or ulcer in the herniated part of the stomach makes surgical repair desirable.

In cases of obstruction, immediate relief of gastric distension is achieved through naso-gastric tube suction. Fluid and electrolytes are provided. Once dehydration and electrolyte imbalance are corrected an operation is performed to reduce the hernia and prevent recurrence.

MIXED HERNIA

The cardia is drawn upwards through the hiatus with the herniated stomach lying along the oesophagus. Symptoms are similar to those in sliding hiatal hernia.

Management and treatment are along the lines indicated for sliding hiatal hernia.

OPERATIONS FOR REPAIR OF HIATAL HERNIA

There are several operations designed to reduce and repair hiatal hernia, including an anti-reflux mechanism when reflux is present but only the principles of these operations will be discussed here.

In most cases a left thoracotomy is performed, access to the abdomen is obtained through the diaphragm. Occasionally, the abdominal approach alone is used.

In all operations the oesophagus is mobilised to some extent. The oesophageal hiatus is cleared of fibro-fatty tissues.

Allison's repair of hiatal hernia

This operation consists of reducing the hernia transthoracically and fixing the phreno-oesophageal ligament below the diaphragm, in order to maintain the reduction and the gastro-oesophageal junction in the abdomen (Fig. 2.10). The widened hiatus is then tightened.

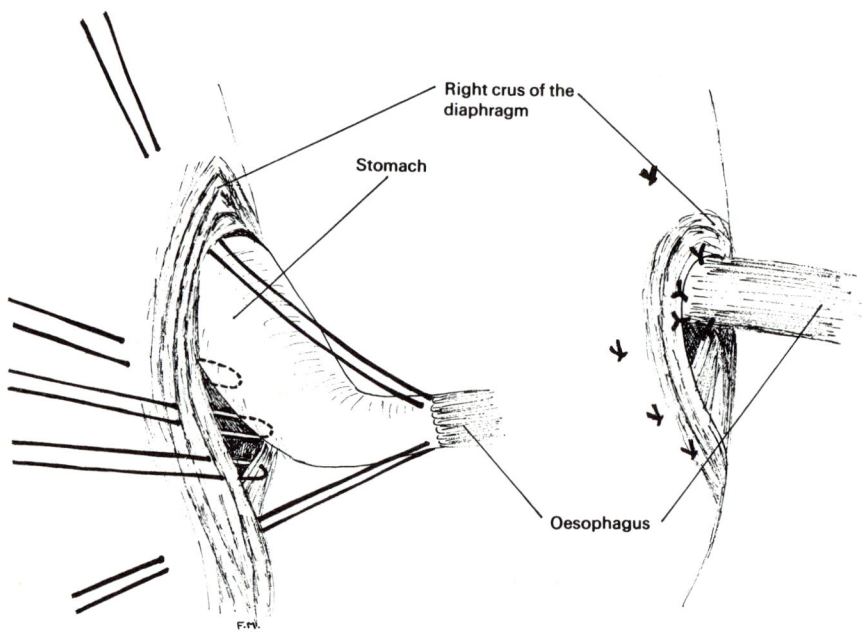

Figure 2.10   Allison-type repair of hiatal hernia.

Nissen-type fundoplication

This consists of wrapping the fundus of the stomach round the lower oesophagus (Fig. 2.11). This inkwell effect acts as an anti-gastro-oesophageal reflux mechanism. The fundus of the stomach and the lower oesophagus have to be fully mobilised to allow the complete wrapping.

Belsey's operation

The principle is similar to that of Nissen repair except that the fundic wrap around the lower oesophagus is incomplete, as can be seen in the illustration (Fig. 2.12).

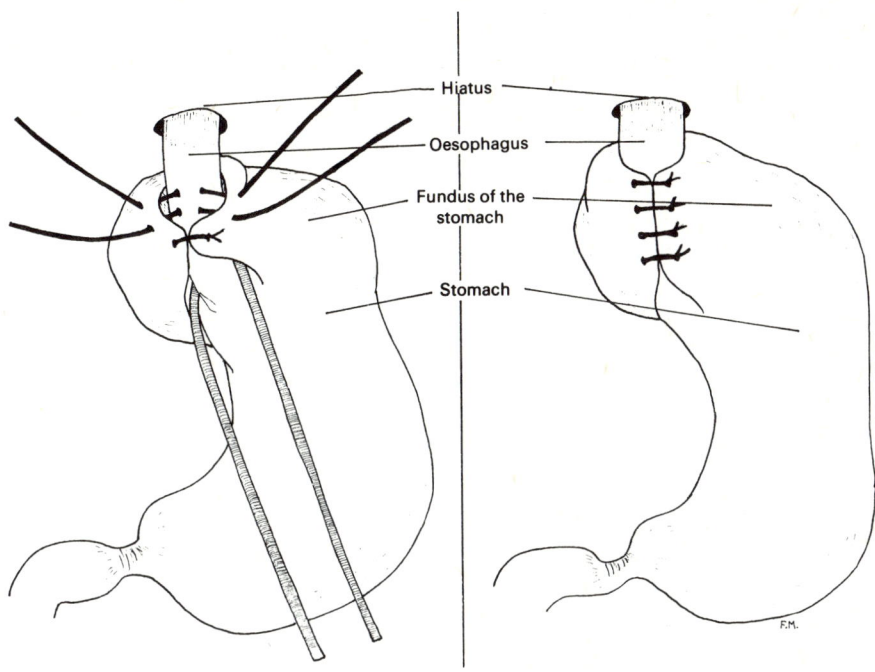

Figure 2.11   Nissen-type fundoplication.

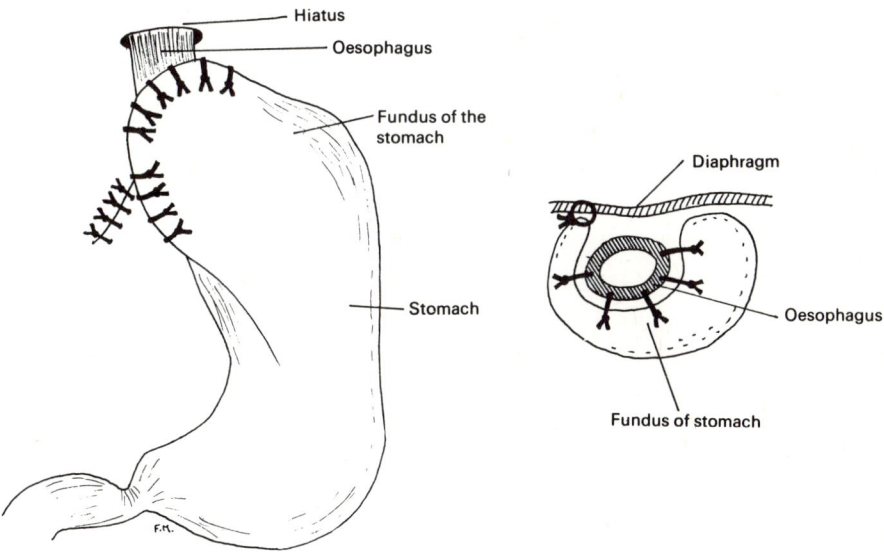

Figure 2.12   Belsey repair of hiatal hernia.

OBSTRUCTIVE LESIONS OF THE OESOPHAGUS

The function of the oesophagus is to provide a channel for the passage of food and to propel the bolus downwards into the stomach. Interference with this function results in dysphagia. In effect obstruction arises as a result of not only a mechanical obstacle, but also functional disorders of the oesophagus. It is therefore appropriate to consider under the same heading all oesophageal lesions which can cause obstruction in its broader sense. A variety of conditions cause obstruction to the bolus, resulting in dysphagia.

PEPTIC STRICTURE (Reflux Stricture)

This type of stricture usually results from long-standing irritation of the oesophagus by gastric juice. In most cases the stricture is caused by gastro-oesophageal reflux associated with hiatal hernia. In some patients there is no demonstrable hiatal hernia; the stricture follows gastro-oesophageal reflux resulting from incompetence of the lower oesophageal sphincter. The initial response to reflux is oesophagitis and oesophageal spasm, followed by ulceration, scarring and fibrous stricture.

Clinical features and diagnosis

The patient seeks advice on account of dysphagia. In many cases heartburn and dyspepsia precede dysphagia. Loss of weight is present when dysphagia is severe and long-standing. Sometimes mild or moderate anaemia and, occasionally, haematemesis are also present.

Barium swallow contrast studies demonstrate the obstruction and its location (Fig. 2.13). Oesophagoscopy and oesophageal biopsy confirm the diagnosis.

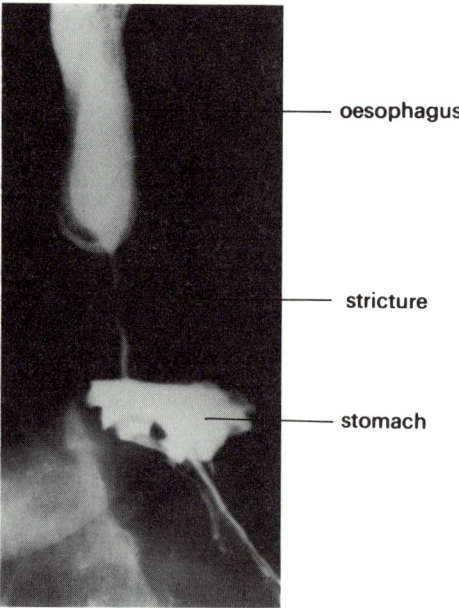

oesophagus

stricture

stomach

Figure 2.13   Peptic (reflux) stricture of the oesophagus.

Treatment
At an early stage the repair of hiatal hernia or an effective anti-reflux operation preventing further gastro-oesophageal reflux arrests the progress of oesophagitis and the formation of stricture. When a stricture is established dilatation will relieve the obstructive symptoms (at least temporarily) but, in the majority of cases, gastro-oesophageal reflux continues and is followed by the reappearance of the stricture and obstructive symptoms.

In most stricture cases operative treatment is advised, particularly when the patient's general condition is suitable for surgery and if repeated dilatations have to be carried out at frequent intervals. Surgical treatment need not be excisional. At present there are generally two surgical methods available:

1. Conservative surgery, where the patient's oesophagus is preserved.
2. Radical surgery. The stricture-bearing area of the oesophagus is resected and the upper alimentary tract is reconstructed (by using a substitute for the oesophagus).

Conservative surgery is based on dilatation of the stricture at operation and, if need be, by transgastric-retrograde route (meaning through a gastrotomy) under vision. This guided dilatation is however one part of the procedure, the other being the provision of an anti-reflux mechanism (repair of hiatal hernia when it is present). In effect the conservative method is an intra-operative dilatation of the stricture coupled with an operation to prevent reflux which had caused the stricture in the first place.

Radical surgery When the stricture is so serious as to require frequent dilatations, when it is judged to be undilatable, or when the oesophagus is irretrievably destroyed, resection and reconstruction of the oesophagus become necessary. In all these cases the stomach is preserved. The part of the oesophagus bearing the lesion is resected. Reconstruction of the upper alimentary tract after resection requires substitution of the resected segment by vascularised transplant of stomach, jejunum or colon (see *Reconstructive surgery of the oesophagus*, p. 209).

Non-operative treatment (dilatation) Occasionally, the patient is in such a poor condition with associated cardio-pulmonary disease that repeated dilatations of the stricture are the only possible therapeutic solution providing relief of obstructive symptoms. Following dilatation of the stricture the patient is advised to sleep in an upright position in order to limit gastric reflux. In addition anti-inflammatory antacid agents are prescribed to reduce oesophagitis.

CORROSIVE OESOPHAGITIS AND LYE STRICTURE
The term 'lye stricture' refers to oesophageal stenotic lesions caused by acid and particularly strong alkali (lye).

Accidental ingestion of acid and alkali by children has become a relatively infrequent occurrence in this country, largely due to precautionary warnings from the media and safety measures used by manufacturers of household products.

The deliberate ingestion of corrosives in adults is encountered more frequently. The injurious effects on the oesophagus depend on the concentration and nature of the ingested substance on the one hand, and the speed and effectiveness of the treatment undertaken on the other. Acids appear to cause less extensive damage than alkalis, mainly because of differing types of necrosis which follow their ingestion.

The early effects of ingestion of caustic substances vary from mild local burns of the mouth and oesophagus to extreme shock, in addition to extensive ulceration or perforation of the oesophagus followed by mediastinitis. The late results, even in the absence of perforation and even when treatment is successfully undertaken, are stricture of the oesophagus and extreme contracture of the stomach with obstruction of the pylorus.

Management
In the early stage anti-shock measures are introduced, parenteral therapy (fluid and nutrition) is commenced and the extent of the damage is assessed by radiological and endoscopical investigations. In the absence of perforation conservative measures have a good chance of success. The late consequence is stricture of the oesophagus. When this is fully formed it can be repeatedly dilated.

Sometimes, however, the conservative approach is unsuccessful and surgical treatment becomes necessary, consisting of resection and reconstruction using a colonar or jejunal substitute (see Chapter 21: *Reconstructive surgery of the oesophagus*, p. 209).

POST-OPERATIVE STRICTURES
Oesophageal stenoses following operation related or unrelated to the alimentary tract are considered here.

Strictures following oesophageal operations
They are anastomotic strictures appearing at the site of oesophageal anastomosis with another organ (stomach, jejunum or colon). They fall into two categories:

1. Some appear *early after operation*, usually a few weeks or a few months later. They are caused by excessive granulation tissues and tissue overgrowth in the line of anastomosis.

2. Others appear *long after surgery* and are usually a recurrence of the stricture due to chronic gastro-oesophageal reflux that the operation has either caused or failed to prevent.

In patients with oesophago-gastric anastomosis following resection of lower oesophageal stricture, continuous post-operative reflux eventually causes a recurrent reflux stricture.

In patients having undergone resection for neoplasm the possibility of recurrence of the tumour should always be considered.

Treatment of these lesions, particularly the late recurrent type, can be difficult and problematic. It is therefore imperative to try and prevent their appearance. The following points should be observed:

1. Patients should be up and about as much as possible.
2. Heavy meals and large amounts of fluids should be avoided before bed.
3. Small and frequent meals should be continued a long time after operation.

4. Bowels should be kept regular.
5. Anti-reflux medication should be prescribed.

When the stricture is fully developed its site and characteristics are investigated radiologically and endoscopically. In some cases, particularly among younger patients, surgery may become necessary.

Strictures following vagotomy and pyloroplasty
Temporary dysphagia after these operations is not infrequent. Persistent dysphagia accompanying a demonstrable stricture of the lower oesophagus is a rare occurrence whose cause remains unknown.

Strictures following abdominal operations
Occasionally oesophageal strictures develop after abdominal surgery. Several factors can be responsible for their development, the most frequent being naso-gastric catheters and post-operative reflux of the gastric contents into the oesophagus.

These strictures can be prevented by avoiding the use of naso-gastric catheters whenever feasible, or by removing them as early as possible, as well as by mobilising patients or at least encouraging them to sit up.

OESOPHAGEAL WEBS AND RINGS
Webs and rings are a fibrous membrane or diaphragm within the lumen of the oesophagus, which reduce and therefore obstruct the passage of food. They are commonly situated in the upper cervical and the lower thoracic oesophagus.

Cervical web and Plummer–Vinson (Paterson–Kelly) syndrome
A cervical web is a thin shelf-like membrane projecting into the lumen of the oesophagus at its junction with the pharynx. The main symptoms in sufferers, who are almost entirely women, is dysphagia. The latter may be associated with glossitis and anaemia, in which case the term Plummer–Vinson (or Paterson–Kelly) syndrome is applied.

Barium swallow examination may fail to show the web, but careful direct endoscopic examination will demonstrate it.

Treatment consists of oesophagoscopy and dilatation of the web (or rupture of the membrane). Anaemia and nutritional deficiencies, when present, are corrected.

Lower oesophageal web (Schatzki's ring)
This web (Fig. 2.14) is found in the lower oesophagus, most typically at or near the junction of the thoracic and abdominal segments. The web is a thin circular membrane attached circumferentially to the oesophageal mucosa. The resulting luminal narrowing causes dysphagia which is the main symptom in this condition.

In many patients the existence of the web is recognised radiologically by a typical annular indentation, or a ring of constriction, visible on a barium swallow film. This was first reported by Ingelfinger and Kramer (1953), then Schatzki and Gary (1953). The condition is known to radiologists and clinicians as Schatzki's ring.

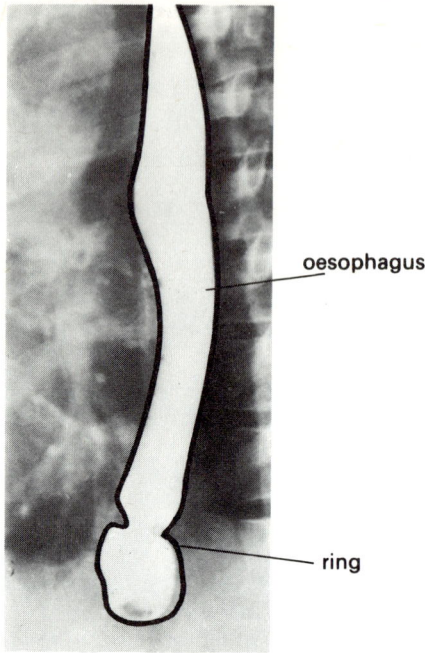

Figure 2.14   Lower oesophagus stricture (Schatzki's ring).

The aetiology and pathogenesis of the condition are not well understood. Because of the occasional association of the condition with a hiatal hernia it is suggested that the membrane may be the consequence of reflux. The most prominent symptom is dysphagia which varies in severity.

Diagnosis is made by barium swallow examination (Fig. 2.14) and by oesophagoscopy with a rigid oesophagoscope.

Conservative treatment consists of endoscopic dilatation which can be repeated.

Surgical treatment consists of excision of the membrane coupled with an anti-reflux procedure, as gastro-oesophageal reflux may play a role in the pathogenesis.

OESOPHAGEAL STRICTURE IN SCLERODERMA

Scleroderma (systemic sclerosis) is a disorder of connective tissues characterised by fibrosis of skin and subcutaneous tissues and peripheral ischaemic changes of Raynaud's syndrome.

Patients with scleroderma suffer frequently from oesophageal disorders. The latter appear to be caused by neuro-muscular disturbances which can produce symptoms ranging from mild dysphagia to total obstruction. Gastro-oesophageal reflux is present in many patients. The stricture is regarded as a type of reflux stricture and is usually treated as such (see p. 183).

ACHALASIA OF THE CARDIA

Achalasia of the cardia (synonym cardiospasm) can be defined as a condition in which the lower part of the oesophagus (cardia) fails to relax in advance of an oncoming bolus which, therefore, cannot enter the stomach. This results in functional obstruction of the lower oesophagus.

It is relevant to remember that the passage of the bolus from the mouth to the stomach through the oesophagus is dependent on a series of co-ordinated muscular activities, called peristalsis, which consist of the relaxation of a section of the oesophagus ahead of the bolus with a simultaneous contraction of the section behind. The contraction behind and the relaxation in front propel the bolus downwards towards the stomach. Lack of relaxation appears to be the abnormality preventing the bolus from entering the stomach. It accounts for dysphagia which remains an important symptom in the patients.

The aetiology of the condition is still unknown. Many patients have a psychologically disturbed background. It is not unusual for a patient to become dysphagic after emotional stress. At structural level degenerative changes can be demonstrated in the nerve plexus (Auerbach's plexus) of the oesophagus. They account for disturbances in peristaltic activities.

Clinical features and diagnosis

The main symptoms are dysphagia which varies in severity, and lower central pain when swallowing. Regurgitation of food into the mouth is a common occurrence. In many patients there is repeated associated chest infection due to accumulation of food debris in the dilated and paralysed oesophagus, followed by regurgitation and inhalation.

Barium swallow examination shows dilation and elongation of the oesophagus reaching enormous proportions in some cases together with the smooth constriction of the cardia allowing a trickle of contrast medium into the stomach (Fig. 2.15).

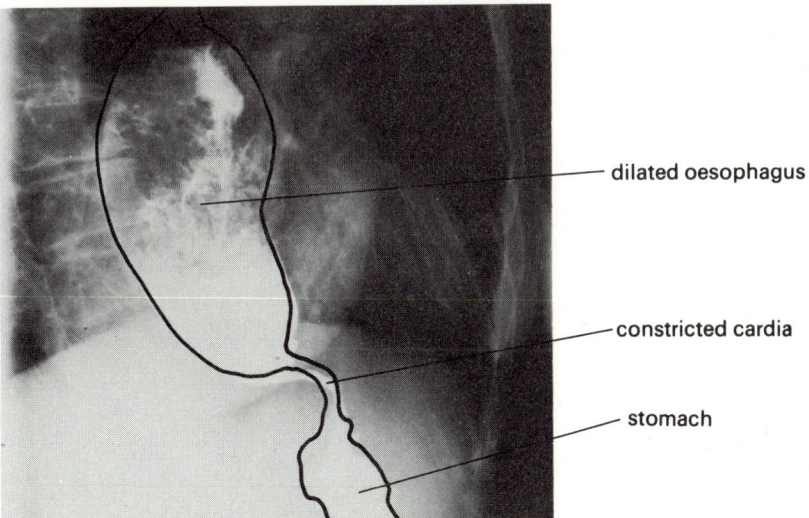

dilated oesophagus

constricted cardia

stomach

Figure 2.15   Achalasia of the cardia.

Oesophagoscopy reveals a dilated oesophagus containing food debris and showing inflammatory changes of the mucosa, but no obstructive organic lesion.

Oesophageal manometric studies demonstrate spasm of the cardia indicated by increased pressure and often complete lack of peristaltic activities in the body of the oesophagus.

Treatment

Conservative treatment consists of endoscopic dilatation of the cardia with bougies or a hydrostatic balloon. This is supposed to disrupt the circular muscle fibres and thus eliminate spasms.

Surgical treatment is considered for younger patients and those not responding to a conservative approach. Prior to surgery any chest infection is treated and nutritional deficiencies are corrected. Lower oesophageal myotomy (Heller's operation) is then carried out. The operation consists of exposing and exploring the oesophagus through a left postero-lateral thoracotomy and carrying out a longitudinal myotomy (Fig. 2.16). The latter is an incision in the muscle layer. Both the longitudinal and the circular muscles have to be incised over 8 to 10 cm on and above the narrow cardiac segment. Most surgeons add an anti-reflux operation as some gastro-oesophageal reflux occurs following myotomy. If not prevented it will cause a reflux stricture.

Post-operatively patients are nourished parenterally for a few days. Fluids, a light diet and then normal solids are gradually introduced. Normal food intake is resumed before discharge.

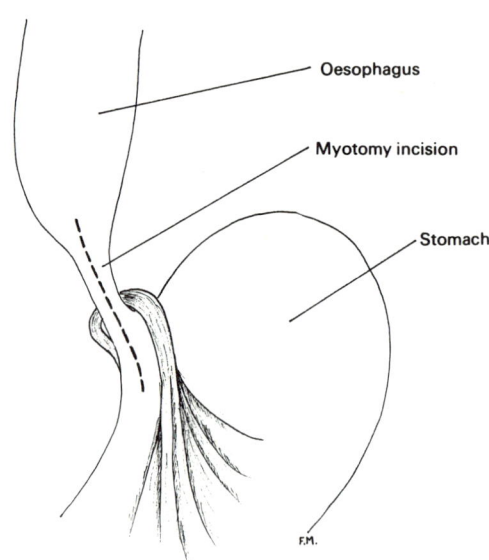

Figure 2.16   Oesophageal myotomy.

OESOPHAGEAL DIVERTICULA

A diverticulum is a mucosal protrusion through a weak area in the oesophageal muscular wall. In effect it is a mucosal cul-de-sac extending out of the oesophageal lumen.

Diverticula develop as a result of either of two mechanisms. First, as a result of increased intraluminal pressure causing mucosal extrusion: they are referred to as pulsion diverticula. Second as a result of an inflammatory process involving the lymph nodes which pull out the mucosa: they are then called traction diverticula.

Anatomically diverticula are situated in:

1. The upper oesophagus at the pharyngo-oesophageal junction (these are pulsion diverticula and by far the most common).
2. The mid-oesophagus (traction diverticula).
3. The lower oesophagus (pulsion diverticula).

Upper oesophagus diverticula (pharyngeal pouch)

A weakness between the oblique and the horizontal portions of the inferior constrictor muscle of the pharynx known as the Killian dehiscence provides a gap through which the diverticulum protrudes into the retro-pharyngeal and retro-oesophageal space (Fig. 2.17). This condition is typically found in the elderly, and more commonly in men than women.

The aetiology of pharyngeal pouches is not clearly understood, though in most cases they result from muscular inco-ordination of the inferior constrictor, leading to mucosal herniation.

The patient usually complains of long-standing dysphagia whose severity can be variable and intermittent. Regurgitation of fluids and food debris into the mouth can occur as the pouch empties. The condition can be complicated by respiratory infection since some of the regurgitated food can be inhaled.

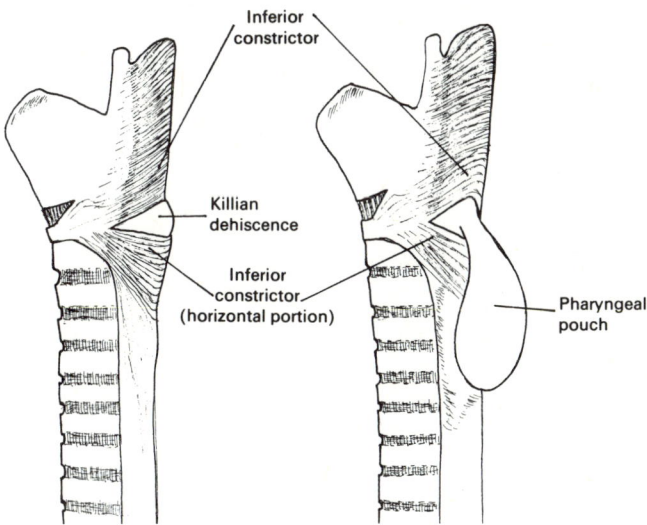

Figure 2.17   Pharyngeal pouch.

Diagnosis is made by barium swallow examination with the contrast medium outlining the pouch. Pharyngo-oesophagoscopy shows the opening of the diverticulum.

Treatment consists of surgical excision of the pouch and repair of the pharyngeal wall. This is sometimes coupled with myotomy of the muscular ring of the crico-pharyngeal muscle (horizontal portion of the inferior constrictor). The operation is carried out through a neck incision.

Following the operation attention is paid to fluid intake and prevention of chest infection. Alimentary tract feeding is resumed a few days after the operation.

Mid- and lower oesophageal diverticula
They are also characterised by variable and intermittent symptoms. In some cases patients remain asymptomatic for long periods.

Diagnosis is established by barium swallow examination which outlines the diverticulum, and endoscopy which shows inflammatory changes (Fig. 2.18).

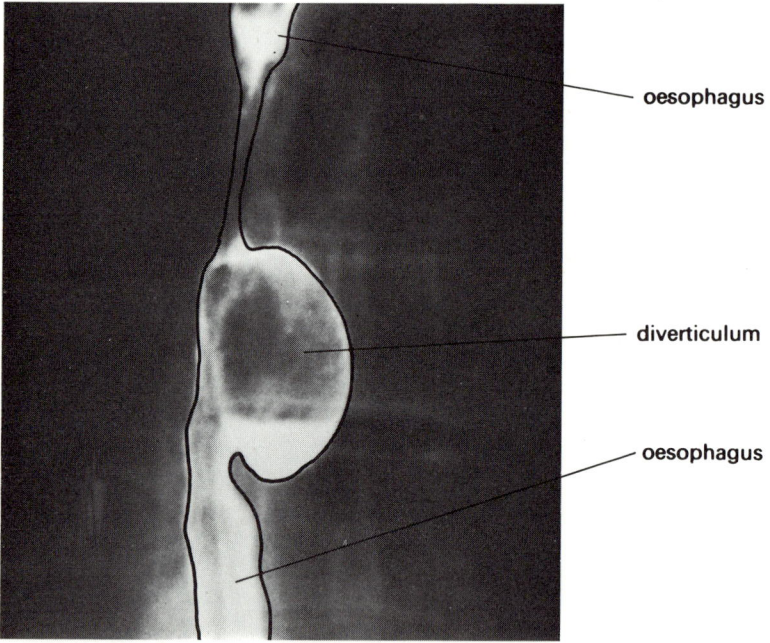

Figure 2.18   Mid-oesophageal diverticulum.

Treatment These diverticula usually respond to conservative medical treatment. *Surgery* may have to be considered in some cases.

CORKSCREW OESOPHAGUS
The condition is so named because of the characteristic appearance of the lower

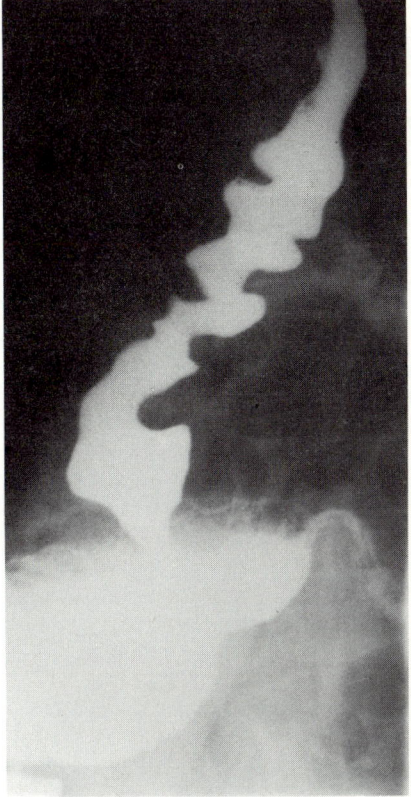

Figure 2.19   Corkscrew oesophagus.

oesophagus on barium swallow examination (Fig. 2.19). The oesophagus displays successive abnormal waves of contraction and relaxation and resembles a corkscrew or a string of pearls.

The aetiology of the condition appears to be related to neuro-muscular disorders of the oesophagus.

The abnormality can be a chance radiological finding or it can be diagnosed after the patient has complained of dysphagia. Severely dysphagic patients require surgical treatment consisting of longitudinal myotomy similar to that for achalasia.

EXTRINSIC OBSTRUCTIONS OF THE OESOPHAGUS

These form a group of heterogeneous conditions, none of them primarily concerned with the oesophagus, but all causing compression on it as a result of their close anatomical relationship to it. Two are of practical importance:

Extrinsic pressure by neoplasms

Neoplastic conditions in the immediate anatomical vicinity of the oesophagus can infiltrate or compress it, causing obstruction to the passage of food. This is particularly common with advanced cancer of the bronchus or the trachea.

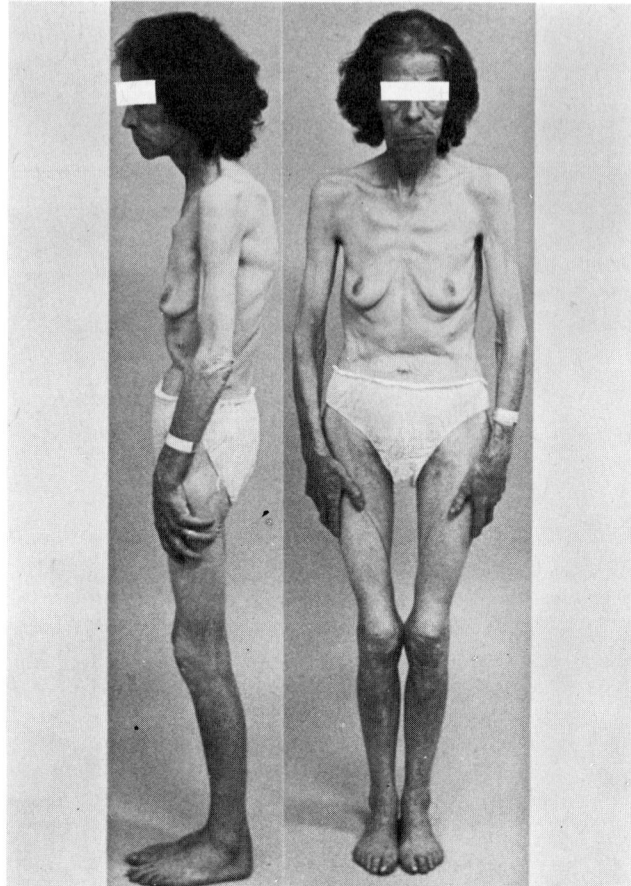

Figure 2.20   Cachetic patient with advanced carcinoma of the oesophagus.

Lymphatic glands surrounding the oesophagus compress it when they become involved by cancer.

Many patients suffering from neoplastic compression of the oesophagus first consult their practitioner when they become dysphagic. It is only in the course of further investigations that the primary neoplasm is discovered.

Management of these patients can be difficult. In many cases when the oesophagus is involved or even simply compressed, surgical treatment of the primary tumour is not possible. Yet the patient has to be offered at least symptomatic relief of the obstruction. Palliation of dysphagia becomes therefore necessary and is carried out in the same way as in cases of advanced and inoperable carcinoma of the oesophagus.

Extrinsic pressure by vascular anomalies

Congenital abnormalities of the aortic arch and its major branches can cause dysphagia. The term *dysphagia lusoria* is applied to the difficulty of swallowing experienced by a patient with these abnormalities.

Aneurysm of the aorta, distorted aorta and left atrial enlargement are known to cause extrinsic compression of the oesophagus.

TUMOURS OF THE OESOPHAGUS

Benign tumours

Benign tumours of the oesophagus are rare, the commonest being leiomyoma. The tumour is usually intramural, originating in the smooth muscle layer of the oesophagus. It can be asymptomatic. When symptoms are present they are generally mild. However, as the growth intrudes into the lumen of the oesophagus or, as is usually the case, when the tumour growth produces an extramucosal compression of the lumen, dysphagia occurs.

Diagnosis This is made from a *barium swallow* which may show a characteristic smooth indentation where the tumour bulges into the lumen of the oesophagus. *Oesophagoscopy* may fail to demonstrate mucosal abnormality but reveals signs related to extraluminal compression and obstruction.

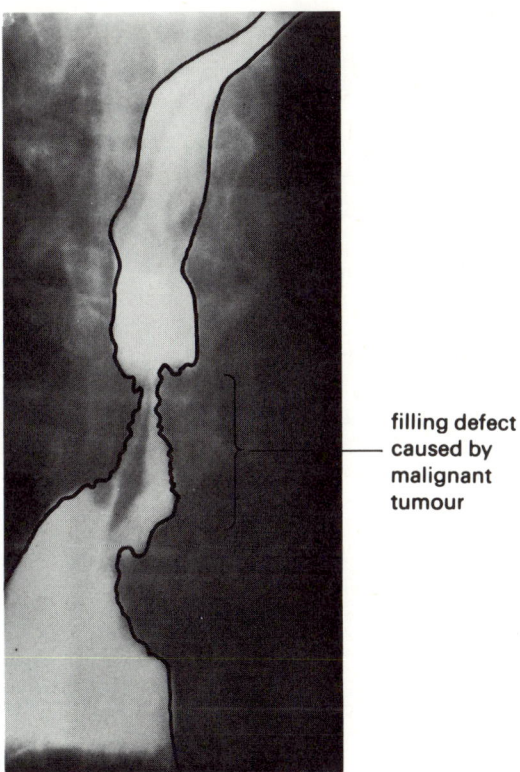

filling defect caused by malignant tumour

Figure 2.21   Barium swallow of the oesophagus.

Treatment The tumour can usually be removed by simple enucleation. Sometimes resection and reconstruction of the oesophagus become necessary.

Malignant tumours

Carcinoma of the oesophagus is the commonest malignant oesophageal tumour, affecting men more frequently than women. In common with many other tumours its aetiology is unknown.

Clinical features and diagnosis   Symptoms are often absent until the disease reaches an advanced stage. Painless dysphagia is frequently the earliest symptom and, at first, is generally to solid foods such as meat (Grade I). As the disease progresses dysphagia becomes more pronounced and extends to semi-solids and purees (Grade II and III). Pain also appears. In extreme cases patients can hardly swallow their own normal saliva. Three modes of treatment are currently adopted: surgery, radiotherapy and a combination of radiotherapy and surgery.

Surgery   Resection of the tumour and reconstruction of the upper alimentary tract are carried out whenever possible. This relieves dysphagia. Although the prognosis is generally poor, surgery offers some chance of a cure.

Radiotherapy is not generally used as the sole method of treatment nor as the first choice in cases suitable for surgery.

Combination of radiotherapy and surgery   In some cases radiotherapy is used pre-operatively, aiming at reducing the size of the tumour and the extent of the lymphatic gland involvement prior to surgery. For resectable cases most centres favour surgery with or without radiotherapy.

Surgical treatment   Resection of the upper, middle and lower portions of the oesophagus is best described under: (1) carcinoma of the cervical oesophagus including the hypopharynx, (2) carcinoma of the thoracic oesophagus, and (3) carcinoma of the lower oesophagus and cardia.

Carcinoma of the cervical oesophagus   Depending on the location of the tumour and the possibility of laryngeal involvement surgical treatment of tumours in the cervical oesophagus can involve total oesophagectomy together with laryng-ectomy. This is followed by the re-establishment of the alimentary tract using the stomach or the colon. A permanent tracheostomy is necessary when the larynx is resected. The operation is best performed by abdominal thoracic and cervical incisions. The abdominal incision gives access to the stomach or the colon which is to replace the oesophagus. The cervical incision is used for excision of the tumour and the reconstruction of the alimentary tract. Through the thoraco-tomy the thoracic oesophagus is resected under vision and the transplanted stomach or colon placed in the posterior mediastinum. Some surgeons prefer not to open the chest. They carry out blind and blunt dissection of the thoracic oesophagus by working through the abdominal and cervical incisions and transplant the stomach or colon blindly within the anterior mediastinum (under the sternum), subcutaneously over the sternum, or in the posterior mediastinum.

Carcinoma of the thoracic oesophagus   The tumour is situated in the oeso-phagus at or near the aortic arch. A right or, rarely, a left thoracotomy approach

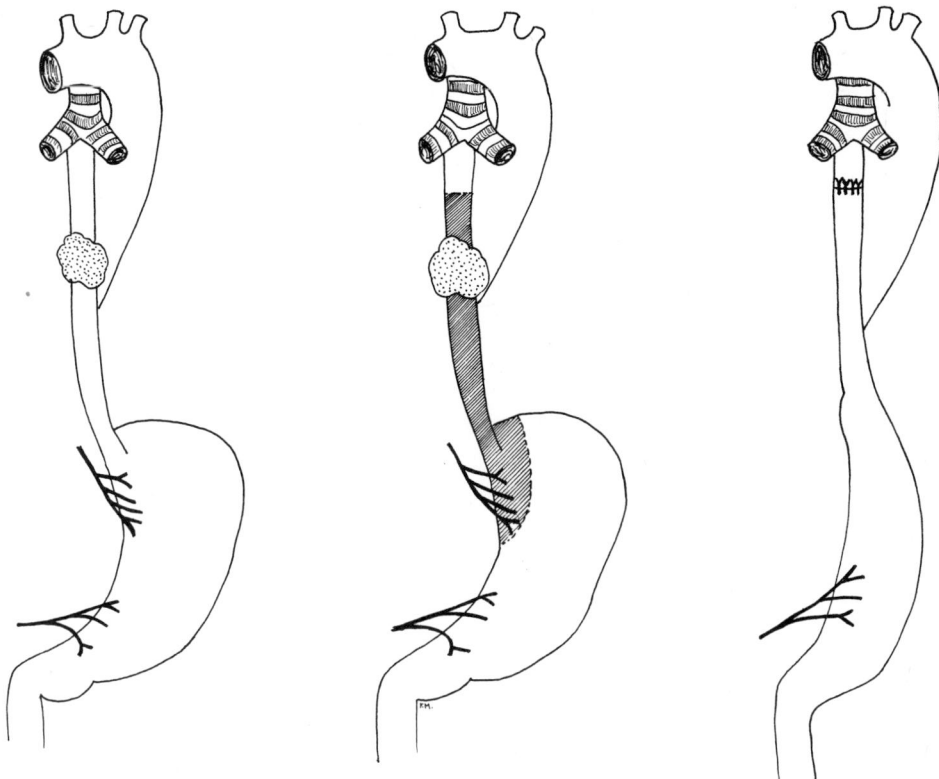

Figure 2.22   Oesophageal resection and reconstruction for mid-oesophageal tumour. Diagram on right shows oesophageo-gastric anastomosis.

is used to excise the tumour and reconstruct the oesophagus. A laparotomy incision is also required to explore the abdomen and to prepare the stomach or the colon to be transplanted. The operation most frequently used in this country is the one pioneered by Ivor Lewis and known as the two-stage oesophagectomy. Both stages are carried out in the same session. In the first stage, with the patient lying flat on his back on the operating table, a laparotomy is performed through an upper abdominal incision. The abdomen is explored and the stomach mobilised. The abdominal wound is closed and the patient is re-positioned for the second stage. For this the patient is placed on his side for right postero-lateral thoracotomy. The oesophagus is explored and mobilised above and below the tumour. The lower mobilisation should involve complete freedom from the hiatal attachment so that the stomach can be drawn into the chest. The portion of the oesophagus bearing the tumour, the whole of the oesophagus below it and a tumour-free portion above it are then excised. An oesophago-gastric anastomosis is carried out (Fig. 2.22).

Carcinoma of the lower oesophagus and the cardia   The tumours of the lower oesophagus and cardia are resected through a left thoracotomy, or a thoraco-

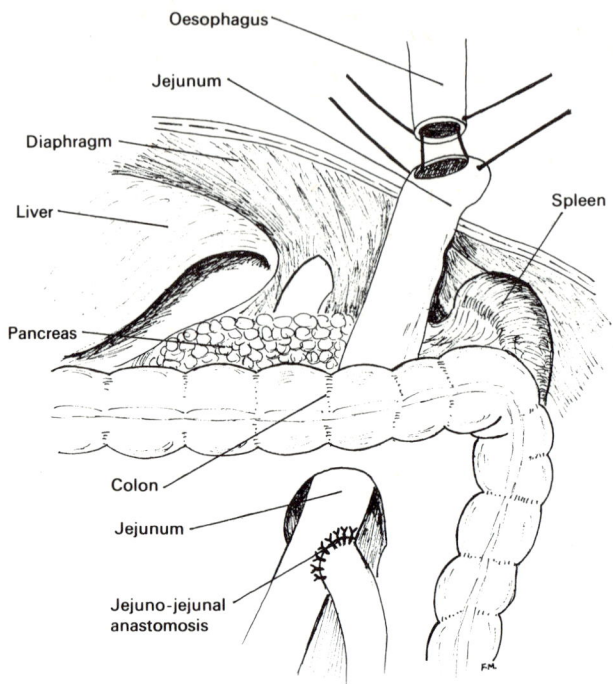

Oesophagus

Jejunum

Diaphragm

Liver

Spleen

Pancreas

Colon

Jejunum

Jejuno-jejunal
anastomosis

Figure 2.23   Roux-en-Y anastomosis.

laparotomy incision. When left thoracotomy alone is used abdominal access is obtained through a diaphragmatic incision. Surgery involves the excision of the tumour-bearing area of the oesophagus together with part of or the whole of the stomach. The reconstruction process depends on whether partial or total gastrectomy is carried out in conjunction with lower oesophagectomy. When partial gastrectomy is carried out an oesophago-gastric anastomosis is established. Alternatively a jejunal or a colonic loop may be transplanted and interposed between the oesophago-gastric remnants. When the whole of the stomach is removed oesophago-jejunal, then jejuno-jejunal, anastomoses are established in the shape of a Y (Roux-en-Y anastomosis) (Fig. 2.23) (see also Chapter 21: *Reconstructive surgery of the oesophagus*, p. 209).

Palliative treatment   When the tumour is unresectable or when the patient cannot be offered excisional surgery on account of his general condition, some palliative method has to be used to by-pass the malignant obstruction. This can be achieved by a by-pass operation or insertion of an indwelling oesophageal tube.

A by-pass operation is particularly suitable for a growth of the lower oesophagus involving the stomach. In this a loop of jejunum is anastomosed to the oesophagus above the growth which remains unresected.

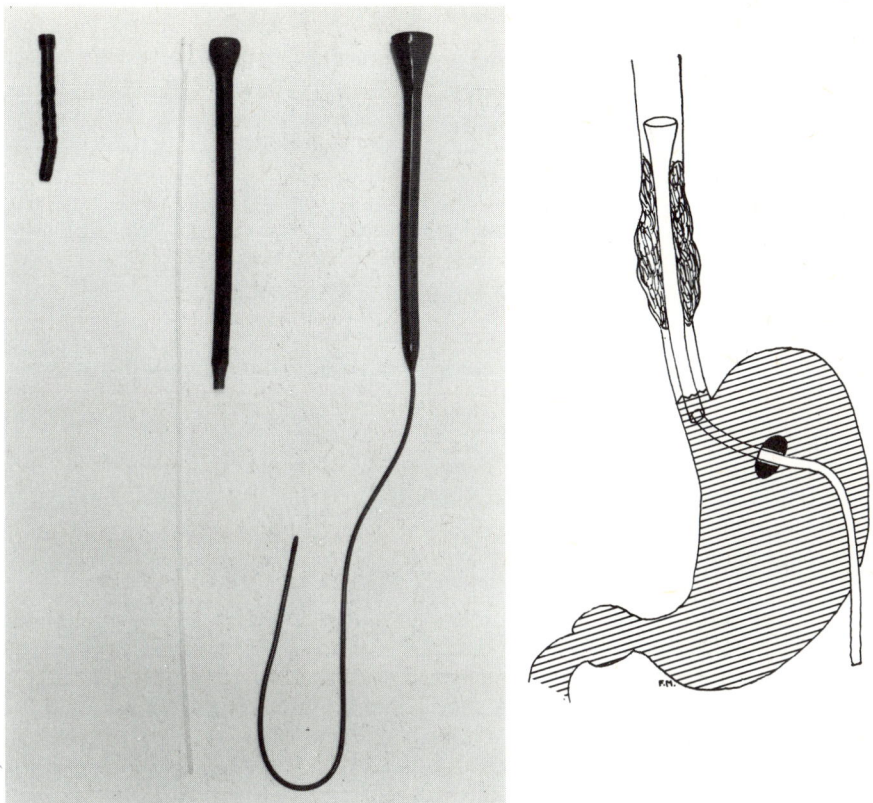

Figure 2.24   (a) Indwelling oesophageal tubes; (from left to right) Souttar, Celestin, Mousseau-Barbin. (b) Position of a Mousseau-Barbin tube by-passing a malignant oesophageal obstruction. The tail section of the the tube is cut-off through the gastrotomy which is then closed.

Insertion of an indwelling oesophageal tube   Three tubes are currently available (Fig. 2.24a): Souttar tube, Mousseau-Barbin tube, and Celestin tube. The basic principle of intubation technique is to place the tube in such a way as to pass through the obstruction with the tube extremities positioned above and below the growth. The bolus thus passes unobstructed through the lumen of the tube. The Souttar tube is a short metal tube, inserted endoscopically. Both the upper and the lower extremities of this tube are positioned within the oesophagus above and below the obstructive lesion respectively. Both the Mousseau-Barbin and Celestin tubes are made of plastic. They are usually inserted by combined endoscopic and surgical techniques through a small laparotomy and gastrotomy. The funnel-shaped upper extremity is positioned in the oesophagus and the lower end adjusted so as to be in the stomach (Fig. 2.24b).

RUPTURE OF THE OESOPHAGUS

Tears and perforations of the oesophagus can be classified under two headings: tears of known and unknown aetiology, commonly referred to as spontaneous rupture.

TEARS OF KNOWN AETIOLOGY

These can occur in many circumstances, most commonly as a result of instrumental perforation, perforation by sharp foreign bodies, or traumatic injuries to the oesophagus.

Post-operative perforations, leaks and fistulae are considered elsewhere (see p. 222).

Instrumental perforation

Though this is a serious complication of oesophagoscopy it is rare when the endoscopist is experienced.

The complication is more likely to arise when a mucosal biopsy is taken, or if forcible dilatation of a stricture is carried out.

When diagnosed early and treated surgically the chances of successful recovery are high. If unrecognised or treated late the outcome is fatal.

Diagnosis and management   The seriousness of instrumental perforation is such that every effort should be made to detect a rupture as early as possible and to prevent further complications arising from the escape of ingested food and fluid into the chest. To this end patients should have a post-oesophagoscopy chest and neck X-ray examination to exclude perforation before being allowed to drink and eat. If a rupture is diagnosed a quick decision should be made about treatment. Perforation can occur in any of the three oesophageal segments, each with distinct signs and symptoms.

Perforation in the neck   This produces severe pain in the neck, surgical subcutaneous emphysema and, after a few hours, cellulitis of the tissue of the neck and muscle contracture. A neck radiograph will indicate subcutaneous surgical emphysema. A day or two after perforation mediastinal cellulitis and abscess formation will result.

Perforation in the mid-thoracic oesophagus   The patient has a severe pain in the back and the chest, usually in the right side. A chest radiograph shows the presence of air in the mediastinal loose tissue and possibly a pneumothorax. If the condition is ignored and left untreated mediastinitis, mediastinal abscess and empyema will follow.

Perforation in the lower oesophagus   The patient complains of severe pain in the lower left chest and upper abdomen. Severe epigastric rigidity, nausea and vomiting can be present. A chest radiograph shows mediastinal emphysema, a left-sided pneumothorax followed by empyema. In order to establish early treatment the nursing staff should be particularly aware of this complication and should notify the medical officer if perforation is suspected. Thorough clinical examination and a chest radiograph are carried out. If a perforation is suspected or confirmed oral food and fluid are withheld. An IV drip is set up and an antibiotic given. Most cases require surgical repair especially when the tear is in the intrathoracic and abdominal oesophagus.

Perforation by sharp foreign bodies
See Chapter 20: *Foreign bodies in the oesophagus*, p. 176.

Traumatic rupture of the oesophagus
Rupture of the oesophagus due to blunt trauma is extremely rare and is a post-mortem finding following severe and fatal injuries.

Rupture caused by penetrating wounds is also rare and usually occurs as the result of stabbing injuries.

Spontaneous rupture
This serious condition occurs without any warning in individuals without any previous history of upper alimentary tract symptoms. The onset is sudden, a bout of vomiting causes excruciating pain in the chest and is followed by persistent pain and dyspnoea.

Typically, the rupture occurs after a heavy meal and the consumption of alcohol. Men are affected more often than women. The tear is usually longitudinal and in the lower 5 to 10 cm of the oesophagus. Oesophageal and gastric contents escape through it into the chest.

Clinical features and diagnosis Sudden chest pain during a bout of vomiting and followed by dyspnoea, especially after a heavy meal, should suggest a possible rupture. On clinical examination surgical subcutaneous emphysema may be noticed in the loose tissues of the neck. There is clinical and radiological evidence of a haemo-pneumothorax. Paracenthesis produces ingested food and fluids.

Treatment Following an early diagnosis surgery is the treatment of choice. A quick but effective pre-operative preparation is imperative. A central venous pressure line is established and dehydration is corrected. A left postero-lateral thoracotomy is carried out. There is usually a great deal of fluid and food debris in the chest. The tear is repaired and the chest drained. Post-operatively fluid, electrolytes and nutrition are given intravenously until healing is complete. Alimentary tract feeding is then gradually resumed.

Incomplete tears of the oesophagus
There are two other varieties of tears which do not involve all oesophageal layers: incomplete or intramural rupture, and the Mallory–Weiss syndrome.

Incomplete or intramural rupture leading to dissection of the oesophagus. In this rare condition the patient develops a double lumen (double-barrelled) oesophagus. The mucosa ruptures and separates from the muscularis, but the latter remains intact. Oesophageal contents do not escape into the mediastinum. The condition is generally treated conservatively. The chest is sometimes drained because of the presence of non-specific pleuritis or pleural effusion. Prognosis is usually good (Fig. 2.25).

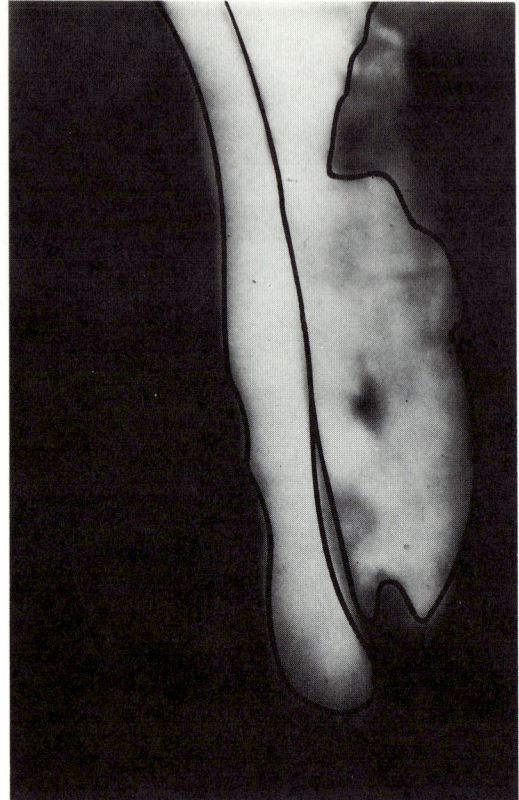

Figure 2.25   Double-barrelled oesophagus caused by intramural rupture.

The Mallory–Weiss syndrome consists of an acute episode of gastro-oesophageal bleeding, presenting itself as massive haematemesis and melena. The condition was first described by Mallory and Weiss (1929) and is caused by a lower oesophageal mucosal tear. The bleeding usually settles after conservative treatment. Occasionally surgery is necessary to arrest the haemorrhage.

OESOPHAGEAL FISTULAE

Congenital tracheo-oesophageal fistula and oesophageal atresia have been discussed in Chapter 20 and therefore only acquired oesophageal fistulae are considered here. They are of particular importance because of their difficult management which involves tedious and painstaking nursing.

Many fistulae are the result of accidental (instrumental) or post-operative perforation. Some follow perforation by a foreign body, others are caused by malignancies. In the latter case fistulae usually communicate with the airways causing severe pulmonary infection. In the other cases fistulae open into either pleural space leading to the escape of air, saliva, fluids and food debris into the chest.

Clinical features and symptoms depend on the location of the fistula, its size, and the presence of an oesophageal obstructive lesion below the fistula. Large tracheo-oesophageal fistulae cause severe aspiration pneumonia and become rapidly fatal. Small fistulae opening into the thoracic cavity present gradual symptoms of empyema particularly when there is no obstruction beyond the opening.

It is convenient to describe fistulae under the following two headings:

FISTULAE BETWEEN THE OESOPHAGUS AND AIRWAYS

They are caused by oesophageal carcinoma infiltrating the trachea or the bronchus and establishing a communication between the alimentary and the respiratory tracts. Alternatively, a malignant tumour of the right or, more often, the left bronchus can invade the oesophagus and create a fistula.

In either case patients are dysphagic and have a productive cough particularly after drinking. Signs of aspiration pneumonia can be clinically and radiologically present. Barium swallow examination, preferably with thin liquid barium or Dianosil, outlines the oesophageal lumen, the fistulous communication and part of the bronchial tree (bronchogram).

Oral feeding and drinking must be stopped as soon as a fistula is suspected. An IV drip is set up, preferably through a central vein. Chest radiography, barium swallow and endoscopic examination confirm the diagnosis, indicate the extent of the condition and therapeutic possibilities. The latter include extensive excision followed by reconstruction, palliative surgery, or non-intervention.

Excision and reconstruction   Oesophago-tracheal (-bronchial) fistulae are very rarely treated by curative surgery which requires excision and reconstruction of the airways and the upper alimentary tract. Definite obliteration of the fistula therefore remains unlikely.

Palliative treatment   It is sometimes possible to offer *palliative surgery*, by-passing the oesophageal fistula. This can be achieved simply through the insertion of a Mousseau-Barbin or Celestin tube in the oesophagus. A more complex approach can be used: the tumour and fistula are left untouched, the oesophagus is anastomosed above the fistula end on with the stomach, or a colonic interposition is used. These palliative measures relieve patients who cough and vomit every time they try to drink.

Non-intervention   This line of management followed in cases of advanced tracheo-oesophageal fistula should not be interpreted as a sign that the patient has been abandoned but as a definite line of management.

Comprehensive nursing care is necessary. This includes full hygiene, prevention or treatment of bed sores, making the patient comfortable, generous use of opiate and cough suppressant. If dysphagia is severe, solids and semi-solids should be avoided. But if dysphagia is mild or moderate the intake of solids should be encouraged as they reach the stomach more safely than less consistent foods and fluids. There should be no restriction as to the quality and type of food.

OESOPHAGO-PLEURAL FISTULAE

These are caused by non-malignant perforation of the oesophagus, mainly as a result of endoscopic accidents and impacted foreign bodies.

If diagnosed early, surgical repair is the treatment of choice. If not, then empyema usually develops. The patient is critically ill and, firstly, requires proper drainage of the empyema together with replacement fluid and electrolytes, plasma and blood transfusion. Subsequent care of the patient includes medical, nursing and nutritional management aiming at closure of the fistula, obliteration of the empyema space and restoration of the alimentary tract function.

Total parenteral nutrition is established through a central vein catheter for long-term intravenous feeding. Drainage volume has to be taken into account in the planning of the daily regime.

Nursing care should include:

1. Strict mouth hygiene, which removes bacteria and keeps the mouth moist.
2. Prevention of chest infection by maintaining the patient in an upright position, and by physiotherapy.
3. Prevention of bed sores, which add to the patient's discomfort but are also a source of loss of protein-rich fluid.

The patient's progress should be regularly assessed. Small fistulae with a limited and well-drained empyema can respond to conservative management. But in many cases, particularly when a stricture is present, reconstructive surgery becomes necessary. Therefore any management of a fistula should also act as possible pre-operative preparation.

21 Surgery of the Oesophagus

This chapter conveniently includes not only surgical procedures, but also preparation, post-operative care and complications of oesophageal surgery. However it should be realised that in many respects these topics cannot be separated from those in pulmonary surgery and therefore it is suggested that the reader also refers to Chapters 14–18, Part 1. Only more specific points are dealt with here.

PREPARATION OF PATIENTS UNDERGOING OESOPHAGEAL SURGERY

Patients undergoing major oesophageal surgery are admitted for pre-operative preparation a few days before surgery. At times it is necessary to admit these patients well before the operation for more elaborate preparation (for example correction of nutritional deficiency).

The preparation of patients can be described under general or special preparation.

GENERAL PREPARATION
This deals essentially with the preparation of patients undergoing any major operation and is similar to that described for lung surgery (see p. 115).

SPECIAL PREPARATION
Simple oesophageal surgery requires an equally simple preparation. However, here we concentrate on the elaborate preparation required by more complex surgery involving resection and reconstruction of the oesophagus, and jejunal or colonic transplant.

Psychological preparation
For many elderly people, eating is one of the few pleasures left. This is denied to oesophageal patients as they are constantly affected by dyspepsia, pain or dysphagia. Many sufferers are depressed and can become mentally unfit for major surgery. Some patients adapt to their alimentary tract problems and may be reluctant to admit them, or seek a remedy.

The nursing staff can do a lot to prepare and comfort the patient. The medical staff can explain the nature of the operation, but nurses should mention some of the necessary but unpleasant post-operative requirements such as intravenous infusion, drainage tubes and naso-gastric catheter. Information should be provided by informal, but informative and clear chats. The object is to reduce fear and secure maximum co-operation after operation.

Hygiene of the mouth and oesophagus

Particular attention should be paid to mouth and dental hygiene before surgery. Repeated antiseptic mouth-wash should be routine. If sepsis is present patients should be referred to a dental surgeon before surgery is undertaken. If nasal and throat swabs have shown the presence of staphylococci, treatment with local nasal antiseptics and appropriate mouth-wash should be prescribed.

In cases of severe dysphagia and oesophageal obstruction the oesophagus can be dilated proximally to the obstructive lesion and can accumulate an enormous quantity of liquid and food debris, forming a pool of stagnant material and pathogenic organisms. Regurgitation and subsequent inhalation (particularly in bed at night and especially during anaesthesia) can cause aspiration pneumonitis and even death by asphyxia (drowning). Furthermore, in the course of oesophageal resection the contents of the oesophagus can easily spill into the chest infecting the suture line and subsequently affecting the patient's recovery. It is therefore important to avoid giving food which cannot be easily swallowed and to carry out oesophageal lavage in severe obstructive lesions. This is done by placing an oesophageal tube and washing the oesophagus using warm saline, twice daily for a day or two (depending on the severity of obstruction) before the operation. In some cases food intake has to be stopped and the patient's oesophagus is given a rest. Parenteral nutrition is then given.

Correction of nutritional deficiencies

On admission many patients are severely dehydrated and are in a marked degree of nutritional deficiency. Some are partially or totally dysphagic. All patients are weighed on admission and regularly thereafter. Their weight is recorded. Patients with complete dysphagia receive intravenous nutrition pre-operatively. Special and appropriate care should be applied to prevent complications and to monitor their progress. Patients not receiving intravenous nutrition are given a high calorie and high protein diet. Their progress is also monitored. Severe anaemia is corrected before the operation.

Treating chest infection

Severely dysphagic patients, particularly the elderly, often suffer from chest infections caused by regurgitation and inhalation of oesophageal contents. Lack of resistance caused by malnutrition, and inability to expectorate contribute to the risk of chest infection. It is important to have a chest radiograph for every patient. It is also important to introduce pre-operative general and chest physiotherapy (see below). A sample of sputum should be sent for microbiological studies and antibiotic sensitivity. It is vital to treat any chest infection before operation.

Physiotherapy

All patients having oesophageal surgery must be given pre-operative physiotherapy and taught to breathe and cough properly. This must involve *general physiotherapy* with active and passive movements, and *specific chest physiotherapy* and breathing exercises, coughing practice, expectoration and postural drainage, using side to side movements, but not the head down (tipping) position.

Bowel preparation

In addition to the usual attention to bowel action and pre-operative enema, special preparation of the bowel is necessary in oesophagectomy patients with colonic substitution. For them the following regime can be used:

1. If the patient is taking food orally a *low-residue diet* should be given for a few days before operation.
2. *Neomycin* is given 1 g/day three times daily starting 72 hours before operation.
3. An enema should be given 72 hours before operation, followed by a twice daily bowel washout.
4. *A final washout* is given the night before operation.

Antibiotics

Prophylactic broad spectrum antibiotics are routine practice in the majority of oesophageal surgical centres. The antibiotics chosen are usually effective against gram-positive and intestinal gram-negative organisms. Patients with pre-operative chest or other infections are given the appropriate antibiotics therapeutically prior to surgery.

Skin preparation

Operations involving the oesophagus can use a thoracic approach alone or a thoraco-abdominal incision. Sometimes separate abdominal and thoracic incisions are made. When the cervical oesophagus is the site of the lesion or when anastomosis involves the cervical oesophagus it may be necessary to have a neck, chest and an abdominal incision. It is therefore important for the surgeon to plan the operation beforehand and inform the nursing staff to prepare the skin accordingly. The following preparation is recommended:

1. Shave the skin on the widest possible area over the chest and the upper abdomen from the shoulders to the umbilicus including the armpits (axillas) and the corresponding area at the back. If surgery is to involve the neck then the latter should be included. It is not necessary to shave the perineum.
2. The night before operation, ensure the patient has a bath.
3. Paint the skin first with a solution of iodine in spirit, then with surgical spirit.
4. Wrap the treated area with a sterile towel (surgical drape); the patient should be sent to the theatre with this towel in position.

Premedication

It is important to check that premedication is written up and administered at the prescribed time.

Collection of documents and case notes

Notes, radiographs, treatment sheets and the signed consent form must be collected in readiness to accompany the patient to the operating theatre.

OESOPHAGOSCOPY

This is a visual examination of the oesophageal lumen by means of an instrument called the oesophagoscope.

THE INSTRUMENT
There are two types of instrument: the rigid, conventional oesophagoscope and the flexible type.

Rigid, conventional oesophagoscope
This type of instrument (e.g. Negus, see Fig. 2.26) consists of a metallic tube with a light carrier which accommodates a fibroptic light attached to a light source by special cable and connector. It allows direct vision of the interior of the oesophagus, therefore localisation of the lesion. It also allows a mucosal biopsy sample to be taken. When necessary bougies can be introduced through the oesophagoscope for dilatation of an oesophageal stricture to be carried out.

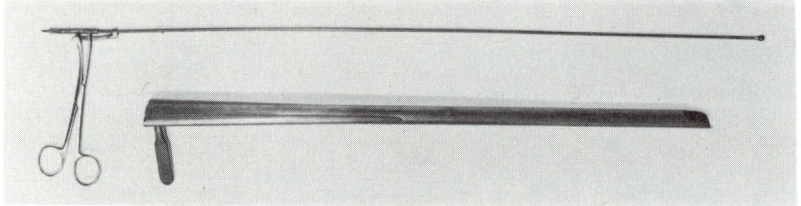

Figure 2.26   *Negus oesophagoscope and biopsy forceps.*

Flexible instrument
This type of instrument (see Fig. 2.27) is a flexible tube carrying within it a fibroptic light and a telescope. It allows indirect (i.e. telescopic) viewing of the oesophageal lumen and can accommodate a pair of very small biopsy forceps capable of providing a sample for histological examination. The flexibility of the

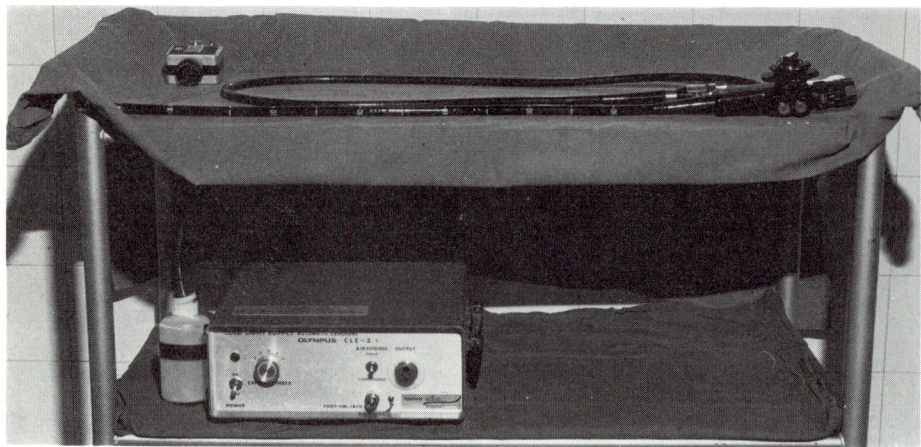

Figure 2.27   *Flexible fibroptic oesophagoscope.*

instrument is particularly convenient for introduction into the stomach thus allowing complete upper alimentary tract examination.

Oesophagoscopy can be carried out under local or general anaesthesia. Whenever possible it is done under general anaesthetic for the patient's comfort.

INDICATIONS FOR OESOPHAGOSCOPY
Indications for oesophagoscopy are:

1. *Diagnostic examination and biopsy.* Either the rigid or flexible instrument is used.

2. *Removal of a foreign body.* This can be carried out successfully through the rigid (conventional) oesophagoscope although in some cases it is done through the flexible oesophagoscope.

3. *Dilatation of a stricture.* Bougies of increasing size are introduced through the rigid hollow instrument and passed through the stricture into the stomach. Dilatation can also be performed using a flexible fibroptic instrument, a guide wire and bougies.

4. *Endoscopic intubation.* Malignant obstruction of the oesophagus can be palliated by endoscopic intubation.

PROCEDURE
The position of the patient depends on the type of instrument used and the surgeon's preference.

The rigid Chevalier-Jackson type of oesophagoscope is generally used with the patient lying flat on his back, the head being straight or slightly flexed. When the instrument is passed through the inlet of the oesophagus the head is then extended.

When the flexible instrument is used the patient usually first lies on his back then is turned over on his left side. Some investigators prefer the patient lying on his back throughout the procedure.

APPARATUS
A complete oesophagoscopy trolley (Fig. 2.28) should have:

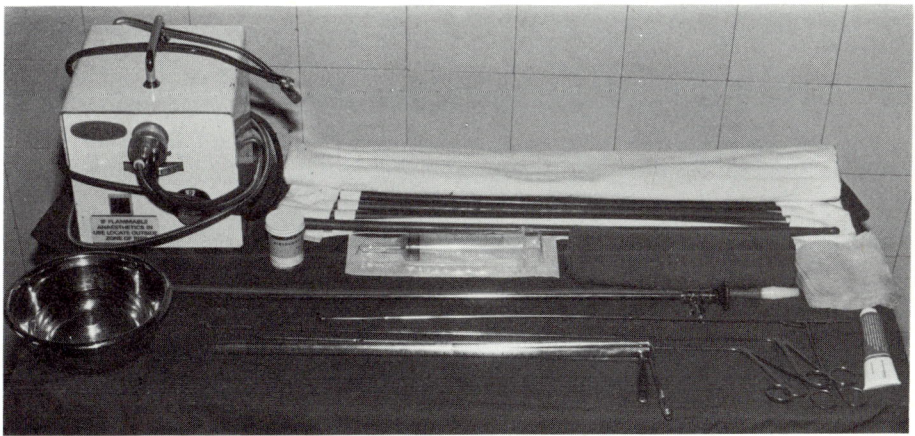

Figure 2.28   Oesophagoscopy trolley. (See text for details.)

1. Oesophagoscope, the size of which depends on the surgeon's preference and the patient's age and sex. This instrument should be checked, particularly the connectors, to ensure it is in good working order.
2. Cable.
3. Light source—fibroptic battery box.
4. Suction machine with suction catheter and connector (and spare suction catheters). The flexible instrument accommodates its own special suction catheter.
5. Biopsy forceps, specimen container and fixative.
6. Telescope (straight).
7. One green towel.
8. 3–4 sterile swabs.
9. Foreign body removal forceps.
10. Gum elastic bougies (full range) or other types. They need not be exposed, just put on the trolley in case they are needed.
11. Bowl containing sterile water or normal saline solution.
12. 500 ml of warm normal saline solution, a bowl and a 50 ml bladder syringe for washing out the oesophagus through the oesophagoscope if necessary. The flexible fibroptic oesophagoscope has its own flushing system.
13. Sterile lubricant.

PREPARATION FOR OESOPHAGOSCOPY

The procedure is explained to the patient who is fasted for general anaesthesia. In cases of longstanding dysphagia or of stricture with the possibility of food debris and liquid in the oesophagus above the stricture, the oesophagus should be cleared of debris and cleaned beforehand by several washouts. This prevents inhalation of regurgitated fluid during the early phase of anaesthesia and allows easy examination of the lumen of the oesophagus. This can be carried out in the ward by introducing a naso-pharyngeal tube and washing out the oesophagus with warm water or saline solution (oesophageal lavage). Suitable pre-medication is given. Radiographs and case notes should be kept ready to accompany the patient to the endoscopy theatre.

OESOPHAGOSCOPY AFTER-CARE

The patient is returned to the ward after full recovery from anaesthesia when the pulse, respiration and blood pressure should be monitored. Particular attention should also be paid to any possible accidental perforation of the oesophagus. This complication is rare, but its seriousness is such that patients should not be fed until clinical and radiological clearance has been given. In all cases an erect, antero-postero chest radiograph—as well as a lateral neck radiograph—should be taken, and subsequently examined by the medical officer, before any fluid or food is given.

COMPLICATIONS OF OESOPHAGOSCOPY

Even in the expert's hands, oesophagoscopy can be complicated by minor and major problems. For instance, following oesophagoscopy, a minor sore throat is often a common occurrence but discomfort can soon be alleviated with the help of washouts. The only real serious complication is *perforation* and if unrecognised or untreated is almost always fatal. It is for this reason that nurses involved in the care of patients undergoing oesophagoscopy must be aware of this complication so as to be able to diagnose it and treat it as soon as possible (see Chapter 20, *Rupture of the oesophagus*, p. 198).

After a biopsy sample, using punch biopsy forceps, minor bleeding may occur but it soon stops. However, more serious haemorrhaging can follow in patients with particular bleeding tendencies or clotting factor deficiencies. Post-oesophagoscopy bleeding should always be reported to the medical officer.

RECONSTRUCTIVE SURGERY OF THE OESOPHAGUS
(Oesophagoplasty)

When a portion of the oesophagus is removed, continuity of the alimentary tract can be established either by joining the remaining two ends together (direct anastomosis), or by bridging the gap with a section of the small or the large intestine (reconstruction by interposition using intestinal transplant). Direct end-to-end oesophago-oesophageal anastomosis is not a practical undertaking but oesophago-gastric anastomosis is possible and has the advantage that the stomach has a particularly favourable vascular anatomy allowing its mobilisation without a great loss in blood supply. There are therefore two principal methods of upper alimentary tract reconstruction following oesophagectomy: reconstruction by direct oesophago-gastric anastomosis; and reconstruction with interposition of an isolated loop of small or large intestine.

SURGICAL APPROACH

As the oesophagus is essentially a cervico-thoracic structure, it can be surgically approached through a cervical or thoracic incision. However, as the reconstructive procedures involved require stomach, jejunum or colon a laparotomy is also necessary. Approach to the cervical oesophagus is effected through a collar type of incision (Fig. 2.29). Approach to the thoracic oesophagus is

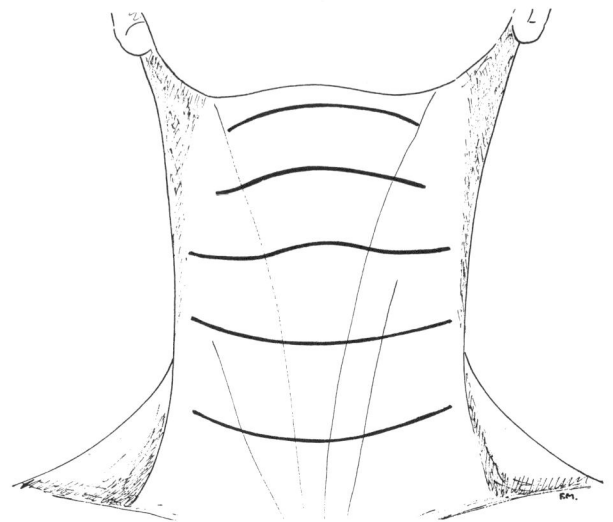

Figure 2.29   Neck incisions at different levels.

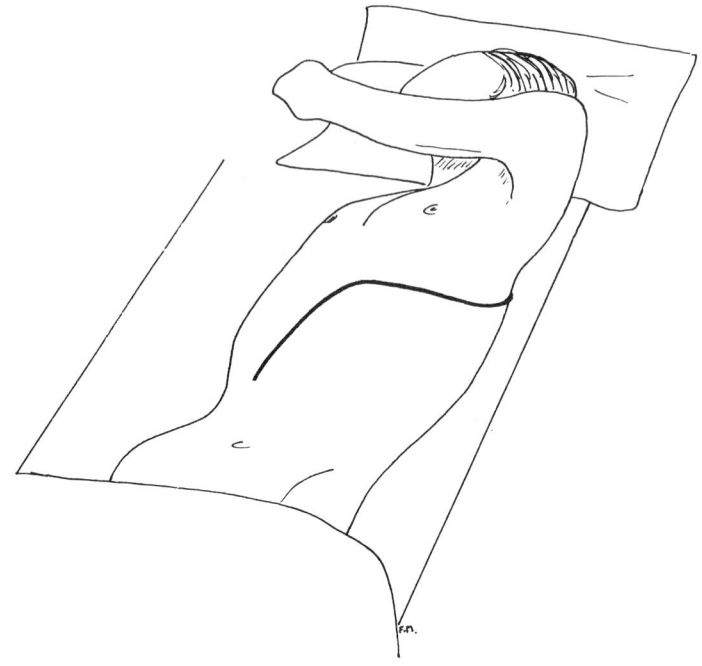

Figure 2.30   Thoraco-laparotomy incision.

effected through a right or a left thoracotomy (Fig. 1.69). Right thoracotomy gives the best access to the upper and mid thoracic oesophagus. Left thoracotomy gives the best access to the lower oesophagus and has also the further advantage of providing access to the oesophageal hiatus and the upper abdomen through the diaphragm.

Access to the abdomen for oesophageal reconstruction purposes can be obtained either by standard upper abdominal incisions or by incision of the diaphragm (left thoracotomy). Alternatively, abdominal access can be obtained through a thoraco-laparotomy (Fig. 2.30) using an extended thoracotomy incision over the upper abdomen with or without division of the costal margin. This provides convenient access to the lower oesophagus as well as the stomach and the upper abdominal viscera.

OESOPHAGECTOMY AND OESOPHAGO-GASTRIC ANASTOMOSIS
The purpose of the operation is to excise a length of oesophagus and to establish continuity by anastomosing the divided end of the remaining part of the oesophagus to the stomach. The choice of surgical approach depends on the anatomical location of the disease and on whether the anastomosis is to be placed in the neck, the upper or the lower chest.

It should be noted that one-, two- or three-stage oesophagectomy does not mean that the operation is carried out on separate occasions, instead it refers to different stages within the same operation involving one, two or three separate surgical approaches.

Based on the above considerations, oesophagectomy and oesophago-gastric anastomosis are carried out using essentially three methods:

1. Resection and reconstruction within the left chest (one-stage oesophagectomy).
2. Resection and reconstruction within the right chest (two-stage oesophagectomy).
3. Resection and reconstruction in the neck (three-stage oesophagectomy).

Resection and reconstruction in the left chest
This operation is carried out for lesions of the lower oesophagus. It is also suitable for upper gastric lesions.

A thoraco-laparotomy approach is necessary to allow (1) sufficient mobilisation of the oesophagus above the lesion and to the level selected for anastomosis, and (2) access to the upper abdomen in order to free the stomach for transplantation into the chest for anastomosis to the oesophagus.

The patient is put into a left oblique or left lateral position. A left posterolateral thoracotomy or left thoraco-laparatomy is carried out. In cases of thoracotomy alone access to the abdominal cavity is obtained by diaphragmatic incision. In either case the stomach is mobilised. Some of the gastric vessels are ligated and divided but the right gastric vessels and the arcade along the greater curvature of the stomach are preserved. The upper part of the stomach is passed through the hiatus after it has been enlarged to allow easy passage. The cardiac end of the stomach is divided and closed. The oesophagus is then divided above the lesion. End-to-side oesophago-gastric anastomosis establishing continuity of the alimentary tract is then performed (see Fig. 2.22). The wound is repaired and a drain placed in the left pleural space.

Resection and reconstruction within the right chest
This operation (see Fig. 2.22) is particularly suitable for neoplasms of the mid-thoracic oesophagus. It was pioneered by Ivor Lewis and is named after him. It consists of two stages carried out sequentially in the course of one operation.

Stage 1 consists of a laparotomy through an upper abdominal incision with the patient in a supine position. The stomach is completely mobilised but not completely devascularised. All the vessels contained within the gastro-splenic and the gastro-hepatic omentum are ligated and divided, as are the left gastric vessels. The right gastric vessels and the arcade running along the greater curvature of the stomach are preserved, as the survival of the mobilised stomach depends on them. Complete mobilisation of the stomach involves freeing the abdominal oesophagus from the hiatal fibro-cellular tissues. The hiatus is enlarged and the abdomen closed.

Stage 2 The patient is turned over to the right for right thoracotomy. The oesophagus is mobilised and the stomach is delivered into the chest. The cardiac end of the stomach is divided and closed. Next, the oesophagus is divided above the oesophageal lesion and anastomosed end-on to the side of the stomach (end-to-side oesophago-gastric anastomosis).

Resection and reconstruction in the neck
This is suitable for the resection of neoplasms of the upper thoracic and lower cervical oesophagus. The operation is carried out in three stages:

Stage 1   Laparotomy is carried out through an upper abdominal incision. The stomach is completely mobilised as in a two-stage oesophagectomy.

Stage 2   A right thoracotomy is carried out with the patient in a right lateral position. The oesophagus is mobilised and the stomach delivered through the hiatus into the chest. The right chest is then closed with a drain left in the pleural space.

Stage 3   The patient is placed back in a supine position. Access to the cervical oesophagus is obtained through a neck incision. The lower cervical oesophagus is mobilised, the whole of the thoracic oesophagus is resected, so is the lesion-bearing section (either thoracic or cervical). An end-to-side oesophago-gastric anastomosis establishing continuity of the upper alimentary is made. The neck space is drained and the wound closed.

RECONSTRUCTION WITH INTERPOSITION
The vascular anatomy of the jejunum and the colon is such that they can be transplanted away from their normal anatomical location yet be attached to their vascular pedicles. They are both supplied by vascular arcades which in turn are supplied by long vascular trunks placed at intervals in a fan shape and converging to the root vessels. This arrangement makes the jejunum and the colon ideal transplant material for oesophagoplasty. The principles of oesophageal reconstruction using jejunal or colonic interposition can be described as follows.

Access to the oesophagus and to the upper abdomen is obtained respectively through a correctly positioned thoracotomy and laparotomy. The choice of surgical approach and incisions depends both on the site of the lesion and on the position of oesophageal anastomosis. With these considerations in mind a one-, two- or a three-stage operation is planned.

A suitable length of jejunum or colon is selected for the transplant, the suitability being dependent on vascular arrangement. This loop is isolated by dividing its proximal and distal ends. The continuity of the bowel is re-established by jejuno-jejunal or colo-colic anastomosis. The cardiac end of the stomach is divided and closed. Resection of the oesophagus is carried out by dividing it above the diseased part. The isolated intestinal loop attached to its vascular pedicle is passed through the hiatus. The proximal end of the loop is anastomosed to the cut end of the oesophageal remains forming an oesophago-jejunal/oesophago-colic anastomosis. The distal end of the loop is then attached to the stomach by jejuno-gastric/colo-gastric anastomosis. The gap between the remaining oesophagus and the stomach is bridged with jejunum (or colon) (Fig. 2.31 and Fig. 2.32).

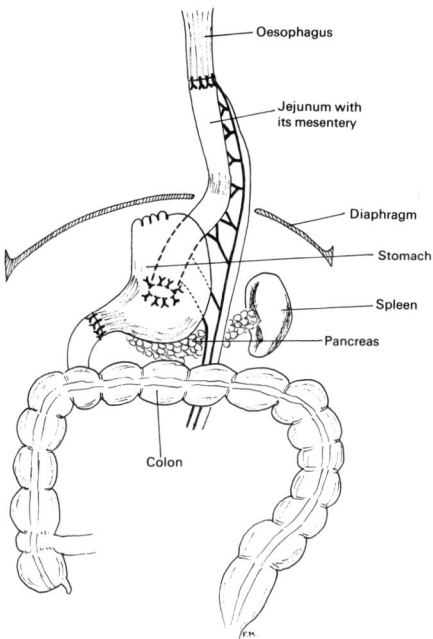

Figure 2.31   Jejunal interposition used in reconstruction of the oesophagus following resection.

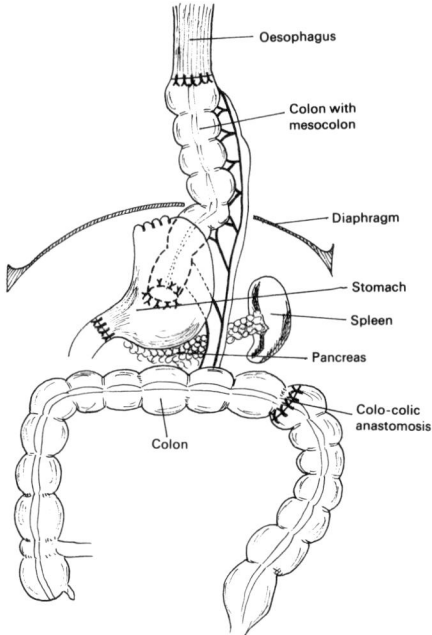

Figure 2.32   Colon interposition used in reconstruction of the oesophagus following resection.

POST-OPERATIVE CARE FOLLOWING
OESOPHAGEAL SURGERY

The success of oesophageal surgery is greatly dependent on (1) post-operative management, (2) co-operation of the patient, and (3) understanding the problems which can arise in this type of operation. Besides the pain and discomfort associated with operative wounds and drainage tubes and the inconvenience of the drips, the patient does not receive food or drink by mouth for the first few days. It is therefore easy to see how some patients can become apprehensive, depressed or even indifferent to their recovery. It is the duty of every one, particularly nurses, to reassure the patient and be well informed about problems in this type of surgery.

Post-operative care aims are to help in the patient's complete recovery, i.e. healing of all surgical wounds and return home as an ambulant and independent individual in good general condition, and to re-establish the full function of the alimentary tract which has been surgically reconstructed. However, the general principles of post-operative care of these patients can best be described under general nursing care, with particular reference to thoracotomy and laparotomy, and special care and nutritional management.

General nursing care includes *early* (the first 48 hours) and *late* post-operative care.

EARLY POST-OPERATIVE CARE

Early post-operative care of oesophageal patients is similar, in many respects, to that of pulmonary cases (see Chapter 17) and should therefore be thought of under the following:

1. Transfer and return to the ward.
2. Initial base-line observations and instructions.
3. Periodic monitoring of vital functions.
4. Early management.

While the monitoring of the patient's progress is always essential to post-operative care as a whole, it cannot be too strongly emphasised that basic nursing care must not be forgotten.

Some aspects of early management are different for oesophageal patients, and these are outlined below.

Additional management

Psychological management   It is important for nurses to establish a good rapport with the patient at all times, particularly in the early post-operative phase when the patient is disturbed by surgical trauma and by numerous tubes and catheters. The presence of a naso-gastric tube and the inability to take fluid by mouth adds greatly to discomfort. It is obviously not possible to eliminate discomfort but doctors and particularly nurses can reduce anxiety and pain. This is one of the nurse's most important tasks.

Sedation, rest and sleep   Once fear and pain are relieved by reassurance and analgesics most patients relax, and require little or no additional drugs. Some individuals, however, may be restless and go through sleepless nights. Before administering more analgesics and strong sedatives attention should be paid first to respiration and the state of oxygenation. It must be ascertained that respiration is not obstructed or hampered. Nurses should also check other possible accessory sources of irritation such as the displaced naso-gastric tube curled up at the back of the mouth, the intercostal drain dragging and hanging down, the drip running under the skin or tissueing. While it is not advisable for patients (particularly elderly ones) to lie in bed and vegetate, it is essential to ensure sufficient sleep and rest. One of the most efficient ways is to prevent noise in the ward.

General hygiene   This is part of basic nursing care and is mentioned here as its importance can never be over-emphasised. Bed-bathing once a day (or more if necessary) is part of the patient's hygiene, adds to his comfort and plays an important part in preventing infection.

Oral hygiene   It is essential to pay particular attention to oral hygiene with regular mouth washes using an antiseptic solution. A mild antiseptic fluid should be provided for mouth rinsing only as patients are not allowed to swallow any liquids. More formal mouth and teeth cleaning is carried out by nurses.

Drains   Abdominal and chest drains should be handled with care and secured. Volume and type of drainage should be recorded. The abdominal drain is usually removed at an early stage (24 to 48 hours). The chest drain is removed when it has stopped draining, which is usually 48 to 72 hours after the operation.

IV catheter   An IV catheter is inserted at the time of surgery or prior to it for supplementary feeding. Special attention should be paid daily to the site of the catheter, and each time the drip set is changed. Any inflammatory changes should be reported to the medical staff. Nurses should take great care in all manipulations connected with parenteral feeding in order to avoid sepsis.

Laboratory procedures

Chest x-ray   A chest radiograph is taken soon after the operation and repeated daily while the drainage tubes are still *in situ*.

Blood test   Blood electrolytes and urea should be estimated daily while intravenous feeding is in progress. Haemoglobin and PCV are estimated frequently.

Sputum   A sample should be sent to the laboratory for bacteriological studies and sensitivity to antibiotics.

Urine   Volume of urinary output is carefully recorded. If there is any suspicion of abnormality of micturition and/or of the urine itself a sample is sent to the laboratory for biochemical and microbiological testing.

LATE POST-OPERATIVE CARE
This deals with the period between the second post-operative day and the patient's discharge from the hospital. Again the aim is to monitor the patient

clinically, radiologically and by laboratory measures to ensure that satisfactory progress is maintained and that complications do not occur.

Clinical management

Temperature, pulse and BP are recorded 2 or 3 times a day. The patient's chest is examined daily by the medical officer to ensure satisfactory expansion of the lungs. The abdomen is examined for evidence of bowel sounds, distension and other physical findings. Micturition is checked and the possibility of residual volume in the bladder, particularly with male and older patients, is kept in mind. Legs and dependent areas are inspected for oedema. Calves are examined for pain; tenderness for early detection of phlebothrombosis. The patient is weighed, daily if possible, but at least every 2 or 3 days, and his weight recorded.

In addition to the recording and analysis of physiological measurements, day-to-day overall observation of the patient provides a clinical impression which is an important evaluation of the progress made. This obviously requires experience and practice, but is largely dependent on knowledge of and interest in the patient. Nurses should realise that in this respect they are very important members of the team.

Particular attention should be focused on:

1. *Naso-gastric tube.* It should not be displaced and should be carefully aspirated as instructed until its withdrawal.

2. *Physiotherapy.* Full chest physiotherapy should be continued during the post-operative period until the patient's discharge.

3. *Hygiene.* Continuous attention should be paid to general and mouth hygiene.

4. *Nutrition.* At some stage, generally about 5 to 7 days after the operation alimentary tract nutrition is resumed (see *Nutritional Management*, below). It is necessary to provide patients, particularly those with oesophago-gastrectomy or oesophago-gastric anastomosis, with frequent small meals. A high calorie and protein diet should be planned.

5. *Bowels.* Some patients develop diarrhoea and pass loose motions after an oesophagectomy. Others experience irregularities to which they are not accustomed. These should be noted and reported to the medical staff.

6. *Mobilisation.* Following early post-operative mobilisation, full mobilisation is encouraged.

Laboratory procedures

A chest radiograph is taken daily while the drainage tubes are still *in situ*, again just after their removal, then repeated at weekly intervals unless otherwise indicated.

Blood tests   As long as the IV drip is the only or main route of nutrition for the patient, a daily blood electrolyte and biochemical profile, particularly urea estimation, should be carried out and deficiencies checked, particularly for potassium. Later estimation is carried out every 5 to 7 days, or more frequently if indicated by abnormal findings. Full blood count, including Hb, PCV estimation and white cell count should be carried out every 4 to 5 days. Patients with total gastrectomy require special estimation and supply of folic acid and vitamin B12.

SPECIAL CARE AND NUTRITIONAL MANAGEMENT

The seriousness of complications following oesophageal surgery, particularly oesophageal resection and reconstruction, is such that every effort should be made to prevent them. The most serious ones are related to anatomical and physiological disorders of the alimentary tract itself, and consequent bio-chemical and nutritional disturbances. It is therefore important to draw up a rational plan of nursing care with full knowledge of the operative procedure and possible complications.

FLUID BALANCE

Daily requirements should be determined and prescribed by the medical team. The task of delivery is left to the nursing staff. Fluid given (or, more precisely, taken by the patient) and fluid lost must be accurately charted. The naso-gastric volume of aspirate should not be forgotten. The patency and position of the tube must be questioned if, in the early post-operative phase, no fluid is aspirated on successive occasions. As long as fluids are solely supplied intravenously, the adequacy of the supply should be checked clinically and by laboratory tests. Electrolyte imbalance judged by serum biochemical profile should be checked daily and reported to the medical staff so that abnormalities may be corrected.

NUTRITION

Nutritional requirements should also be precisely evaluated and prescribed by the medical staff. It must be realised that even without any complications patients will require a high-calorie and high-protein diet taking account of pre-existent deficiencies as well as of post-operative increased demand, in addition to the individual's basic requirements. Experience has shown that in un-complicated cases 40–45 kcal/kg b.w. and 0.20–0.25 g N/kg b.w. are adequate amounts following oesophagectomy (see Chapter 29).

Accurate delivery of intravenous nutrients, which in the first post-operative days are the patient's only food supply, is the responsibility of the nursing staff.

When alimentary tract feeding is resumed four aspects of food should be constantly checked: consistency; volume taken at each meal, and frequency of meals; quality; total intake.

Consistency of food

The aim of reconstructive surgery of the oesophagus is to re-establish swallowing of normal-consistency food. After operation this is achieved by gradually increasing the consistency of food. The patient is on IV fluids and nutrition for the first 5 to 7 post-operative days following which a liquid diet is gradually introduced. Supportive intravenous feeding is gradually withdrawn until complete independence from parenteral nutrition is achieved. Consistency is then gradually increased to solids.

The following pattern is characteristic:

Grade I — Liquid diet (2 to 3 days).
Grade II — Pureed and liquidised food (2 to 3 days).
Grade III — Semi-solids (2 to 3 days).
Grade IV — Solid diet.

Many patients are eager to eat and to move to Grades II and III, but are frightened to eat solids as a result of pre-operative dysphagia. Some will swallow normal-consistency food while in hospital but return to soft food 'as a preventive measure' as soon as discharged.

Particular attention has to be paid to this aspect of post-operative feeding.

Volume of food taken at each meal

In many patients the reconstruction of the alimentary tract has been done with the stomach (see *Reconstructive Surgery of the oesophagus*, p. 209). In such cases the stomach has become more of a food duct and less of a food container. It is therefore not difficult to realise that these patients cannot accommodate a large volume (quantity) of food. Daily requirements and intake should be divided into five or six meals instead of the customary three.

Quality of food

Digestion and absorption of food are adversely affected by resection and reconstruction of the oesophagus. During the late post-operative phase, and even after discharge, diet should be high in proteins and calories. Vitamins and minerals should not be forgotten. A dietitian should be involved in the design of meals.

Total intake

While guide lines have been published on the calorie and protein requirements of patients just after surgery, little attention has been paid to the convalescing period. The nurse in charge should, with the help of the medical staff and the hospital dietitian, take the responsibility of establishing a diet designed for each patient.

PREVENTION OF DISTENSION

Whatever substitute is used to replace the oesophagus the reconstruction of the alimentary tract requires one or more anastomotic procedures. It is important to prevent distension of the alimentary tract, particularly distally to the anastomosis. The collection of fluid and gases distally to the anastomosis has several deleterious effects. Firstly, the suture line is strained. Secondly, distension interferes with the blood supply of the substitute and therefore affects the site of anastomosis, which is the most vulnerable part. Thirdly, the distended bowel interferes with fluid and electrolyte exchange and creates imbalances which, if not checked, lead to disturbances of body fluid generally and eventually the patient's biochemical death.

There are many ways in which bowel distension can be prevented. For example, in many instances, a naso-gastric tube is placed at the time of operation. In the early post-operative phase it is aspirated regularly. In between aspirations the tube should not be clamped or spigoted as it is important to allow constant escape of the gas which can cause distension. One method is to connect the open end of the tube to a 20–50 ml syringe from which the plunger is removed, and fix it in a vertical position to the patient's pillow, allowing sufficient free length of tube for the patient's movement.

Particular attention should also be paid to the bowels' peristaltic activities. Alimentary tract feeding should therefore not be resumed before definite bowel sounds are heard and peristaltic functions are evident. Additionally, among electrolytes, potassium has a particular importance in relation to neuro-muscular activity of the bowel. Serum potassium level should be checked regularly (this should be done daily whilst the patient is receiving total parenteral nutrition). Abnormality of serum potassium should be corrected promptly.

PREVENTION OF REGURGITATION

When part of stomach is used as a substitute for the oesophagus the stomach as such no longer exists to accommodate normal food volume. The lower portion of the oesophagus with its sphincteric action is also resected. With it the mechanism responsible for the prevention of gastric juice into the oesophagus disappears. The relevant consequences of this are:

1. Regurgitation of gastric contents into the oesophagus, with an accompanying sensation of nausea or vomiting, particularly when the patient is in a reclining position.

2. Reduction of effective gastric capacity with consequent rejection (vomiting), when too much food is taken at once or when passage through the pylorus is delayed as usually is the case temporarily after an oesophagectomy (which includes vagotomy).

It therefore follows that particular attention should be focused on (1) provision of small meals at frequent intervals, (2) early mobilisation of patients and propping up while in bed, (3) checking that intestinal movement is taking place, and (4) prescribing anti-reflux drugs.

CONSTIPATION AND DIARRHOEA

The majority of patients after oesophagectomy tend to develop constipation. Some patients, particularly after gastrectomy, develop diarrhoea. The absence of stomach, direct entry of food into the jejunum and rapid transit are the main contributing factors. Changes in bowel habits should be observed and noted by the nursing staff. They can be prevented to some degree by regular, small and frequent meals. Constipation can be prevented by attention to dietary intake, but, if persistent, as the last resort it can be treated by suppositories, small enemas, and aperients. Diarrhoea can similarly be prevented by careful attention to the diet and by smaller and more frequent meals.

Medication such as Codeine Phosphate may be necessary in some cases. If diarrhoea persists, a sample of stools should be collected for microbiological studies.

CORRECTION OF ANAEMIA

As the absorption of vitamin B depends on the intrinsic factor of the stomach, patients undergoing total gastectomy should be given a regular supply of this vitamin intra-muscularly in order to prevent macrocytic (pernicious) anaemia. Anaemia of microcytic type can be present in other patients. This is most likely due to insufficient absorption of iron which is dependent on the acid gastric juice.

COMPLICATIONS OF OESOPHAGEAL SURGERY

One of the aims of post-operative care is to prevent complications which could jeopardise recovery or at least delay it. Most post-operative complications set in gradually and are therefore easily detectable in their early phase when proper post-operative monitoring is carried out.

Some complications are similar to those following any major surgery, pulmonary surgery in particular (see Chapter 18). Others are specific to oesophageal surgery and are discussed under the two headings of (1) early complications arising within the first 48 hours, and (2) late complications developing after two days.

EARLY COMPLICATIONS

Shock

Oesophageal resection and reconstruction entail extensive surgery, often in elderly patients who are likely to develop post-operative shock. The cause of shock should be investigated and early treatment applied (see Chapter 18).

Haemorrhage

Bleeding can be external or internal. Intrathoracic bleeding is usually detectable from recovery of blood in the pleural drains whose patency and working order must be constantly checked. Abdominal haemorrhage can be intraperitoneal or intraluminal. The latter can be diagnosed from constant recovery of blood in naso-gastric aspirate. At all times in the post-operative phase signs and symptoms of haemorrhage, viz. air hunger, pallor, increased pulse rate and lowering of arterial and central venous pressure must be kept in mind. When bleeding is suspected the medical officer should be summoned (see Chapter 18).

Respiratory complications

These complications can occur in the following circumstances:

1. Difficulty of effective spontaneous breathing immediately after operation is usually due to extensive surgery and interference with thoracic, abdominal and diaphragmatic muscle mechanisms in an often elderly and emaciated patient.

2. Respiratory failure in patients suffering from bronchitis and emphysema.

3. Retention of excessive normal or abnormal broncho-pulmonary secretions causing atelectasis and hypoxia.

Particular attention should be paid to early post-operative chest physiotherapy and monitoring of respiration.

Subcutaneous surgical emphysema

This is a rare complication in this type of surgery. Its presence indicates malfunctioning of the pleural drainage tube.

Cardiac complications

Many oesophageal patients are frail, elderly and often with latent heart disease. Some are manifestly hypotensive, others suffer from myocardial ischaemia. Dysrhythmic complications, particularly atrial fibrillation and ventricular extrasystoles, can develop soon after surgery. Proper monitoring of heart rate and rhythm is essential in these patients. Blood biochemical profile with particular reference to potassium level should not be forgotten in patients most likely totally dependent on intravenous infusion. A number of patients require prophylactic or therapeutic digoxin (see Chapter 18).

Urinary retention, anuria and early renal failure

Retention of urine, particularly in elderly patients, after extensive surgery of any type is not unusual. It gives discomfort and affects renal performance. It should be avoided and, if necessary, relieved by catheterisation.

Oliguria and anuria are diagnosed only when urinary catheterisation proves low output or absence of production of urine. Even transient oliguria should be notified to the medical staff since renal failure occasionally occurs as an oesophageal complication. When renal failure is fully developed dialysis has to be considered with all the risks involved (see Chapter 18).

Iatrogenic complications

They arise because of nursing mismanagement. It may be surprising to find them listed here as, strictly speaking, they should not occur. However, as they do occasionally happen, they should be mentioned in order to prevent them.

Intravenous infusion complications Early in the post-operative phase intravenous infusion of fluid, blood and nutrient solutions are essential. In most cases central venous catheterisation is carried out before or during operation to establish post-operative IV infusion. Sometimes a more peripheral vein is used.

Extrusion of the IV catheter not only deprives the patient of essential requirements but also increases morbidity through extravasation of fluids into the tissues. The patient is put through unnecessary additional discomfort when the catheter is re-inserted. When this complication arises the drip should be stopped, the medical officer summoned, the time and cause of catheter displacement noted, and the IV infusion drip re-established. Occlusion of the catheter occurs occasionally. It is unlikely to happen if continuous flow of the infusion is ensured, and the intravenous set and infusion bottles changed with due care. When the catheter is blocked the medical officer should be informed. It is sometimes possible to unblock the catheter without replacing it.

Naso-gastric tube complications After major oesophageal resection and reconstruction many surgeons insert a naso-gastric tube. This is kept in position for the first few post-operative days with the object of periodic aspiration of stagnant fluid or gases collected in the upper alimentary tract. The catheter should not fall out or be accidently withdrawn. Should this occur, it must not be re-inserted by nurses without the knowledge of the medical staff.

The naso-gastric tube may become blocked. Beside causing unnecessary discomfort to the patient blockage leads to misleading calculations of fluid balance.

LATE COMPLICATIONS

This group of complications occurs after the first two post-operative days.

Because they arise late in the post-operative phase their development can be prevented or aborted by early diagnosis and correct therapy.

Pulmonary complications

Sputum retention, pulmonary collapse, chest infection and even lung abscess are constant problems requiring particular vigilance. Effective physiotherapy and antibiotics given prophylactically and therapeutically can prevent them to a large extent. Sputum must be sent to the laboratory for macrobiological studies.

Cardio-vascular complications

Atrial fibrillation   It is not uncommon in elderly patients. A post-operative ECG is carried out on all patients which indicates the nature of dysrhythmia.

Phlebothrombosis and pulmonary embolus   They are prevented by early mobilisation and the prophylactic administration of anti-coagulants pre- and post-operatively.

Oedema   Post-operative general and peripheral oedema in patients undergoing oesophagectomy used to be common. This complication is nowadays infrequent because attention is paid pre- and post-operatively to nutrition, blood protein and albumin. Most cases of oedema are caused by hypoproteinaemia (see Chapter 18).

Alimentary tract complications

These complications are obviously important in cases of oesophagectomy and oesophageal reconstruction.

Ileus   Relative or complete lack of peristaltic activity results in abdominal distension, vomiting and copious aspirate from the naso-gastric tube. Electrolyte imbalance often accompanies the condition. Ileus can be averted or treated early through attention to details such as regular abdominal examination for bowel sounds, check on fluid and electrolyte balance.

Irregular bowel action   Constipation in some patients and diarrhoea in others are not infrequently observed when alimentary tract feeding is resumed. Constipation is prevented and treated by attention to diet and by assistance in the form of suppositories or small enemas; laxatives are avoided. Diarrhoea is particularly common following total gastrectomy. Codeine phosphate for a few days is the usual remedy. Infective diarrhoea must be recognised and treated accordingly. The medical officer's attention should be drawn to it before the patient becomes dehydrated.

Anastomotic leaks and fistulae

These are serious complications whose treatment requires patience and care on the part of the medical and nursing staff. Fortunately they are now uncommon. Apart from faulty surgical techniques the cause can be malnutrition, pulmonary collapse and infection.

Malnutrition   The importance of nutrition in oesophageal surgery cannot be overemphasised. It should be noted that many dysphagic patients are undernourished and that increased post-operative demands should be met with an increased supply of both calories and proteins.

Lung collapse   Maintenance of expansion should be checked clinically and radiologically. Chest physiotherapy is carried out throughout the post-operative period.

Infection   Prophylactic and therapeutic antibiotics are necessary to prevent infective complications which are a major contributory factor to leaks.

Diagnosis of a leak can be confirmed by (1) presence of purulent effusion in the chest, (2) radiological examination: the site of leak and/or fistula is outlined on the X-ray plate by the swallowed radio-opaque medium, and (3) swallowing methylene blue (10 ml ampoule in 20 ml water) when the drainage tube is still *in situ*. The dye is recovered in the drainage bottle when a leak is present.

When diagnosis is confirmed every effort should be made to achieve closure, either surgically or conservatively. Staff should prepare themselves and the patient for a long period of intensive and tedious care. Many leaks and fistulae can be satisfactorily closed provided there is no distal obstruction, and provided malnutrition, fluid imbalance and infective elements are kept under control. The policy with regard to the treatment of such complications is determined by the surgeon in charge of the case.

Infective complications

These complications can be conveniently classified as wound sepsis, chest infection (i.e. pulmonary infection and pleural empyema), urinary infection, abdominal subphrenic abscess, and septicaemia.

Every precaution should be taken to avoid infective complications by observing general principles of asepsis and eliminating known risk factors.

Once infection is fully developed the following steps should be taken:

1. Identification of the site of infection.
2. Identification of the pathogenic organisms and of their sensitivity to antibiotics (samples of pus, discharge and blood are sent for culture and sensitivity testing).
3. Drainage of pus if it collects (e.g. in empyema and subphrenic abscess).
4. Correction of anaemia and nutritional deficiencies.
5. Appropriate antibiotic therapy.

It must not be forgotten that intravenous infusion is a likely route for introducing micro-organisms into the body and that nutrient solutions are perfect media for the proliferation of organisms. It is also important to remember that lowering of resistance following major surgery leads to greater susceptibility to infection (see also Chapter 18).

Anaemia

It is not uncommon for oesophagectomy patients to become anaemic during the late post-operative phase. Blood count should be checked every three to four days and anaemia corrected, usually by blood transfusion.

Late malnutrition

Some patients deteriorate in the late post-operative phase. They lose their appetite. Loss of weight, general asthenia and hypoproteinaemia soon follow. If this is ignored they are likely (particularly when they are elderly) to deteriorate further, to become bed-ridden and die.

Their nutritional needs should be attended to as soon as they start showing a slight deterioration. Supplementary parenteral or enteral feeding should be re-introduced as a means of breaking a vicious circle.

Bed sores

Many patients with carcinoma of the oesophagus have lost a considerable amount of weight and are in a severe state of nutritional deficiency on admission. They are likely to develop bed sores post-operatively. Bed sores are painful and distressing and should be prevented by early mobilisation and extra nursing care, when fully developed joint medical and nursing efforts should be concentrated on their treatment.

Part 3
The Diaphragm, Mediastinum and Trachea

This section deals with three specific topics not covered in Parts 1 or 2: Diaphragm, Mediastinum and Trachea. All these topics are either directly connected with, or the pathological condition become part of, the mediastinum.

22 The Diaphragm

The diaphragm is the main inspiratory muscle. It is a double domed-shaped musculo-tendinous structure separating the abdominal and the thoracic cavities (Fig. 3.1). It is formed by a club-shaped tendon, the central tendon, into which are inserted muscle fibres, arising from the lowest six ribs, the bodies of the first, second and third lumbar vertebrae and the sternum.

The muscle fibres arising from the lumbar vertebrae form two distinct muscular pillars known as the crura. The oesophagus passes through an

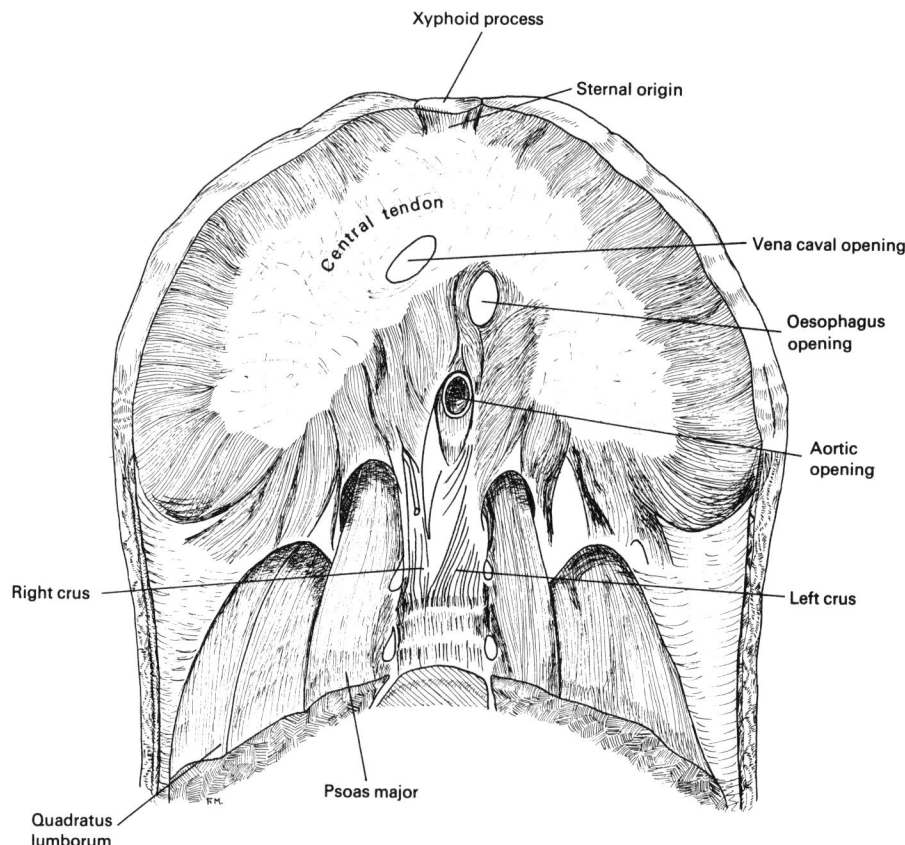

Figure 3.1 Diaphragm viewed from its abdominal aspect. Note *encircling fibres of the right crus round the oesophageal hiatus.*

226

opening produced by the looping fibres of the right crus. This is known as the oesophageal hiatus. The tendinous part of the diaphragm has an opening for the inferior vena cava. Other openings in the diaphragm allow the passage from the thorax to the abdomen behind the crura. The diaphragm is innervated by the phrenic nerves with some contribution from spinal nerves.

INVESTIGATIONS OF DIAPHRAGMATIC DISEASES

In view of its anatomical position the diaphragm is liable to be affected by thoracic and abdominal diseases. It therefore follows that clinical manifestations of diaphragmatic involvement may not be due to primary diaphragmatic conditions.

SYMPTOMS
Diaphragmatic diseases give rise to very few specific symptoms, but pain and dyspnoea are worthy of special mention.

Pain
Pain in the lower chest to the tip of the shoulder is typical of diaphragmatic involvement. The pain is within the distribution of the phrenic nerve whose fibres innervate the diaphragm and whose roots are derived from the cervical spinal nerves (principally the 4th). The latter also provides sensory nerves to the skin of the shoulder thus accounting for shoulder pain of the phrenic nerve.

Dyspnoea
This condition is always present when the diaphragmatic function is seriously interfered with by whatever changes.

RADIOLOGICAL INVESTIGATIONS
Radiological investigations are particularly relevant for elucidation of diaphragmatic diseases. These include:

1. *Antero-posterior and lateral chest radiography* indicates the position (e.g. elevation) and the anatomical integrity of the diaphragm.
2. *Screening* (fluoroscopy) is useful for checking on the evidence of movement of the diaphragm.
3. *Barium examination* of the gastro-intestinal tract demonstrates displacement of the viscera below the diaphragm, herniation through it and other diaphragmatic abnormalities.
4. *Pneumo-peritoneum* (i.e. air in the peritoneal cavity. In this case, air is introduced for diagnostic purposes, and is then re-absorbed by the body), followed by an appropriate X-ray film of the lower chest and upper abdomen, can demonstrate the diaphragmatic domes on each side between two air-filled spaces, namely the lungs above and the air contained in the abdomen below.

CONGENITAL DIAPHRAGMATIC HERNIAE

They result from congenital diaphragmatic defects whose understanding becomes clearer with some preliminary knowledge of the development of the diaphragm.

The separation of abdominal and thoracic cavities in the embryo follows the formation of the diaphragm from the fusion of several components, four of which are particularly important:

Septum transversum   A mesodermal septum appearing ventrally (anteriorly) and separating the pericardium from the peritoneal cavity. This becomes the central tendon and anterior part of the diaphragm. The septum transversum grows dorsally (posteriorly) to meet the dorsal mesentery.

Dorsal mesentery of the foregut (mesentery of the oesophagus and stomach) is joined by muscles fibres forming the crura and the postero-central part of the diaphragm.

Muscle fibres originating from primitive body wall muscles (myotomes) attach themselves to the part mentioned above. In this manner the partition becomes complete except for an area of the postero-lateral circumference on either side of the chest. Through this area called the pleuro-peritoneal canal the abdomen is connected to the chest.

Pleuro-peritoneal membrane   A pair of structures (one on either side) forms the postero-lateral part of the diaphragm and completes the partition by closing the pleuro-peritoneal canal.

HERNIA THROUGH THE DIAPHRAGMATIC DOME
In this condition, a portion or an entire hemi-diaphragm may be congenitally absent. Complete absence of one diaphragmatic leaf (dome), usually the left, is a serious anomaly in which there is gross herniation of upper abdominal viscera in the chest. The hernia is usually diagnosed at birth because of its presentation as a respiratory distress syndrome.

Diagnosis is confirmed radiologically and surgical repair undertaken urgently. Meanwhile decompression by naso-gastric tube aspiration is carried out as a life-saving measure.

POSTERO-LATERAL DEFECT HERNIA (Synonym Bochdalek)
This occurs through the postero-lateral defect which is a vestigal embryonic pleuro-peritoneal canal (Fig. 3.2). It is normally closed before birth by the pleuro-peritoneal fold on each side, completing the separation of the thoracic and abdominal cavities. The hernia is usually discovered during infancy or childhood. Pain, respiratory distress and bouts of vomiting are the main symptoms. Chest radiography and barium contrast studies usually confirm diagnosis.

Treatment consists of surgical reduction of the hernia and repair of the defect.

ANTERO-LATERAL DEFECT HERNIA
This hernia (synonym substernal or sub-sternocostal or Morgagni's hernia) occurs through an antero-lateral defect situated behind the sternum and the

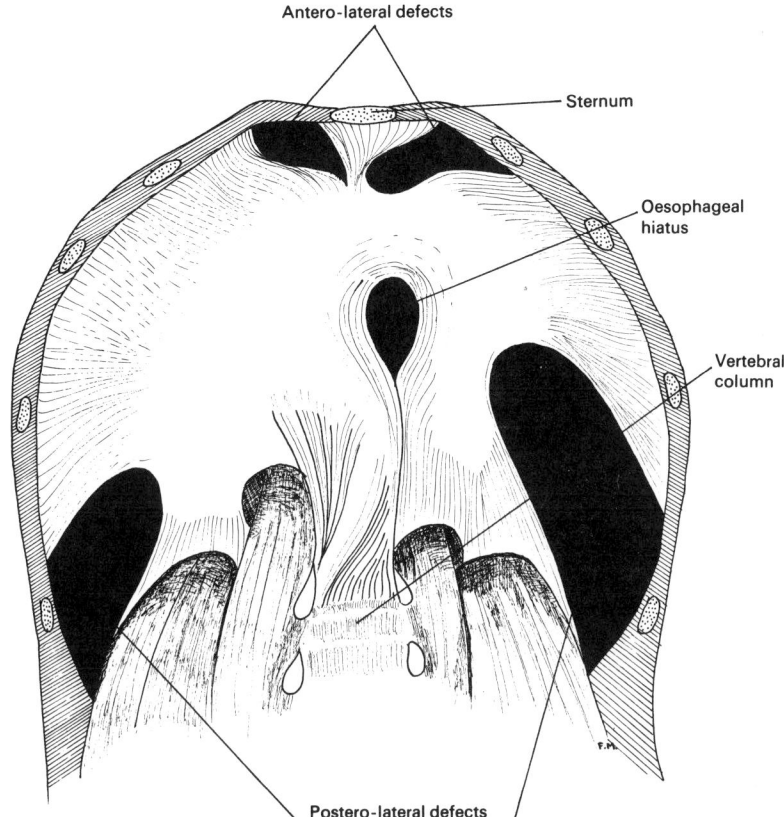

Antero-lateral defects

Sternum

Oesophageal hiatus

Vertebral column

Postero-lateral defects

Figure 3.2 Diaphragmatic congenital deficiencies providing passage for diaphragmatic herniae. Diaphragm is viewed from its abdominal aspect.

costal margins and is due to the absence of sterno-costal diaphragmatic fibres (see Fig. 3.2). A sac which can contain the omentum, stomach and colon is herniated into the chest.

The patient can be asymptomatic and remain undiagnosed for many years. Sometimes there are mild symptoms of discomfort and epigastric pain. Exceptionally there are symptoms of acute pain and vomiting. A chest radiograph and barium contrast studies confirm the diagnosis of obstruction. Surgical repair is done either through an upper abdominal laparotomy or, preferably, through thoracotomy. The hernia is reduced and the defect closed.

PRINCIPLES OF NURSING MANAGEMENT IN DIAPHRAGMATIC HERNIA

Some patients with congenital diaphragmatic hernia will be emergency admissions requiring surgery soon after their arrival. In these circumstances little time may be available for investigations and preparation. It is important to pay particular attention to the following:

1. To place a naso-gastric tube and aspirate gastric contents to reduce distension and obstructive symptoms.

2. To establish an intravenous drip to replace the fluid loss which is the consequence of vomiting and dehydration.

3. In severe cases shock may be present and a central venous pressure line should be inserted to assess the extent of fluid loss.

4. Serum electrolytes should be estimated and a sample of blood should be sent to the laboratory for Hb and PCV estimation, blood grouping and cross-matching for the operation.

Post-operatively the maintenance of fluid and electrolyte balance, and the expansion of the lungs are of particular importance (see Chapter 17).

EVENTRATION OF THE DIAPHRAGM

This is a condition in which one leaf of the diaphragm is abnormally high and thin. The upper abdominal organs are displaced upwards. The condition may be congenital or acquired as a result of phrenic nerve involvement in disease process. In the latter case the diaphragm is paralysed.

In infants and children eventration can cause respiratory difficulties. In adults they are less frequent. Upper gastro-intestinal symptoms can be present. When an operation is indicated it is performed through the appropriate thoracotomy. Plication and re-inforcement of the diaphragm with fascia or a prosthesis may be required.

TRAUMATIC INJURIES OF THE DIAPHRAGM

Blunt trauma and more rarely penetrating injuries are the cause of laceration and rupture of the diaphragm with herniation of the intra-abdominal viscera.

Pain, dyspnoea and shock followed by obstructive gastro-intestinal signs are usually present. A chest radiograph shows collapse of the lung and herniation of viscera into the chest.

When the tear is on the left side and hollow viscera protrude into the chest, radiography readily establishes the diagnosis (Fig. 3.3).

Tears on the right side and those accommodating the omentum may not be so readily diagnosed. Occasionally a ruptured diaphragm can escape immediate recognition.

Treatment consists of the appropriate thoracotomy, replacement of the intra-abdominal viscera, and repair of the diaphragm. This is usually carried out as soon as the patient is prepared and after anti-shock treatment, blood transfusion and introduction of a naso-gastric tube and evacuation of stomach contents.

MANAGEMENT

The patient is admitted following a chest injury and is examined radiologically. As many patients with diaphragmatic rupture are shocked, anti-shock measures should be applied. A central venous pressure catheter should always be inserted. Besides venous pressure monitoring it is used for fluid, plasma or blood

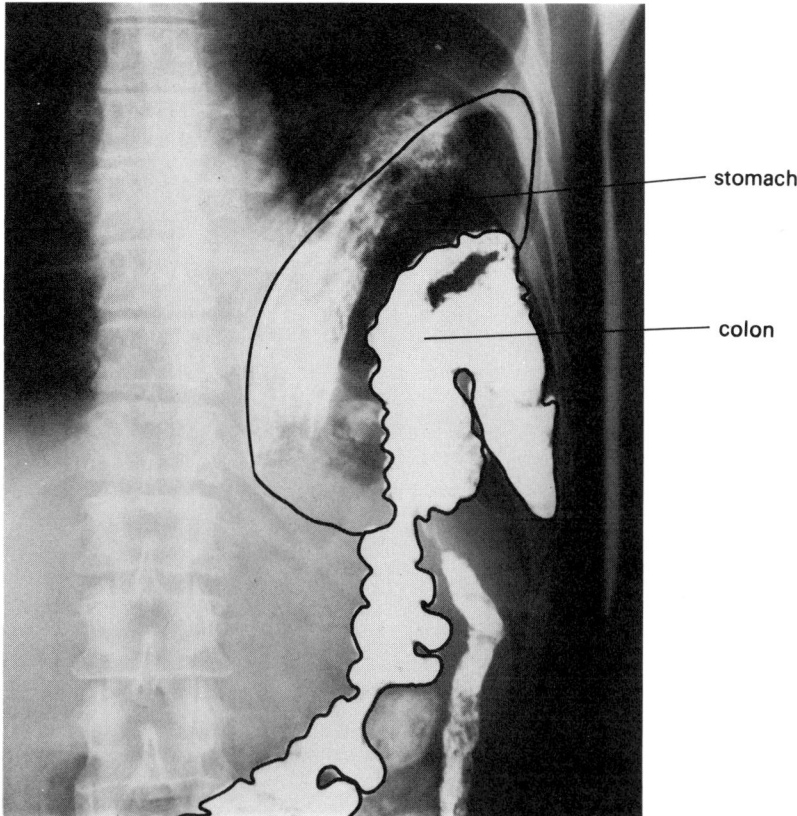

stomach

colon

Figure 3.3 Traumatic rupture of the diaphragm showing the stomach and part of the colon herniating into the chest.

transfusion. Many patients are grossly dyspnoeic because of the distended stomach within the chest and resulting pulmonary collapse. A naso-gastric catheter is inserted and aspirated.

When diagnosis is in doubt the patient should be monitored by frequent recordings (at the beginning half-hourly, then depending on progress) of arterial and venous blood pressure, pulse and respiration. The naso-gastric tube is aspirated intermittently. In the interval it is left open into a bag to allow escape of air and excess fluid only.

When immediate operation is indicated the patient is prepared for surgery through a right or left thoracotomy as indicated.

In an uncomplicated rupture the herniated abdominal viscera are reduced into the abdomen and the diaphragm is repaired. In a diaphragmatic tear complicated by intra-thoracic or abdominal visceral injuries appropriate measures have to be taken in addition to the above repair and reduction. This may in rare cases involve extending a thoracotomy incision and performing a laparotomy in order to obtain suitable surgical access.

Following operation the general care for thoracotomy patients should be applied (see Chapter 5, *General Care of Pleural drains*, p. 48). Expansion of the lung by physiotherapy and proper management of chest drains prevents complications. Particular attention should be paid to provision of intravenous water, electrolytes and nutrition until establishment of oral feeding and adequate intake. Fluid balance should be carefully monitored taking into account urinary output, naso-gastric suction volume and pleural drainage, when present. Serum electrolyte should be estimated daily and abnormalities corrected.

23 The Mediastinum

The space in the middle of the chest situated between the two pleural cavities is known as the mediastinum (Fig. 1.2a,b, p. 3). It is occupied by the heart, the great vessels, the thymus gland, the trachea and oesophagus and extends from the sternum anteriorly to the vertebral column posteriorly. Its superior boundary is indicated by a line drawn between the first thoracic vertebra and the upper border of the sternum. The diaphragm forms the inferior boundary. Laterally the mediastinum is separated from the left and right pleural spaces by the mediastinal pleurae.

For descriptive purposes the mediastinum can be divided into four compartments, i.e. the anterior, middle, posterior and superior.

The anterior mediastinum is situated in front of the heart and pericardium, and contains the thymus gland, pericardial fat and the lymphatics.

The middle mediastinum is the space occupied by the heart and its pericardial covering.

The posterior mediastinum is situated behind the heart and pericardium and accommodates the oesophagus and the aorta, the thoracic duct, the azygos system of veins and the vagus nerves.

The superior mediastinum is that portion above the pericardium which accommodates (1) the thymus gland (or its remnants), (2) superior vena cava and the innominate veins, (3) arch of the aorta and its major branches, (4) trachea and its bifurcation, (5) upper part of the oesophagus and (6) thoracic duct.

It is important to appreciate that the superior mediastinum is continuous with the anterior and posterior mediastinum and that the tissue spaces of the superior and posterior mediastinum communicate with the neck spaces in front of the trachea and behind the oesophagus, respectively. Therefore an infection in the neck behind the pharynx and oesophagus can easily spread into the chest.

In this chapter we deal with the mediastinum and some of its contents, with the exclusion of the heart and the great vessels. The oesophagus is described on p. 166.

METHODS OF STUDY

The anatomical position of the mediastinum and its close relationship with the structures within this space are such that one may refer to the mediastinum as the crossroads of the chest. Conditions affecting the structures within the mediastinum can manifest themselves in a variety of ways. Mediastinal pathology can be investigated radiologically and endoscopically.

RADIOLOGY

An antero–posterior and lateral chest X-ray shows abnormalities of the mediastinum without indicating the precise nature or position of the disease. However, some specific pathological conditions, tumours in particular, can cast a shadow on the chest X-ray film in a definite compartment of the mediastinum, thus facilitating diagnosis.

More specialised and sophisticated radiological investigations are necessary to indicate pathological conditions associated with specific structures. These include tomography, barium swallow, aortography, pulmonary angiography and caval venography. These investigations are helpful as pathological changes affect the normal anatomical arrangements and relationships of these structures within the mediastinum.

ENDOSCOPY AND BIOPSY

Bronchoscopy and oesophagoscopy aid diagnosis of mediastinal pathology in view of the anatomical position of the trachea, the main bronchi and the oesophagus within the antero-superior and the posterior mediastinum respectively. Mediastinoscopy and biopsy of the mediastinal glands provide a more precise diagnosis.

MANIFESTATIONS OF MEDIASTINAL LESIONS

Many mediastinal lesions, in particular benign tumours and cysts, may be discovered in the course of a routine X-ray. The manifestations of a mediastinal condition depend on the size, nature and anatomical situation of the lesion. When the structures of the superior mediastinum are primarily affected the presenting symptoms are respiratory and venous compression. Cough, dyspnoea and stridor are usually present. This may be particularly pronounced in children and infants. Venous congestion and progressive oedema of the face and neck indicate innominate vein and superior vena caval compression. When the posterior mediastinum is involved oesophageal compressive symptoms are prevalent.

SUPERIOR MEDIASTINAL (superior vena caval) SYNDROME

This condition, which when fully developed is characterised by dyspnoea, cyanosis and oedema of the face and neck with grossly congested veins, is very distressing for the patient. At times, the whole of the upper part of the body is oedematous and displays prominent veins.

These signs are more prominent on waking in the morning and indicate compression of superior vena cava and interference with venous return to the heart.

Symptoms such as pain in the chest and hoarseness indicate the involvement of the sensory and laryngeal nerves. The involvement of the inferior cervical and superior thoracic sympathetic ganglia produces symptoms and signs known as Horner's Syndrome. This consists of ptosis of the eyelid, enophthalmos and a contracted pupil, together with warm and dry facial skin on the affected side.

The superior mediastinal syndrome is in effect a manifestation of compression of structures within the upper thorax. In almost all cases the compression is caused by a malignant tumour (usually bronchial carcinoma).

DIAGNOSIS AND MANAGEMENT

Clinical examination alone confirms the compression syndrome. Further specialised investigations are necessary to determine the aetiological diagnosis. These include radiological and endoscopic investigations. Superior caval venography outlines the site of the venous obstruction and in particular the anatomy of the venous system within the thorax (Fig. 3.4).

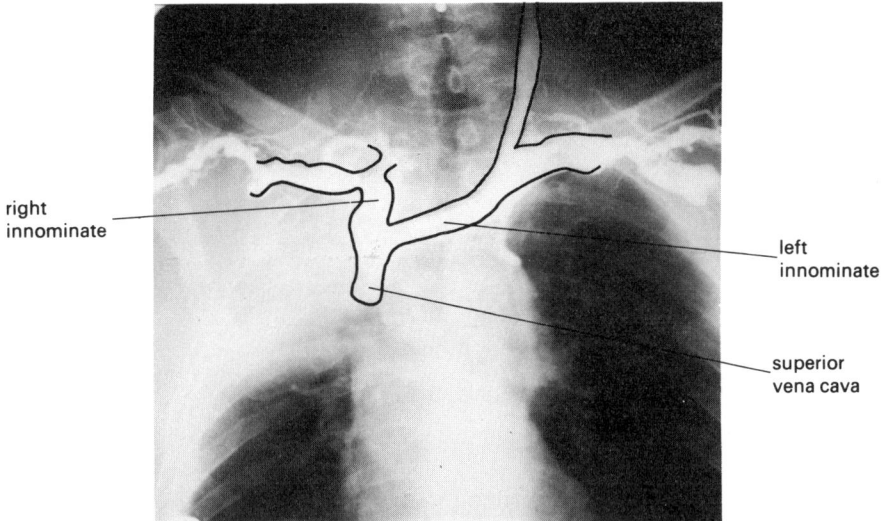

right
innominate

left
innominate

superior
vena cava

Figure 3.4   Superior caval venography showing complete obstruction of the superior vena cava by a tumour involving the mediastinum.

Management of these patients is difficult because the obstructive syndrome can progress rapidly and the primary cause, which in the majority of cases is extensive malignant neoplasia, is difficult to treat. By the time the obstructive syndrome becomes apparent the neoplasm is often unresectable. The obstructive symptoms and signs can be temporarily alleviated by diuretics and other symptomatic treatment.

When venography shows an obstructed vena cava but a patent left innominate vein symptomatic and palliative surgical treatment is possible. This consists of a superior vena cava by-pass graft which diverts the venous blood from innominate veins to the right atrium. Palliative radiotherapy is used for the treatment of the primary cause in most cases since compression arises from an extensive carcinoma of the bronchus which is usually unresectable. Nevertheless, in some cases of thymic tumours excision of the growth is possible. In practice most patients with superior mediastinal syndrome can only be offered temporary relief with radiotherapy, only a minority derive long lasting benefit from surgery and/or radiotherapy.

MEDIASTINITIS

An inflammation of the cellular tissues of the mediastinal spaces indicates mediastinitis. As an inflammatory condition it is not strictly surgical although surgery is involved in its treatment. It is important to recall two anatomical characteristics of the mediastinum:

1. The division of the mediastinum into compartments and spaces is empirical and for descriptive convenience. In practice spaces communicate. This is of major importance in the posterior mediastinum which is in direct communication with the retro-oesophageal neck space. Because of this communication inflammation in one compartment of the mediastinum easily spreads to another.

2. The mediastinum is separated from the pleural spaces by the mediastinal pleura, a barrier which is easily broken by spreading infection. Therefore inflammation or infection can extend to the pleural spaces.

Because of these anatomical characteristics mediastinitis is a serious condition as any infection of the mediastinal spaces can give rise to widespread infection extending right through the chest.

CLINICAL FEATURES AND DIAGNOSIS
In the majority of cases the cause of mediastinitis is oesophageal perforation, sometimes following operation. The patient looks very ill and toxic, and has a raised temperature and pulse rate. Shock is often present. A chest radiograph generally shows a hydro-pneumothorax (pyo-pneumothorax). Additional laboratory, radiological and endoscopic examinations are required to confirm diagnosis and give the aetiology.

MANAGEMENT
Depending partly on the cause of mediastinitis, and partly on the condition of the patient when first seen, the principles of treatment are:

1. To establish a central venous pressure line which, in the acute cases, monitors the venous pressure and can be used for parenteral nutrition.

2. To provide fluid, plasma and blood transfusion as required to replace losses.

3. To supply adequate nutrition taking into account the higher level of calorie and protein requirements in patients with extensive infection.

4. To drain the mediastinum and the pleural spaces adequately and as appropriate.

The patient's progress is carefully monitored.

TUMOURS AND CYSTS OF THE MEDIASTINUM

Though different pathological entities, mediastinal tumours and cysts may be described together because they can have similar clinical and radiological presentations—some share the same origin—and only the more common lesions are considered here.

Specific types of tumour have a fairly definite topography within the mediastinal spaces: some are found in the superior mediastinum others in the anterior or posterior mediastinum (Fig. 3.5).

TERATOMAS (Dermoid cysts)
A teratoma is defined as a tumour composed of multiple tissues foreign to the part

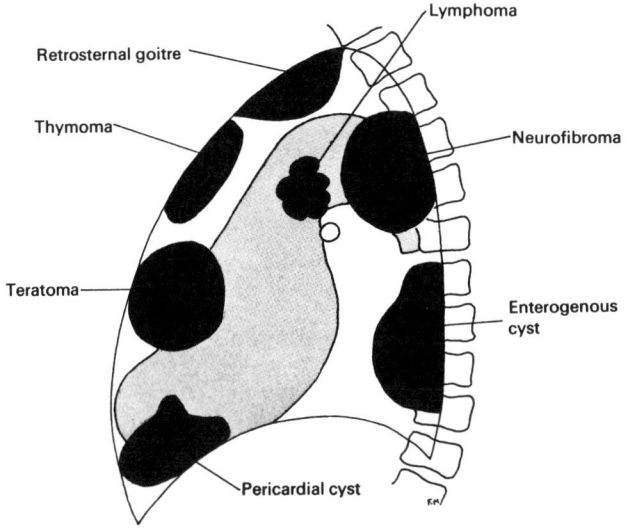

Figure 3.5 Lateral aspect of the mediastinum showing topography of tumours and cysts within the mediastinal spaces.

in which they are found (Willis). When teratomas are cystic they are referred to as dermoid cysts. The tumour or the cyst can contain elements of one, two or all three germinal layers, that is hair, bone, and muscle tissues. In the chest they occur in the anterior mediastinum.

In the absence of complications, these cysts cause no symptoms and are often only discovered in the course of chest radiography for an unrelated condition. The most important complications are infection within the cyst causing re-current fever, and rupture of the cyst delivering its contents into the media-stinum or into the bronchus, thereby forming a fistula.

In the case of rupture into the bronchus the patient expectorates the contents and the condition can lead to chronic bronchial fistula.

Malignant changes occur in about 15–20% of all teratoid tumours.

All teratomas and dermoids are removed surgically when discovered.

THYROID TUMOURS AND CYSTS (Retro-sternal goitre)
These type of tumours are mediastinal extensions of thyroid tumours of the neck descending retro-sternally to the chest. They are almost always situated in the superior mediastinum in front of the trachea. Only very rarely do they extend into the posterior mediastinum.

They cause compression symptoms related to the trachea and the major veins in the superior mediastinum.

Diagnosis of retro-sternal thyroid tumour is not usually problematic. Clinical examination shows the extension of the tumour from the neck down to the thorax. A chest radiograph, barium swallow and endoscopic examination outline the tumour and the extent of displacement in neighbouring structures. The tumour is usually removed surgically through a standard thyroid (collar) incision. However, preparation should be made for sternal split (sternotomy) in case the cervical approach is found to be inadequate for excision of the tumour.

NEUROGENIC TUMOURS (neurofibromas)

The majority of neurogenic tumours are benign and arise from the nerve sheath. Neurofibromas and neurilemomas are encapsulated tumours found in the posterial mediastinum. Malignant neurofibromas are rare (sarcomatous degeneration).

They can either remain asymptomatic for a considerable time or their growth can affect the surrounding structures and produce symptoms. They are treated by surgical excision through a postero-lateral thoracotomy.

LYMPHATIC TUMOURS

Secondary lymphatic tumours are often found in the mediastinum. Occasionally lymphomas present themselves primarily as mediastinal tumours with no evidence of lesion in other sites.

Not uncommonly the mediastinum is the primary site of Hodgkin's disease. Signs of mediastinal compression can be present in these conditions.

OTHER MEDIASTINAL CYSTS

These cysts have different origins, but all share some characteristics. They are benign, generally asymptomatic and are usually discovered in the course of a chest X-ray; true diagnosis can only be done at thoracotomy. They are:

1. Bronchogenic cysts (cysts of bronchial origin) found in the superior mediastinum.
2. Para-oesophageal or enterogenic cysts, in the posterior mediastinum.
3. Pericardial cysts containing clear fluid and known as 'spring water cysts'.
4. Lymphatic cysts (cystic hygroma).

VASCULAR ANOMALIES, TUMOURS AND ANEURYSMS

In addition to haemodynamic implications, tumours manifest themselves as mediastinal masses. Given their location they can produce pressure syndromes affecting surrounding structures. On rare occasions an aneurysm leaks or is frankly ruptured. The outcome is fatal. Aneurysm of the thoracic aorta, in particular can compress the trachea or the oesophagus thus drawing attention to its existence. The only effective treatment is surgical excision.

SURGERY OF MEDIASTINUM

Surgery of mediastinum involves access to the mediastinal spaces, together with necessary excisional and/or reconstructive procedures.

SURGICAL ACCESS

Access to the mediastinum can be obtained by a number of surgical approaches. The choice of a surgical approach depends mainly on the structure and the mediastinal space which has to be exposed for surgical operation.

Anterior approach and sternotomy

Anterior vertical, or transverse incision with median (see Fig. 1.72, p. 129) *or transverse sternotomy* (see Fig. 3.6) Median sternotomy is the more commonly

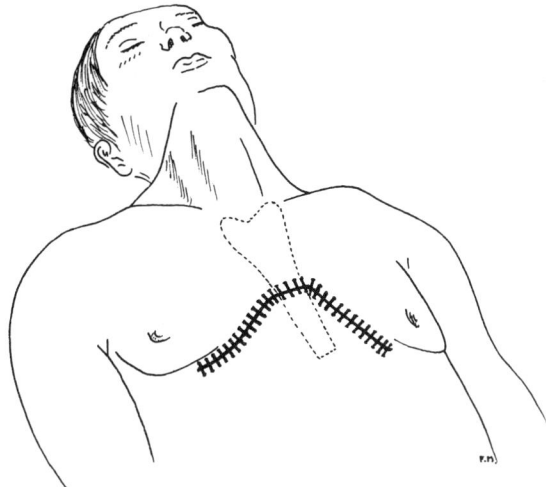

Figure 3.6   Access to the mediastinum through transverse sternotomy incision.

used and provides good access to the anterior and superior mediastinum and the structures within them. The repair of the surgical wound involves the approximation of the two halves of the sternum by stainless steel wire (or other) stitches.

Postero-lateral thoracotomy   Right or left standard thoracotomy incision (see Fig. 1.69, p. 127) is used to gain access to the posterior mediastinum and its contents. Right thoracotomy is used for structures in the posterior and superior mediastinum, left thoracotomy for those in the posterior and inferior mediastinum. In addition right or left thoracotomy is used when a lesion predominantly projects into one or the other side.

DRAINAGE

Every drain placed in the mediastinum should follow the principles of closed underwater sealed drainage system (see Chapter 5) as the mediastinum follows pleural pressure changes. In practice the anterior mediastinum is drained by a superior and an inferior mediastinal drain placed in the mid-line. If the pericardial cavity is entered this is drained as well. When a pleural space is opened in the course of a median sternotomy the space which is opened is also drained.

In a standard right or left thoracotomy the pleural space is drained. It is important to label the drains so that they can be identified.

THYMUS GLAND

The thymus gland is a bilobed gland situated partly in the anterior mediastinum and partly in the neck. It is relatively large at birth, but shrinks during childhood and adolescence. In adults the glandular element is greatly reduced and replaced by fibro-fatty tissues situated over the pericardium and forming part of the pericardial fat.

The thymic lobes are formed by numerous lobules each of which contains a number of follicles made of lymphoid and reticulo-endothelial tissues. The function of the thymus is related to its lympho-reticulo endothelial structure and is believed to be concerned with the immunological response of the body.

ROLE OF THE THYMUS IN MYASTHENIA GRAVIS
The exact role of the thymus and its pathological changes in myasthenia gravis is uncertain. In some myasthenic patients the thymus presents histo-pathological changes. They can be no more than minimal and non-specific, or as much as a definite tumour. What is well known and documented is that thymectomy leads to a considerable improvement in many myasthenic cases.

MYASTHENIA GRAVIS
This is a condition in which there is increased fatiguability of some muscles leading to their weakening. Muscles principally affected are those concerned with movements of the eye, mouth, and swallowing. Diplopia, ptosis and dysphagia are therefore the presenting symptoms. Respiratory and limb muscles can become involved causing dyspnoea, chest infection and inability to undertake any physical work.

The cause of the disease is unknown, but the condition appears to be caused by a failure in the transmission of nervous impulses to muscles. The defect is at the neuro-muscular·junction, presenting itself as a block in the neuro-muscular transmission. There is rapid improvement of symptoms in response to the injection of drugs influencing neuro-muscular transmission, such as Neostigmine and Edrophonium (Tensilon).

Medical treatment generally consists of the use of anti-cholinesterase drugs, such as Neostigmine and Pyridostigmine (Mestinon), which can have undesirable side-effects (e.g. salivation and colic, particularly when Neostigmine is used subcutaneously). These side-effects may be checked by Atropine Sulphate. In progressively resistant cases with repeated respiratory symptoms, thymectomy is undertaken.

THYMIC TUMOURS
Thymic tumours are generally found in adults. They can be asymptomatic and discovered in the course of a chance radiological examination. In some cases myasthenic symptoms can be present, in others signs of mediastinal compression (see p. 234) becomes apparent.

Histologically thymomas are epithelial, lymphoid or lymphoepithelial tumours. Many are frankly invasive and malignant. Some lead to secondary deposits in distant sites. The majority remain confined to the mediastinum and the thorax but enlarge and expand to involve surrounding structures (Fig. 3.7). Only a few remain truly benign.

Precise diagnosis of thymomas is rarely made prior to surgical excision. In the absence of specific signs radiological and endoscopic investigations used for mediastinal tumours are made, principally to exclude other intra-thoracic neoplasia. It is occasionally possible to obtain diagnosis by histological examination of a sample of tissue taken at mediastinoscopy.

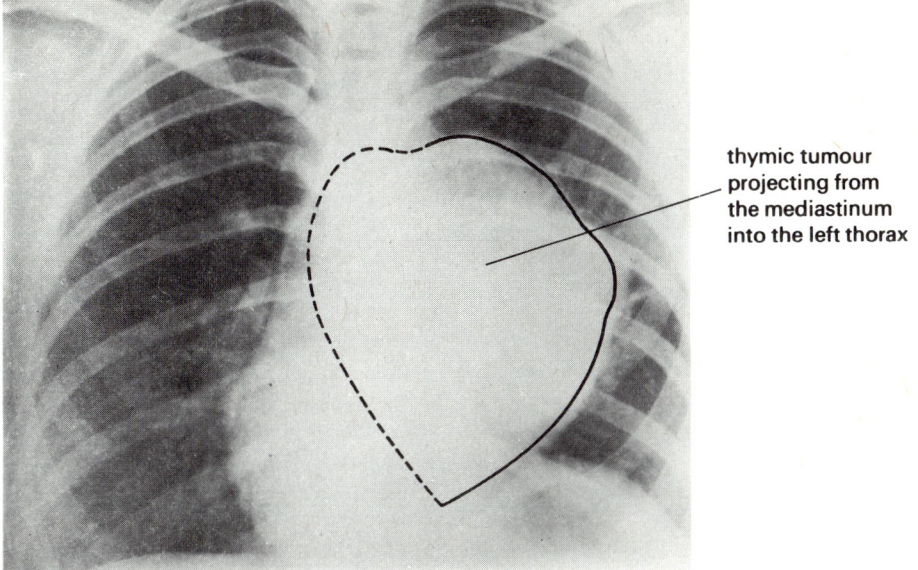

thymic tumour
projecting from
the mediastinum
into the left thorax

Figure 3.7   Antero-posterior chest radiograph of a patient with malignant thymic tumour.

The mainstay of treatment is surgery when possible. Benign and locally invasive tumours are excised, usually with the underlying pericardium. Radiotherapy is indicated in cases when there are no distant secondaries, and particularly when there are signs of mediastinal compression.

SURGERY OF THE THYMUS
Surgical excision of the thymus (thymectomy) is undertaken principally in cases of thymic tumours (thymoma) or in cases of myasthenia gravis. The surgical approach is through a median sternotomy incision (see Fig. 1.72, p. 129). When thymectomy is carried out in myasthenia gravis every fragment of the thymus, extensions and pericardial fat is removed. In cases of thymic tumours the pericardium may have to be excised if attached to the tumour or involved by neoplasia.

The mediastinum is drained and the wound closed.

POST-OPERATIVE FOLLOWING THYMECTOMY FOR MYASTHENIA
Immediately upon return to the ICU/High Dependency Unit the patient is made comfortable. The number and position of drains are noted. The usual recording or base-line observations related to vital functions are made (see Chapter 17). The patient's progress is monitored.

Not all myasthenic patients benefit from thymectomy. In those who do, improvement may be very gradual, taking a few weeks or even months. It is therefore important to monitor and observe these patients very closely in the immediate post-operative phase and continue to supply an anti-myasthenic drug in appropriate doses. The patient should be placed in an intensive care or a high dependency unit where there are facilities for urgent endo-tracheal intubation and ventilatory assistance should the need arise. The most difficult aspects of post-operative care relate to:

1. Establishing an optimum regime for the adequate supply of Neostigmine/ Mastinon together with Atropine Sulphate.

2. Close surveillance of respiration and recognition of early signs of respiratory difficulties.

3. Close observation of the patient without undermining his self-confidence, particularly when drug therapy has been altered.

Establishing an optimum regime
Patients differ greatly in their response to drugs. Nursing staff should receive clear instructions about the frequency and the dose of drugs. They should also be prepared to give an additional dose of Neostigmine (and Atropine) in very urgent cases. They must be instructed to recognise the signs indicating the need for additional supply and its dose.

Early signs of respiratory difficulties
It should be noted that although the drug regime may have been clearly indicated and followed, the patient's response may not be as expected. An additional dose should be given when there are signs of (1) shallowing of respiration, which becomes rapid, (2) weakening in the movements of mouth and eye-lids, and (3) difficulty of swallowing saliva as noticed or expressed by the patient.

Many patients feel and express the need for anti-cholinesterase in rapidly developing or extreme cases. Cyanosis develops with respiratory arrest, requiring resuscitative measures.

Observation and physchological management
Many myasthenic patients have experienced such unpleasant symptoms, with associated fright, that they become anxious and continue to remain so for a long time after operation. This and the close surveillance they have had in the immediate post-operative period in the ICU make their late post-operative management in a general ward difficult. It is important for them to regain their confidence. They should be given increasing dependence while being watched carefully and discreetly.

24 Trachea

The trachea or wind-pipe is the part of the respiratory tract dealing with the passage of air from the larynx to the bronchi. For an anatomical description of the trachea see Chapter 2.

The trachea lies superficially in the neck and can be palpated. It bends behind the sternum at the junction of manubrium and the body and divides into two bronchi. During its course from the neck to the chest it is closely related to the oesophagus posteriorly, and anteriorly it comes into contact with the isthmus of the thyroid gland, the innominate artery and vein.

OBSTRUCTIVE LESIONS OF THE TRACHEA

Tracheal surgery is largely concerned with the obstruction of this tube and resulting respiratory distress. The commonest causes of obstruction are:

1. Obstruction by foreign body.
2. Post-intubation tracheal stenosis.
3. Obstruction due to benign and malignant tumours.

TRACHEAL OBSTRUCTION DUE TO IMPACTED FOREIGN BODY

Occasionally a large foreign body becomes impacted in the trachea and presents an urgent and serious problem. In almost all cases the foreign object descends into the bronchial tree where it finally lodges. A history of foreign body inhalation, acute dyspnoea and cyanosis leave little doubt as to diagnosis.

Sometimes, however, the history of inhalation is not provided. Acute respiratory distress in otherwise healthy infants and children is commonly caused by inhalation of a foreign body and should be treated as such unless otherwise disproved. As only radio-opaque objects show on X-ray films radiological investigations should not deter from removing the object endoscopically. However in some exceptions it may be necessary to resort to surgical removal. (See also Chapter 10, *Foreign Bodies in the Airways*, p. 84).

POST-INTUBATION TRACHEAL STENOSIS

Infective strictures have practically disappeared since the advent of anti-tuberculous drugs and effective control of tuberculosis.

The majority of strictures result from complications of trans-laryngeal endo-tracheal intubation (tracheostomy) for ventilatory assistance.

Treatment

In recent years the frequency of post-intubation tracheal stenosis has been greatly reduced due largely to a better understanding of its pathogenesis.

Factors responsible for ulceration and stricture formation following intubation are numerous. They include (1) faulty surgical techniques, (2) pressure by the cuff of the tracheostomy tube, (3) ulceration caused by the distal end of the tube, (4) trauma inflicted by suction catheters, and (5) sepsis. Individually, or collectively, these factors can lead to stricture formation. The resulting stricture can be situated at the level of the tracheostomy opening or at any level below it.

Detailed studies suggest that these lesions are preventable if attention is paid to details of nursing care, selection of equipment and prevention of infection. It is therefore appropriate to point out that the staff who are nursing patients that require mechanical respiratory assistance should aim at preventing stenosis.

When stenosis is established, conservative or radical treatment becomes necessary.

Conservative Treatment consists of dilatation of the stricture, disinfection of the airways by bronchoscopic lavage and administration of appropriate antibiotics.

Radical Treatment consists of resection of the stenosed segment of the trachea, followed by reconstruction.

OBSTRUCTION DUE TO BENIGN AND MALIGNANT TUMOURS

Benign tumours of the trachea are rare. Fibromas, adenomas (cylindromas) and hemangiomas are occasionally seen. Among them cylindromas are the commonest. Although benign they are potentially malignant.

Malignant tumours of the trachea are also rare, the commonest being squamous cell carcinoma. Secondary tumours of the trachea are more common particularly those involving the lower trachea as an extension of a bronchial carcinoma. Carcinoma of the oesophagus, the thyroid and the larynx can involve the trachea by direct extension and produce obstruction with respiratory embarrassment.

Investigations and diagnosis

At an early stage the condition may be asymptomatic, but later on wheezes and noisy breathing develop progressing to definite stridor; blood-stained sputum and haemoptysis can also be present.

A chest radiograph can be entirely normal. Tracheal tomography and tracheography show the presence and the extent of the obstructive lesion. Endoscopic examination, namely tracheo-bronchoscopy, is the most useful investigatory method. It reveals the type and extent of the lesion and provides biopsy material for histological studies.

Treatment of tracheal tumours

Surgical treatment is undertaken for all resectable tracheal tumours. Even benign tumours have to be resected because of their obstructive nature. For them resection is limited and reconstruction of the airways can be achieved by end-to-end anastomosis.

In primary malignant tumours suitable for surgery resection followed by reconstruction is undertaken. In cases not suitable for surgery radiotherapy can be offered although results are often disappointing. In,many patients treated by radiotherapy the distressing symptoms remain or soon recur.

In secondary malignant tumours resection (though palliative in many cases) is undertaken whenever possible in order to relieve the obstruction. Tracheal involvement by bronchial and laryngeal carcinoma is particularly suitable for resection.

Surgical approach

Cervical, cervico-mediastinal and right thoracotomy approaches are used to gain access to the cervical, cervico-mediastinal and the thoracic trachea respectively.

Cervical approach is gained through a suitably placed neck incision (see Fig. 2.29, p. 209). In the cervico-mediastinal approach a T-shaped incision is made over the neck and the chest with the patient in a supine position. The sternum is incised in the middle (median sternotomy). This incision provides good access to the cervical and the superior mediastinal parts of the trachea.

Right postero-lateral thoracotomy incision gives access to the thoracic trachea, carina, right and even left main bronchus.

PRINCIPLES OF TRACHEAL RESECTION AND RECONSTRUCTION

Resection of the trachea is undertaken for all obstructive lesions, inflammatory and post-intubation stenosis, benign and malignant tumours. Following resection the airways have to be reconstructed. End-to-end anastomosis is the ideal method of reconstruction and one which gives constantly good results. But recently some success has been recorded in tracheal reconstruction in selected cases using prosthesis. Surgical access to the trachea is obtained through the most suitable incision for the site of the lesion. The trachea is exposed and mobilised. This involves separation from the oesophagus, freeing from the great vessels and, at times, mobilisation of the carina and two main bronchi. One important technical consideration in tracheal reconstruction is the maintenance of ventilation and anaesthesia during an operation requiring the excision and anastomosis of the tracheal tube. The technique is illustrated in Figure 3.8 and described as follows:

1. Incision of the anterior aspect of the trachea while the trans-laryngeal tube is in place.
2. Withdrawal of the endo-tracheal tube (T_1) to below the larynx to allow introduction of another endo-tracheal tube (T_2) by the surgeon through the anterior tracheal incision. This tube (T_2) is connected to the anaesthetic apparatus which now provides the patient with anaesthesia and ventilation.
3. The diseased portion is removed and the posterior wall of the trachea is reconstructed.
4. The tube (T_2) is removed and the trans-laryngeal tube (T_1) is advanced by the anaesthetist allowing continuation of anaesthesia and ventilation through it. Anterior wall reconstruction is then carried out.

When direct anastomosis for reconstruction is not possible and when the gap to be bridged is wide, a prosthesis (e.g. Marlex Mesh) is used. It can be used as patch graft or as circumferential replacement.

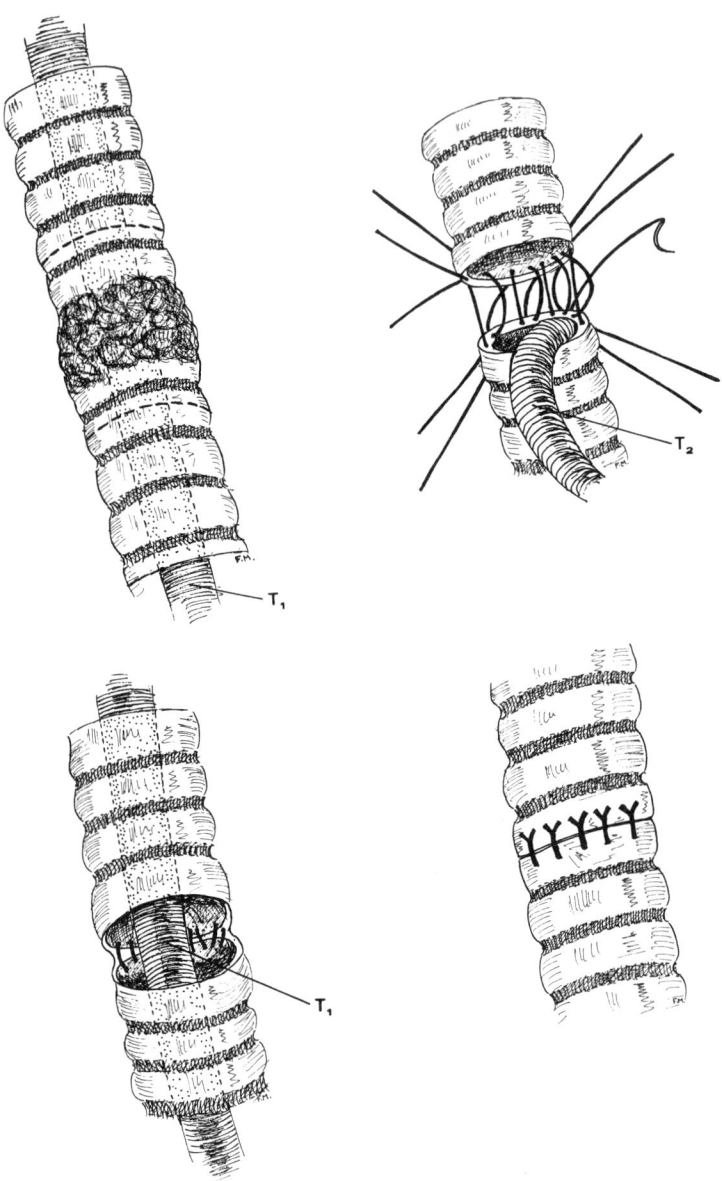

Figure 3.8   Steps in reconstruction of the trachea. (See text for details.)

POST-OPERATIVE MANAGEMENT

Post-operative management of patients following resection and reconstruction of trachea can be discussed under: general and special post-operative management.

GENERAL POST-OPERATIVE MANAGEMENT
Basic post-operative monitoring and care are applied and management is essentially similar to that for patients undergoing major lung surgery (see Chapter 17).

SPECIAL POST-OPERATIVE MANAGEMENT

Drains
These may be situated in the thorax, mediastinum or neck. In principle all drains should be treated as being intrathoracic and subjected to the underwater sealed drainage method as the neck spaces communicate freely with the mediastinal spaces and, therefore, follow intrathoracic and pleural pressure changes (see Chapter 5).

Physiotherapy and expectoration of secretion
This should be particularly attended to. In patients with circumferential tracheal excision and end-to-end anastomosis generally, and particularly those with any sort of prosthesis, expectoration is difficult. Humidification of air and a mucolytic agent should be provided. Tenacious secretions may have to be aspirated by suction bronchoscopy. A sputum sample should be sent to the laboratory for microbiological studies and sensitivity to antibiotics in order to provide the patients with a suitable antibiotic if necessary.

Tracheostomy
If a temporary tracheostomy is left for the immediate post-operative period, extreme care should be applied to aseptic techniques of aspiration and handling.

Resection of trachea
When extensive resection of the trachea has been carried out, in order to achieve direct anastomosis without undue tension the patient's head is flexed. This position should be maintained for a few days post-operatively.

TRACHEOSTOMY

Tracheostomy is an artificial opening in the trachea. The operation may be carried out under local or general anaesthetic in the operating theatre, an intensive care unit, or the ward. A tracheostomy is best carried out as a planned procedure, in the operating theatre, under general anaesthesia. However, a thoracic surgical ward should envisage the possibility of a tracheostomy being performed under local anaesthetic in the ward in an emergency situation.

It must be realised that many patients are extremely frightened and upset about loss of voice and the inability to talk resulting from tracheostomy. It is therefore essential to explain fully to the patient before the operation the necessity for and the results of the tracheostomy. This must also be explained to the patient's relatives.

It is important to make a writing pad and pencil available to the patient to enable him to communicate with staff and relations.

INDICATIONS FOR TRACHEOSTOMY

Tracheostomy is carried out for a variety of unrelated purposes which can best be described under the following headings. They are as follows:

1. *For by-passing laryngeal obstructions*, e.g. obstruction by foreign bodies and tumours, inflammatory lesions or oedema.

2. *For ready access to the trachea and the bronchial tree.* For instance, the removal of excess and abnormal bronchial secretions (e.g. post-operative sputum retention).

3. *For the supply of oxygen.*

4. *For reducing the respiratory dead space.*

5. *For assisted ventilation* using intermittent positive pressure ventilation.

TRACHEOSTOMY TUBES

There is a variety of tracheostomy tubes on the market that fall into three groups: cuffed tracheostomy tubes (plastic or rubber); uncuffed tracheostomy tubes (plastic or rubber); silver tracheostomy tubes (Chevalier Jackson), consisting of an introducer, a removable inner tube and an outer tube. Different sizes are available in each group.

THE OPERATION

In the operating theatre the patient is placed flat on his back, head extended, with a sand bag under his shoulders. In an emergency, or when there are contra-indications for moving the patient, the operation can be carried out in the ward, with the patient lying flat or sitting upright in bed, but always with the head extended.

The incision may be transverse or vertical, over the anterior aspect of the neck (Fig. 3.9). In urgent or emergency cases the vertical incision is usually preferred.

The opening in the trachea is usually made at the level of the 2nd and 3rd cartilaginous ring. After the opening is prepared the tracheostomy tube is introduced as the anaesthetist withdraws the endotracheal tube (i.e. if the operation is performed under general anaesthesia). The tracheostomy tube should be fixed *in situ* by two tapes tied at the side of the neck. The tapes should be tight enough to hold the tube in position.

MANAGEMENT OF TRACHEOSTOMY

This is discussed under two headings: (1) care and management of the tube and its complications, and (2) tracheal suction and humidification.

Care and management of the tube and its complications

During the early hours following tracheostomy, it is important to ensure that the tracheostomy tube is in the trachea and has not slipped into the peritracheal tissue, and that breathing is unobstructed and the tube not blocked. The younger the patient, the narrower the tube and the more likely that this will happen. Figure 3.10 illustrates a tracheostomy tube almost completely blocked by

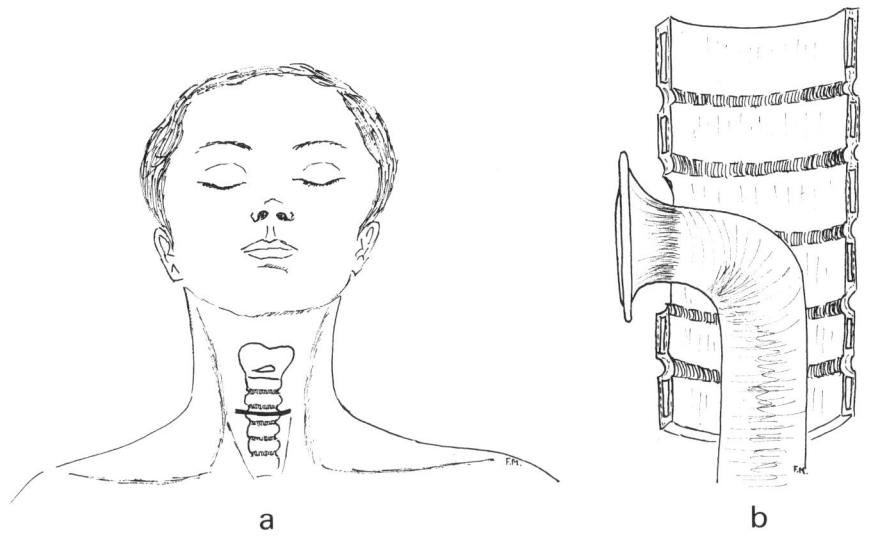

a b

Figure 3.9   (a) Tracheostomy incision and (b) tracheostomy tube in situ.

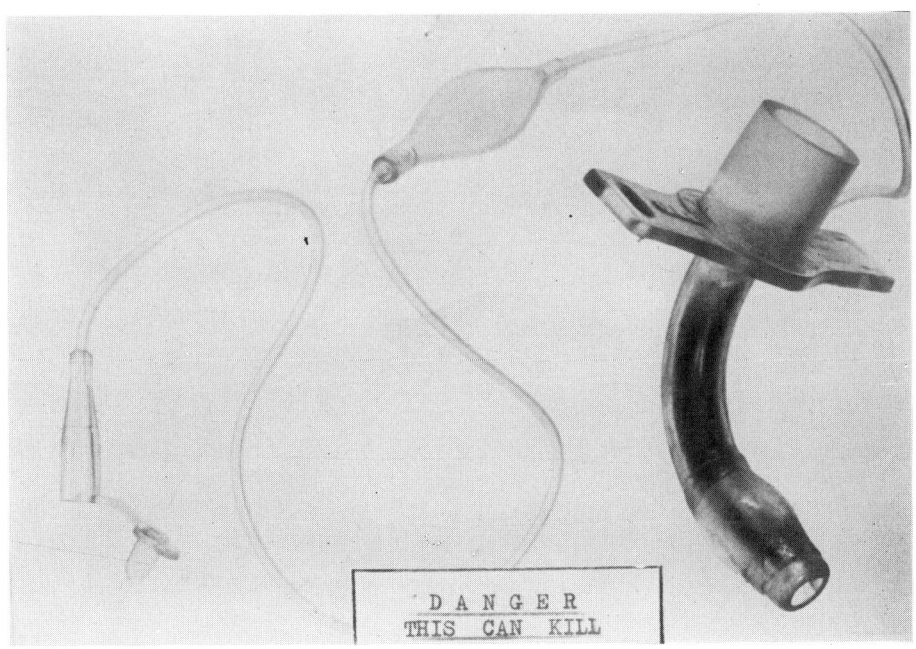

Figure 3.10   Tracheostomy tube obstructed by inspissated secretions and fibrin clots.

secretions. In this case the tube was *in situ* for 24 hours and was hourly sucked out. When the patient's breathing became laboured, the blockage was discovered. A check should also be made to ensure there is no haematoma or surgical emphysema of the neck.

Additionally, the tube should be changed regularly or, in the case of a silver tracheostomy tube, the inner tube replaced. When a cuffed tracheostomy is used, the cuff should be released for 2 or 3 minutes in every hour in order to prevent tracheal necrosis. The opening of the tube should also be safeguard by placing a gauze swab (one layer) over it. This will prevent any foreign particles entering the tube.

Equipment for changing a tracheostomy tube is illustrated in Figure 3.11 and is as follows: (1) a suitably-sized sterile tracheostomy tube, similar to the one being changed; (2) two tapes; (3) a pair of scissors; (4) a sterile tracheal dilator; (5) sterile gloves and mask; (6) a sterile gown. If a cuffed tube is being used then a pair of artery forceps (Spencer Wells) and a sterile 10 ml syringe is additionally required.

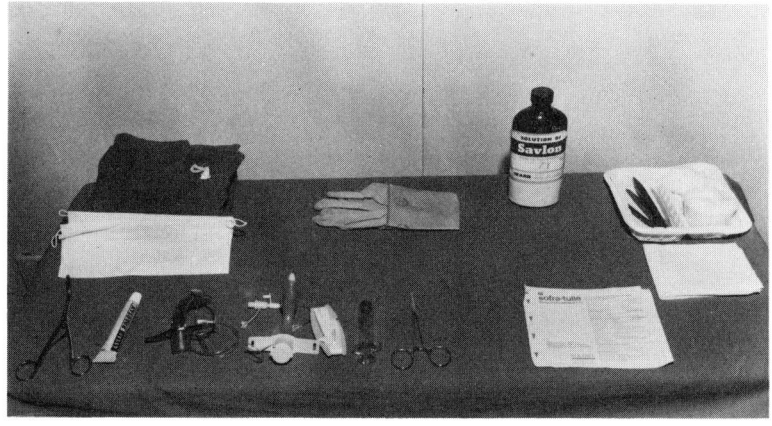

Figure 3.11   Equipment for changing tracheostomy tube. (See text for details.)

Tracheal suction and humidification

The removal of secretions involves the introduction of a catheter into the trachea through the tracheostomy tube, and suction via a machine or central piped vacuum (Fig. 3.12). The following principles must be observed:

1. The procedure must be aseptic, with precautions against contaminating the inner tube or trachea.

2. The suction must be brief (5 to 10 seconds) and effective and should not be performed at too frequent intervals.

3. For suction to be effective it is necessary to have good humidification and effective chest physiotherapy.

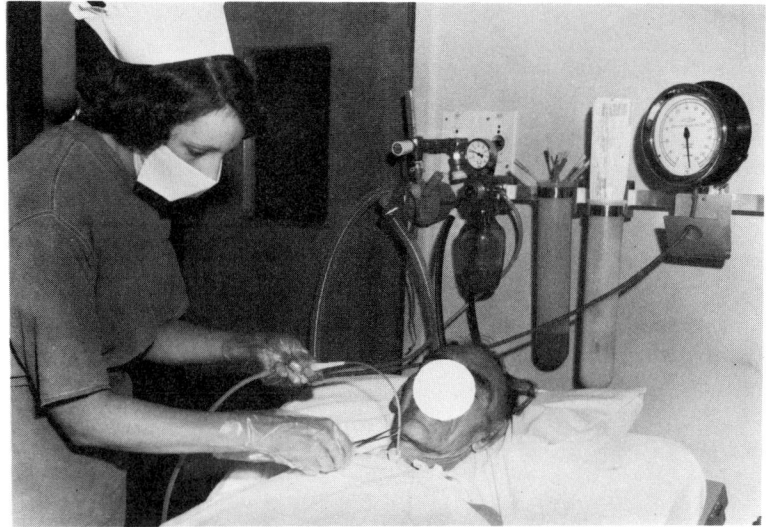

Figure 3.12   Tracheal suction.

Equipment for tracheal suction   The equipment to have near the patient for this is as follows: (1) suction catheters (sterile, disposable catheters are now available) that should not be too sharp-lipped or rigid as this can traumatise the tracheal mucosa; (2) Y-connector or similar device to connect the suction catheter to the suction tube and allow controlled aspiration by the operator; (3) suction tube and machine or central piped suction; (4) disposable sterile gloves (e.g. disposable polythene gloves) and mask; (5) sterile gown; (6) container for water (or mild antiseptic); (7) pair of dissecting forceps.

The procedure is as follows:

1. Wear a mask and gown.
2. Scrub hands thoroughly then put on sterile gloves.
3. Explain the procedure to the patient (i.e. that you are about to suck inside the tube, which will make him cough).
4. Connect the sterile suction catheter and its Y- or other connector to the suction tube and machine.
5. Withdraw the catheter from its container or sterile sheath, making sure that the distal tip does not touch the outside of the tube.
6. With one hand hold the proximal part of the catheter with a finger over the open end of the Y-connector to control the suction power. With a pair of dissecting forceps in the other hand, hold the distal part of the catheter, guiding and introducing it through the tracheostomy tube into the trachea.

Suction should be carried out in the following order:

1. The pharyngeal pool, i.e. the mouth and the pharynx above the tracheostomy. Change the catheter. Do not use the catheter used previously for the pharyngeal pool inside the trachea.

2. Suck the trachea through the tracheostomy tube and direct the catheter into the right and left main bronchi.

3. Flush the catheter by dipping it into the sterile water (with suction on 1).

4. If necessary repeat the suction.

When a cuffed tracheostomy tube is used, the cuff should be released as instructed. Before doing so, however, suction of the pharyngeal pool and the trachea is undertaken as above. The cuff is then inflated and the trachea once more sucked through the tube.

Humidification   One of the problems arising from the by-passing of the naso-pharyngo-laryngeal passage in tracheostomy is the lack of humidification of the air breathed through the tracheostomy tube. This results in thick and sticky secretions difficult to dispose of by suction. Artificial humidification of the air or gases entering the tracheostomy tube is necessary. Many types of humidifiers and nebulisers are available. In addition to these the regular instillation of 1–2 ml of normal saline or aqueous solution of hibitane 1 in 5000 into the tube is helpful.

Bacterial monitoring of secretions

Bacteriological study of tracheo-bronchial secretions should be taken as an important routine investigation of tracheostomy patients. Every day a sample should be forwarded to the bacteriology department for identification of organisms and their sensitivity to antibiotics. When secretions are not abundant the tip of the suction catheter can be sent to the laboratory after use.

Further management of tracheostomy

When tracheostomy is to be discontinued the removal of the tube is very simple. After the final tracheal toilet the tube is removed, the wound cleaned with a disinfectant such as aqueous Hibitane solution and a dressing applied. Within a few days the tracheostomy wound will close and heal.

COMPLICATIONS OF TRACHEOSTOMY

It is important to have a clear knowledge of complications of tracheostomy in order to prevent or to diagnose them early. In the majority of cases the danger of complications arises from the obstruction of the airways.

Obstruction

It can be caused by the displacement of or a kink in the tube. A well-placed tube can be blocked by plugs of mucus, blood clot and fibrin (see Fig. 3.10).

It is obviously very important to remove the obstruction, which would otherwise result in asphyxiation.

Haemorrhage

It can present itself on the surface at the edges of the wound, in the peri-tracheal neck tissue or in the tracheal lumen itself. Haemorrhage in or out of the lumen will obstruct the airways, the second less directly than the first. In either case the medical staff should be summoned.

Surgical subcutaneous emphysema

Escape of air under the skin and subcutaneous tissue is caused by displacement of the tube particularly when a ventilator is in use. Sometimes air escapes from a tube not fitting properly in the trachea.

Infective complications

Infective complications, due to aspiration of contaminated secretions and debris, can be prevented by observing strict aseptic techniques in handling the tracheostomy tubes and by providing suction and chest physiotherapy.

Pulmonary collapse

Pulmonary collapse (segmental, lobar and sometimes whole lung) can occur due to the accumulation of tenacious, dried up and inspissated secretions which cannot be removed with a tracheostomy suction catheter. Efficient tracheo-bronchial suction together with effective physiotherapy and humidification of inspired air can often prevent this complication. Sometimes, however, it is necessary to carry out a preventive or therapeutic suction bronchoscopy.

Post-tracheostomy tracheal stenosis

This complication is often the result of long-standing and complicated tracheostomies when there is infection, ulceration and scarring. In many cases resection and reconstruction of the trachea becomes necessary (see p. 245).

Part 4
Topics in Chest Surgery

This section consists of heterogeneous topics which are extremely important in chest surgery. None can be left out or ignored by the practising nurse in a thoracic surgical ward.

25 Radiology

X-rays are fundamentally similar to light rays, that is, they are part of the same electro-magnetic spectrum and have the same basic characteristics as light. They differ only in their wavelength and penetrating power.

PRODUCTION OF X-RAYS

X-rays are produced when electrons travelling at high velocity collide with atoms. An X-ray tube, therefore, must provide a source of electrons, the means of accelerating them to a high velocity and a target for them to strike.

The electron source is a heated filament (cathode), and the target is called the anode. These are enclosed in a tube containing a vacuum.

A small current is passed through the filament to heat it (the current is measured in milliamperes or mA). The heat in the filament causes its atoms to vibrate, and electrons are released. A very high voltage, in the order of 50–100 kilovolts (1 kV = 1000 volts), is passed across the tube and this accelerates the electrons from the cathode to the anode, with which they collide, producing X-rays (Fig. 4.1). The characteristics of the X-rays can be altered by varying the voltage, current and the time during which the current flows. A higher voltage applied across the tube causes the electrons to travel faster and the X-rays produced have a shorter wavelength, with more penetrating power.

The number of electrons leaving the cathode can be increased by either increasing the filament current or prolonging the time for which it flows. The more electrons produced, the greater the amount of X-rays, hence, when X-raying the chest of a breathless patient, the exposure time is kept very low, say

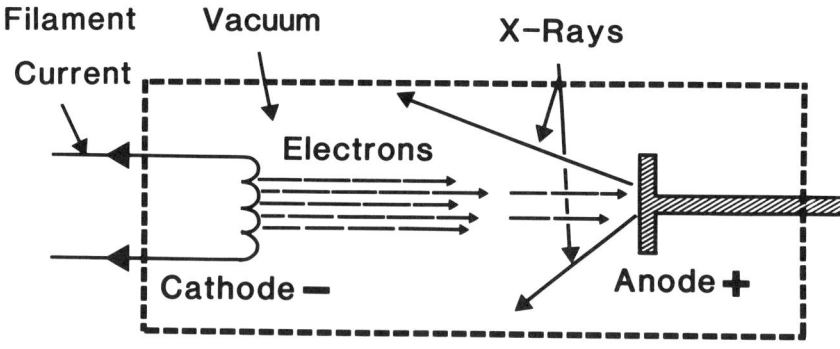

Figure 4.1   Diagram of X-ray tube.

0.2 of a second, and the current is correspondingly increased. The actual exposure is usually measured in mAs (the product of mA × seconds), and either can be varied according to the circumstances to produce the exposure required.

RECORDING THE IMAGE

X-rays were discovered because they affected photographic film. Photographic film is still used today to record the X-ray image. However, most X-rays will pass through the film without being absorbed and are therefore wasted.

In order to utilise this 'waste' radiation, the X-ray film is placed in a cassette between intensifying screens. These intensifying screens are coated with a substance which fluoresces when bombarded by X-rays. This fluorescence is in the form of visible light. The X-ray film is therefore affected both by the X-rays and by the light from the fluorescent screens. Using the intensifying screens enables the dose of radiation required for a given examination to be reduced.

COMMON THORACIC SURGERY X-RAY EXAMINATIONS

POSTERO-ANTERIOR CHEST

The postero-anterior view of the chest is taken with the patient's back to the X-ray tube, and the front of the chest against the X-ray film. The distance between the tube and the film is 6 feet (1.83 metres). This is the standard X-ray examination of the chest.

Figure 4.2 shows a labelled chest film taken in the postero-anterior (PA) projection. Note that the markings seen in the lungs in a normal subject are virtually all due to blood vessels and not the air passages.

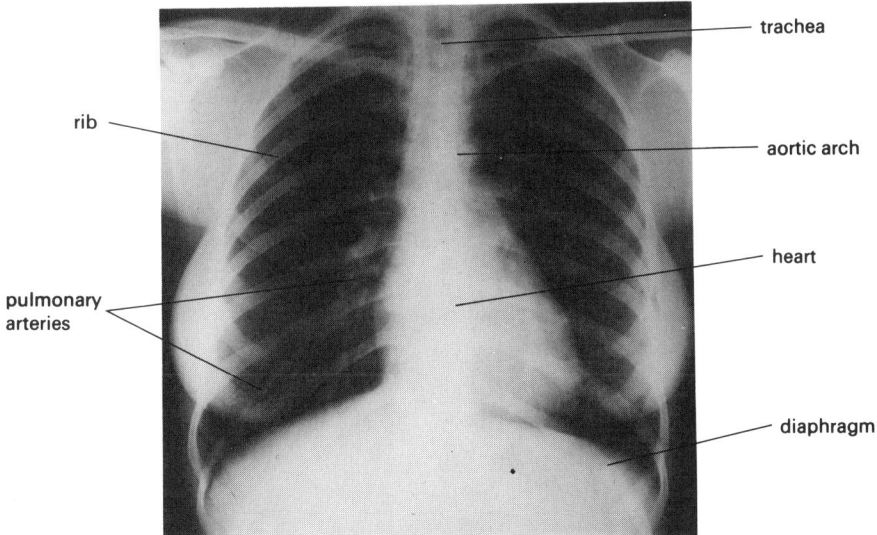

Figure 4.2   Normal postero-anterior chest.

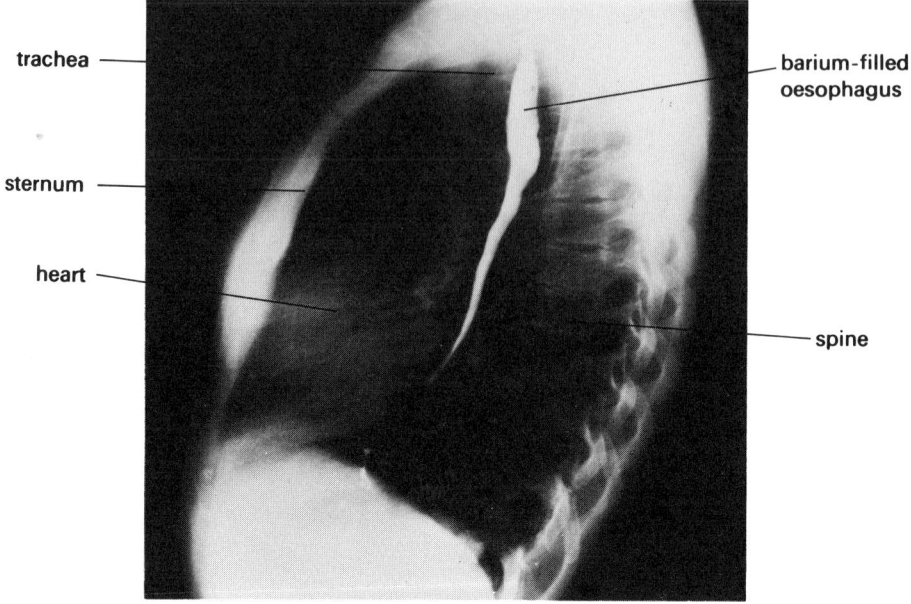

trachea

barium-filled
oesophagus

sternum

heart

spine

Figure 4.3   Normal lateral chest and barium-filled oesophagus.

LATERAL CHEST X-RAY
This is again taken at a distance of 6 feet. A right lateral has the right side of the chest against the film and a left lateral the converse. Figure 4.3 shows a labelled lateral X-ray.

BRONCHOGRAPHY
In order to demonstrate the bronchi, it is necessary to introduce some form of contrast medium that will adhere to the bronchial wall and cause it to be visualised on the X-ray.

There are several ways of instilling the contrast medium. This may be done at bronchoscopy, by running it down the bronchoscope. A tube may be passed through the nose down into the bronchi, or a needle may be passed through the crico-thyroid membrane into the larynx. The contrast is instilled and the patient turned into different positions in order that all the bronchi may be filled. Films of the chest are then taken in PA and oblique positions. Figure 4.4 shows a PA film of a normal bronchogram.

TOMOGRAPHY
This is a method of enhancing structures seen on plain X-rays. By moving the X-ray tube and the X-ray film parallel to each other but in opposite directions, it is possible to blur out structures in front and behind the area of interest (see Fig. 4.5). Figure 4.6 illustrates how only the structures in the plane of the pivot point are always projected onto the film, and other structures blurred out.

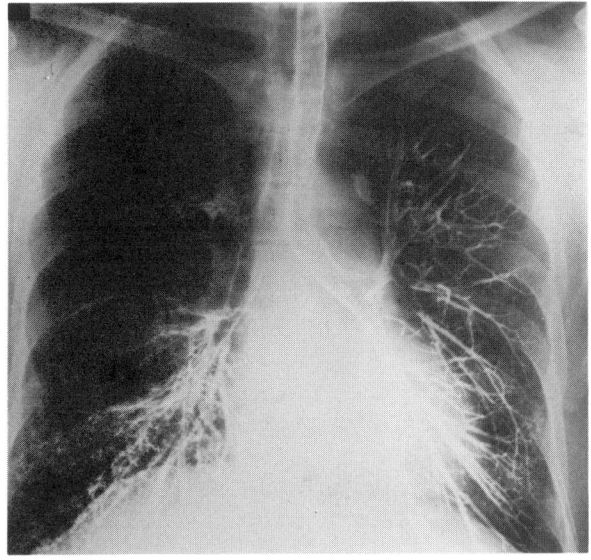

a

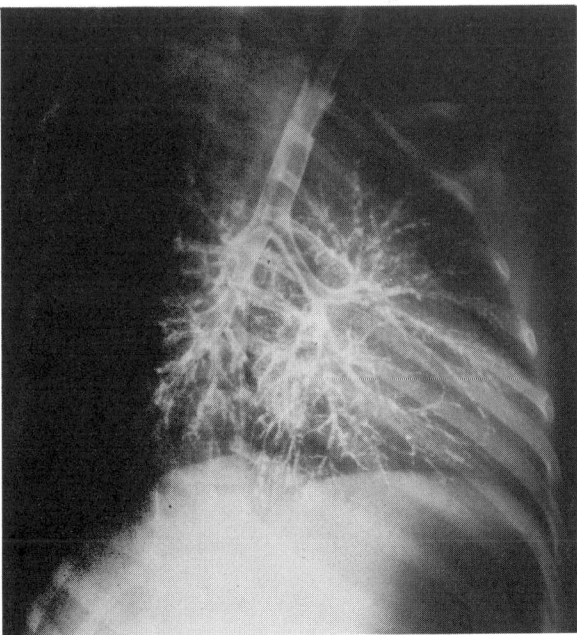

b

Figure 4.4   Normal bronchogram. (a) Antero-posterior and (b) left oblique view.

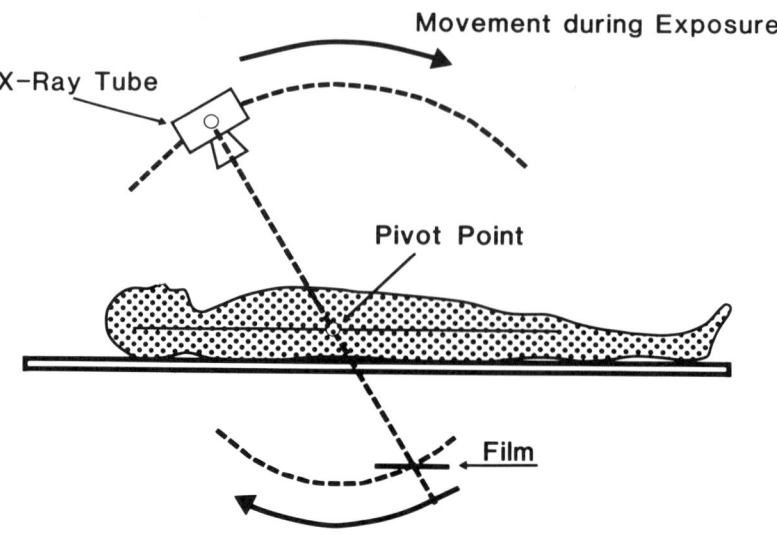

Figure 4.5   Principles of tomography.

BARIUM SWALLOW

In barium studies of the oesophagus, the passage of the barium down the oesophagus is watched on a fluoroscopic screen. A fluoroscopic screen is composed of a substance (mixture of zinc sulphide and cadmium sulphide), which glows when bombarded with X-rays. This screen is then viewed through an image intensifier which enhances the image produced, and this is finally displayed on a television screen. The barium sulphate used is very dense and hence absorbs most of the X-rays and therefore appears on the fluorescent screen as a dark area (i.e. few X-rays striking the screen), in contrast to the surrounding areas.

The passage of barium down the oesophagus is observed and films are taken to show areas of interest. The films are negatives, and therefore the barium appears white on them (see Fig. 4.3).

It is also possible to record the barium swallow on video-tape or in cine film, and this is particularly useful when it is necessary to study oesophageal function rather than anatomy.

ANGIOGRAPHY

It is possible to demonstrate the arteries and veins inside the thorax by injecting contrast directly into the blood stream. The contrast medium used is an organic iodine-containing compound. This has the same property as the barium in that it absorbs the X-rays and so appears black on the fluoroscopic screen, and white on X-ray film.

The contrast medium is injected into the blood vessel, as near as possible to the area of interest. In the case of vessels inside the thorax, this may mean passing a catheter either through a vein or artery in the arm or in the leg, and negotiating it through the vessels into the thorax. When the catheter lies as near as possible

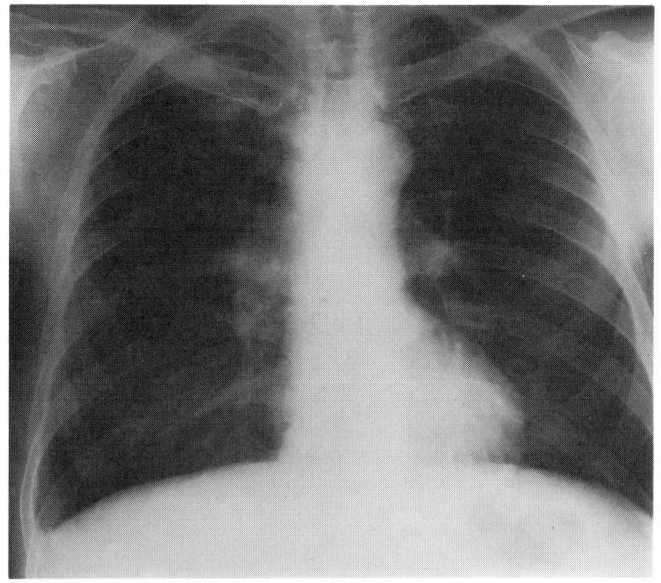

a

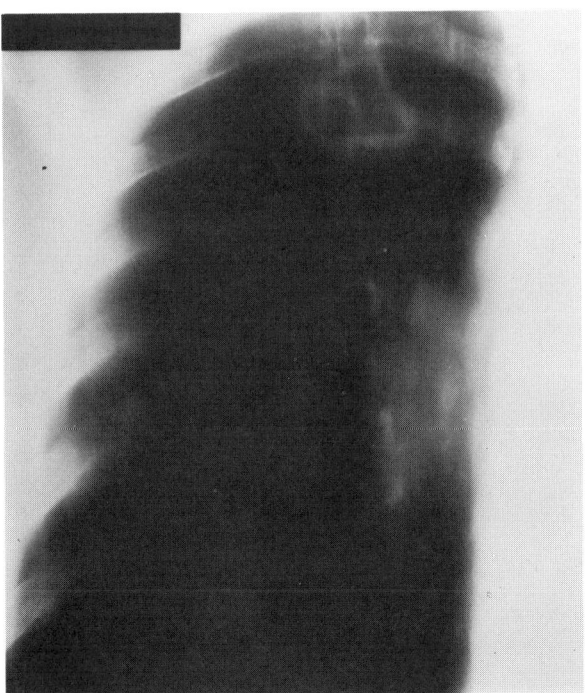

b

Figure 4.6 (a) *Chest X-ray showing a vague lesion in the right upper lobe.* (b) *Tomography of the same lesion.*

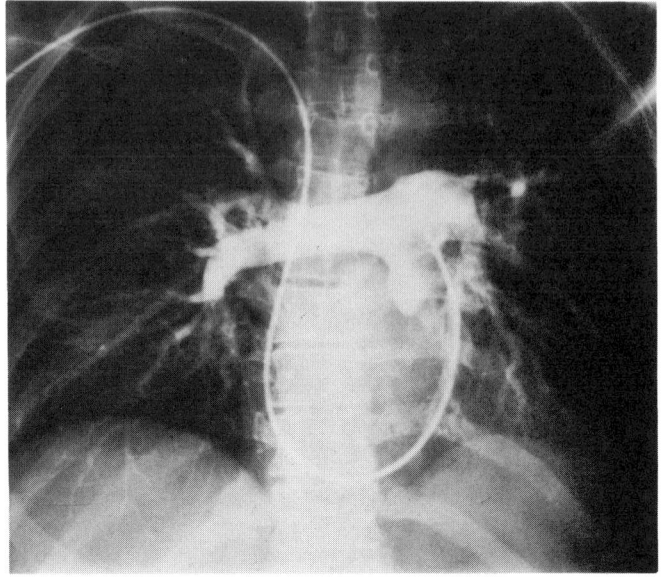

a

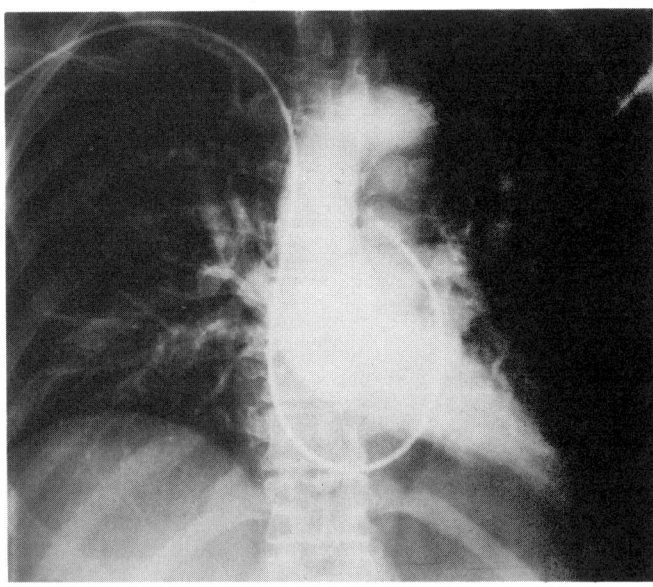

b

Figure 4.7   (a) Arterial phase of a pulmonary angiogram. (b) Venous phase of a pulmonary angiogram.

to the area under investigation, the contrast medium is injected through it, using a pressure pump, and films are taken in rapid sequence (Figs. 4.7a,b).

MOBILE X-RAY UNITS

Mobile X-ray units are available for X-raying patients on the ward who are too ill to be moved to the X-ray department. They do, however, have serious drawbacks and should only be used in these circumstances. These units are of low power and can only be used for certain examinations. Because the patient is usually X-rayed in bed, the chest film is an AP film and there is considerable magnification of the heart and mediastinum. The unit is not powerful enough to enable satisfactory films to be obtained of bones and of the abdomen.

CONTRAST MEDIA

As previously mentioned, the contrast media used in radiology absorb the X-rays and therefore cause a shadow on the X-ray film.

BARIUM SULPHATE
This is a suspension of fine particles of barium sulphate in water. It is a good contrast medium for use in the alimentary tract because it adheres well to the mucosa, is very dense and is not absorbed.

GASTROGRAFIN
This is a hypertonic water soluble contrast medium containing organic iodine and may also be used to examine the alimentary tract. It is less dense than barium and adheres less well to the mucosa. Its main use is in conditions where a perforation of the oesophagus is suspected, as any contrast leaking out of the alimentary tract will be observed. It must not be used if there is any danger of aspiration into the bronchial tree, as being a hypertonic solution, it attracts water, and therefore causes pulmonary oedema.

DIONOSIL
This is an iodised oil. Its main use is in bronchography as it is slowly absorbed from the bronchi without causing pulmonary oedema. It should also be used to examine the oesophagus if aspiration is a possibility (e.g. in suspected oesophageal atresia in infants).

ANGIOGRAPHIC CONTRAST MEDIA
These are water soluble organic iodine compounds. Because they are injected directly into the blood stream, it is important to ascertain whether or not the patient has any allergies, particularly to previous injections of contrast media, as cases of anaphylaxia and death have occurred due to injections of contrast medium.

RADIATION PROTECTION

All radiation is dangerous and its effects are cumulative. No nurse should be working in an area where X-rays are being taken unless it is absolutely necessary. If this is unavoidable, then the nurse must wear suitable protection (lead rubber apron). If possible, nursing staff should not hold patients who are being X-rayed. Again, if this is unavoidable, they must wear lead aprons and gloves, and must not stand in the primary X-ray beam.

Remember, there is considerable scatter of X-rays, both from the X-ray apparatus and the patient, so persons standing close by will also be irradiated.

It cannot be too strongly emphasised that radiation is dangerous and no member of staff or patient should be unnecessarily exposed to irradiation. In particular, any female member of staff who may be pregnant should leave the room when X-rays are being taken.

26 Physiotherapy in Chest Surgery

The value of breathing exercises in chest diseases has been recognised for a considerable time. The development of chest surgery has re-emphasised the importance of physiotherapy in patients undergoing an operation.

At the present time, the physiotherapist is considered as an integral member of the thoracic surgery team along with the medical and the nursing staff. Whilst the nursing staff are not expected to undertake the functions of trained and professional physiotherapists they should be familiar with the principles of chest physiotherapy. There are two reasons for this. Firstly, a team can only operate as a functional unit when each of its constituent members understands the contribution made by the other members to the work of the team. Secondly, compared with the nursing staff the physiotherapists can spend relatively little time with patients. Therefore, nurses can help with informal physiotherapy between formal sessions: they can ask the patient to 'take a deep breath' or 'give a good cough'. This may appear trivial, but when repeated often it will go a long way towards effective respiration and airway clearance.

The principal aims of chest physiotherapy are:

1. To upgrade the efficiency of respiration generally and of ventilation in particular.

2. To prepare the patient pre-operatively with a disciplined and yet relaxed attitude to expectorating secretions in order to prevent post-operative respiratory complications.

3. To help the patient with his breathing, expectoration and posture in the post-operative period and to participate in the recovery from operation and the return to active and normal life.

These aims can be fulfilled providing there is all-round co-operation between the physiotherapist, the patient and the nursing staff.

As early as possible after admission to the Unit the patient is introduced to the physiotherapist who initiates him in the elements and the aims of the treatment. Nurses should co-operate with the physiotherapist to create a relaxed, and fear-free atmosphere when physiotherapy is in progress. It is also the responsibility of the nurse in charge to allocate time to the physiotherapist for treatment in the daily schedules of the ward. In turn, the physiotherapist must appreciate the routine of a particular ward. The Sister in charge should introduce the layout of the ward and in particular the resuscitation equipment to a new physiotherapist.

Four aspects of physiotherapy are particularly relevant to patients undergoing chest surgery. These are (1) breathing exercises, (2) coughing practice, (3) postural drainage, and (4) postural training and general exercise.

BREATHING EXERCISES

The object of the exercises is to establish breathing control particularly deep diaphragmatic breathing. The real value of this is to permit a greater tidal volume without a change in the dead space, and therefore an increase in the 'effective tidal volume' (see Chapter 3: *Lung volumes and capacities*, p. 28).

In addition, deep breathing helps to open up some of the swollen bronchioles and alveoli which may be collapsed and airless, and improves the perfusion/ventilation ratio. Although this is of particular value in the post-operative phase it is in the pre-operative period that controlled breathing must be mastered.

COUGHING PRACTICE

Through coughing the airways are cleared of excessive normal or abnormal secretions which can then be expectorated. In order to achieve expectoration, the cough has to be effective and 'organised'. Practice of effective coughing by the patient pre-operatively helps its continuation post-operatively. Effective coughing and expectoration is helped by gentle but firm pressure applied to the chest by the physiotherapist in the 'explosive' expiratory phase of the cough.

POSTURAL DRAINAGE

The basic principle of postural drainage consists of placing the patient in positions which permit direct bronchial drainage. The segmental bronchi are directed towards at least six points: anterior, posterior, medial, lateral, superior and inferior (see Fig. 1.14). Taking into account the fact that there are two lungs (i.e. two bronchial trees), it is easy to see that if the drainage of secretions has to be effected entirely by reliance on posture, the patient has to be placed in several different postions.

Postural drainage is carried out regularly in patients undergoing surgery for bronchiectasis or in those having a large volume of secretions. Pre-operatively, postural drainage gets rid of infected secretions, and post-operatively it keeps the airways clear. Postural drainage should be carried out with care and discretion. It should not be practised rigorously in patients with conditions other than those mentioned above. Complete postural drainage, with patients placed in all positions is contra-indicated in oesophageal surgery such as oesophagectomies and oesophageal reconstruction, and in very sick individuals. However, modified postural drainage such as lying on the side with head up or level should be used. At all times care should be taken to have a relaxed and pain-free patient. The intercostal drains and the intravenous drips should not be disturbed and pulled out accidentally when the position of the patient is changed. The nurse in charge of the ward, guided by the medical staff, must indicate to the physiotherapist any reason why a patient should not have postural drainage. The present tendency is to use a modified form of postural drainage with care and discretion.

POSTURAL TRAINING AND GENERAL EXERCISE

The maintenance of good posture is one of the aims of chest physiotherapy. Operative pain, pulmonary excision and interference with the chest wall are all factors contributing towards a bad posture and balance seen in some patients following chest surgery. Children, and those undergoing extensive chest wall surgery, such as thoracoplasty are particularly at risk. In such cases the patient's chest becomes flatter on the operated side, and there is a tendency to scoliosis and shoulder drop resulting in distorted posture. In severe cases, there are definite spinal and chest deformities with the patient standing and walking with distorted posture. Patients' attention must be drawn to bad postural tendencies before definite deformities are developed. Postural training should start pre-operatively and continue after operation. Remedial exercises must be introduced at the slightest indication of bad posture becoming a habit and when there is a developing deformity. The use of a mirror helps the patient by enabling him to visualise his posture and carry out exercises in front of it.

The vicinity of the thoracotomy wound to the muscles involved in shoulder movements and the pain arising from muscular actions can establish a fear of moving the shoulder on the operated side. The result is restriction of shoulder movement post-operatively. If this is allowed to continue, a rigid and 'frozen shoulder' will be the result.

After operation, shoulder exercise is encouraged. Even when patients are in bed the arms can be moved and the patient should be asked to practise arm movements.

General exercises start early after operation with the patient sitting out of bed with the drain *in situ*. After the drains are removed, walking and more active exercise and group physiotherapy are resumed.

27 Anaesthesia in Chest Surgery

The success and rapid development of thoracic surgery in recent years has been due, in no small measure, to a parallel development in anaesthesia. Prior to the Second World War such surgery was relatively uncommon and confined for the most part to operations on the chest wall. These operations were carried out under local or general anaesthesia, using anaesthetic gases with the patient breathing spontaneously and inhaling the gases. When such a general anaesthesia was administered for abdominal or limb surgery the risks attached were primarily those of overdosage and toxicity. When administered for thoracic surgery, while those risks were still present, there were other more urgent and life-threatening complications. Many of these complications were the direct result of the 'open chest' and related to the anatomo-physiological peculiarities of the thorax (see p. 20 and p. 32) notably the sub-atmospheric intrathoracic (intrapleural) pressure.

It is relevant to discuss some of the following problems associated with general anaesthesia specifically in chest surgery. These are (1) pneumothorax and problems of open chest, (2) bronchial secretions, and (3) one lung anaesthesia and ventilation.

PNEUMOTHORAX AND PROBLEMS OF THE OPEN CHEST

In normal circumstances and/or when an individual is anaesthetised but breathing spontaneously, the opening of the chest results in the collapse of the lung on the open side. In addition other complications follow in these circumstances, such as paradoxical respiration and swinging of the mediastinum resulting in the respiratory gases passing from one lung to the other. The overall result is anoxia, carbon dioxide retention and cardio-vascular disturbances.

The development of intravenous anaesthetic agents, endotracheal intubation and controlled respiration using muscle relaxants has solved this particular problem which had been for many years the biggest single factor preventing advances in chest surgery.

BRONCHIAL SECRETIONS

Secretions in the bronchial tree could, and often did, spell disaster for the patient in the early years of chest surgery. Such secretions can be mucoid, purulent, or blood with tissue debris and vomitus. In addition the handling of the lung by the surgeon can suddenly express large quantities of material into the bronchial tree, leading to obstruction of the airways and asphyxiation. Several methods have been used to deal with bronchial secretions.

POSTURE AND POSITIONING OF THE PATIENT ON THE OPERATING TABLE

The patient is positioned on the operating table so as to allow secretions to gravitate to the trachea, avoiding spillage into the healthy opposite side. Prone position thoracotomy is an example of drainage position and is still used in many centres, particularly in patients with bronchiectasis.

SUCTION

Endotracheal intubation and suction of the trachea by a catheter through the tube can keep the airways clear.

BRONCHIAL BLOCKERS

These consist of special tubes used to confine secretions to the diseased lobe or lung, until the thoracotomy is carried out. The surgeon can then clamp the affected bronchus and effectively close the thoracotomy side preventing it from discharging its contents into the trachea.

ONE LUNG ANAESTHESIA AND VENTILATION

ENDOBRONCHIAL CUFFED TUBES

The principles of the use of these tubes is to allow 'one lung' anaesthesia and ventilation, that is to collapse the affected lung whilst the operation is going on, with the ventilation carried out entirely by the healthy lung. This not only blocks off the bronchial tree on that side, thus preventing secretions from spilling over, but the collapse of the lung also helps the surgical procedure.

There are a variety of these tubes but generally they have a single or a double lumen.

DOUBLE LUMEN TUBES

The most popular of these tubes at present are Robertshaw's, Carlen's and Green's double lumen tubes. They are manufactured in various sizes and are designed to be placed into the right or left bronchus (Fig. 4.8a,b). They are, in essence, two tubes in one and when they are correctly inserted and positioned it is possible to isolate and remove secretions from either lung or main bronchi. In addition the lung on which the operation is carried out can be collapsed, while permitting ventilation of the opposite lung. The collapse of the lung facilitates the surgeon's work within the chest, for pulmonary and other types of chest surgery.

SINGLE LUMEN TUBES

These tubes are similar to but larger than the ordinary cuffed endotracheal tubes. The Macrae tube is a prototype of this kind of tube and has a shortened cuff designed to fit the right or the left main bronchus (Fig. 4.9). Such tubes can be positioned, blindly or under direct vision, by means of an introducer. When positioned the ventilation is carried out through one lung, namely the one into which the tube is introduced. The opposite lung on the operated side then collapses. Secretions from the operated side gravitate down the tube into the trachea and can be aspirated out.

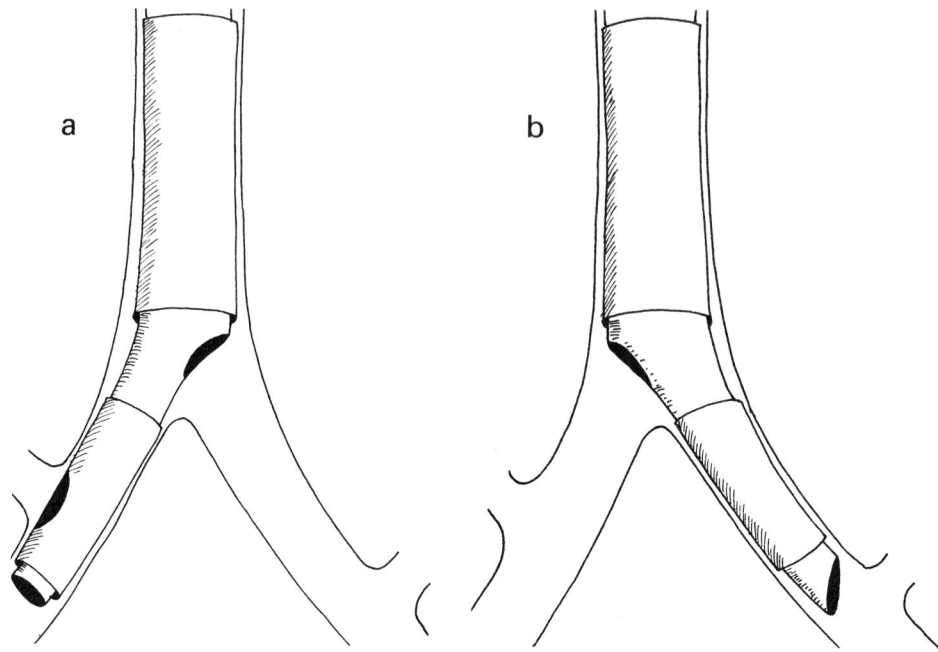

Figure 4.8   Robertshaw's (a) right and (b) left double lumen tubes.

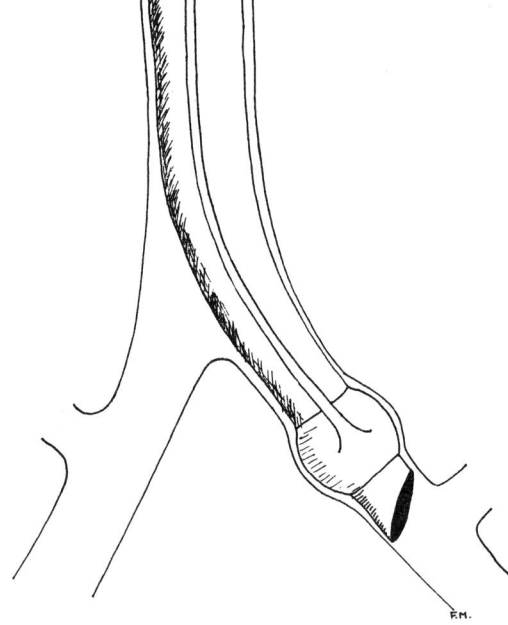

Figure 4.9   Macrae's tube in left bronchus. Right lung is not ventilated until the cuffed tube is pulled into the trachea.

GENERAL CONDUCT OF ANAESTHESIA IN CHEST SURGERY

Apart from the above-mentioned characteristics related to the thoracotomy, there is in essence no difference between anaesthesia for chest and abdominal or limb surgery.

PREMEDICATION

Prior to any surgical intervention it is the usual practice to administer sedative and 'drying' drugs to the patient. The objective in so prescribing is as follows:

1. To allay fear, anxiety and to bring the patient to the theatre in a calm and relaxed mental state.
2. To reduce secretions especially saliva and mucus in the respiratory tract.
3. To counter the vagotonic effects of the anaesthetic agents.
4. To counter nausea and vomiting.

Heavy premedication is usually avoided because of the added risks of respiratory depression at the end of the operation. Many new drugs have been introduced in recent years with less depressing effects than the older narcotic agents.

GENERAL ANAESTHESIA

General anaesthesia consists of three stages: induction, maintenance and recovery.

Induction

A butterfly or other needle is introduced into the vein and sleep or narcosis is induced by injecting the appropriate quantity of the chosen drug, usually a barbiturate, although there are many new non-barbiturate agents.

Following induction an injection of a short-acting muscle relaxant such as succenylcholine is given and intratracheal or endobronchial intubation is performed to meet surgical requirements.

Maintenance

The muscle relaxant produces a paralysed apnoeic patient and consequently oxygenation must be maintained both before and after intubation. Pure oxygen or a nitrous oxide and oxygen mixture can be used with at least 40% oxygen. This is conveyed by means of a semi-closed circuit with high flow rate or a closed circuit with a low flow and with a soda lime absorber unit in the circuit (either a circle or a 'to and from' system).

After a few minutes the short-acting muscle relaxant drug wears off and spontaneous respiration returns. The way the anaesthesia is handled now depends on whether there is a need for muscular relaxation and controlled ventilation, in which case the patient will receive an additional muscle relaxant, this time a longer-acting one. Ventilation is continued by squeezing a bag or by use of a mechanical ventilator. While the nitrous oxide and oxygen mixture has analgesic properties it must be reinforced by additional agents given intravenously. At the end of the operation the muscle relaxant will be wearing off and the return of spontaneous and active respiration is encouraged by injecting an anti-cholinesterase drug along with atropine.

Recovery

On termination of surgery the recovery phase begins with the return of spontaneous respiration. Controlled ventilation should be continued for a variable time post-operatively until full recovery of respiration.

Before the endotracheal or endobronchial tube is removed a bronchial toilet is carried out.

The patient is transferred from the theatre to a post-operative recovery or surgical intensive care unit.

ARTIFICIAL VENTILATION

Since the development of the technique of endotracheal intubation and controlled respiration, it has been possible to offer ventilatory assistance to patients with respiratory insufficiency. A comprehensive and detailed survey of the care of patients on assisted ventilation or of the apparatus used is not within the scope of this book, and the student should refer to the appropriate literature on the subject. It is, however, relevant and desirable to present an outline of the essentials of artificial ventilation with special reference to chest surgery.

The basic principles of artificial ventilation as practised at the present time consist of the provision of an intermittent positive pressure flow of air delivered into a tube which is placed into the trachea. Tracheal intubation is carried out through the larynx or via the tracheostomy (see Chapter 24: *Tracheostomy*, p.

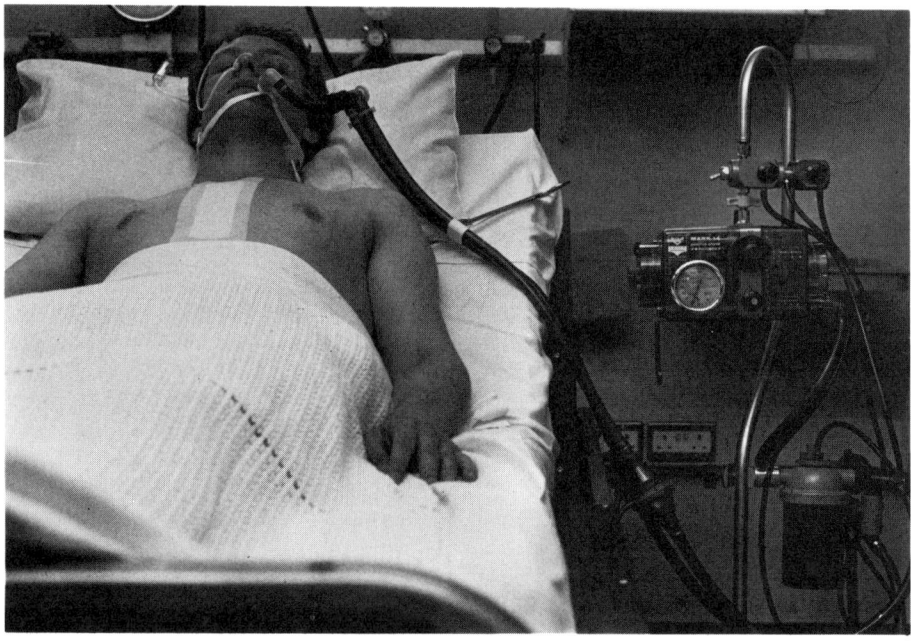

Figure 4.10   Patient on a pressure-controlled ventilator. Note the way the endotracheal tube is fixed on the pillow.

247). In either case the tracheal tube must be of a cuffed tube variety with the cuff inflated when breathing is controlled.

It is obvious that controlled ventilation except for a short period such as in an emergency situation, necessitates the use of a mechanical ventilator. Functionally speaking, a ventilator must be capable of inflating and deflating the patient's lungs, corresponding to the inspiratory and expiratory phases of breathing. It must also have a mechanism allowing for the change-over from inspiratory to expiratory phase and vice versa.

The manufacture of many ventilators, which can be classified in various ways, has been based on these principles. The driving force of ventilators can be taken as a basis for their classification, e.g. whether they are driven by electricity or compressed gas. On the other hand, ventilators can be classified according to their cycling mechanism which means the way they are preset to provide cyclic breathing. According to the latter classification which is commonly used, ventilators are of two principal types: volume-cycled and pressure-controlled ventilators (see Fig. 4.10).

Volume-cycled ventilators (Synonym: low generators or volume-controlled ventilators) This type of ventilator delivers a predetermined volume of gas into the lungs following which the inspiratory phase (or cycle) ends, irrespective of pressure changes in the machine or the lungs.

Pressure-controlled ventilators (Synonym: pressure-cycled ventilators or pressure generators) In these the preset pressure determines the flow of the gas, which is delivered into the lungs and the inspiratory cycle ends when the pre-determined pressure within the machine and the airway tube system is reached, irrespective of the volume of gas delivered.

It should be appreciated that in the volume-cycled ventilators the cyclic changes of breathing are determined by the volume of gas received in the lungs, whereas in the pressure-cycled ventilators the cyclic changes are governed by the pressure (and therefore resistance) which is reached within the system. Many of the present-day ventilators have both mechanisms incorporated within their system.

MONITORING OF ARTIFICIAL VENTILATION
In an artificial system, such as that of controlled ventilation incorporated in a biological system it is essential that careful monitoring of the machine, as well as its effect on the body as a whole, is undertaken. In this respect, the following are therefore important:

1. The mechanical working of the machine and its driving force must be known and checked regularly during its usage.

2. Measurement of the tidal volume delivered to the patient must be carried out intermittently whilst the machine is in use. This can be done using ventilation meters such as Wright's respirometer.

3. Clearance of air-conducting tubes must be assured and checked at all times.

4. Humidification of air driven into the lungs and prevention of drying of secretions must be assured. This can be achieved using a variety of humidifiers

which are available and/or by the simple method of water instillation into the airways directly by syringe or even a drip.

5. The effectiveness of artificial ventilation is monitored by the measurement of pH, PO_2 and PCO_2 in the arterial blood.

6. Microbiological monitoring, that is the determination of pathological micro-organisms and their sensitivity to antibiotics, is carried out regularly.

ESSENTIAL POINTS FOR THE NURSING CARE OF PATIENTS ON A VENTILATOR

It is important to appreciate that controlled and assisted ventilation requires care of the patient by a team of medical, nursing and laboratory personnel. No benefit will be gained by simply connecting a patient to a ventilator without careful assessment and monitoring; indeed definite harm will be the result of such action. Some of the essential points about the nursing care of these patients are:

1. Patients, if conscious, must be psychologically prepared. All procedures and manipulations must be explained to the patient, and should be carried out with utmost gentleness, accuracy, and by a trained individual.

2. A patient on a ventilator must not be left unsupervised, not even for one minute.

3. The nurse who is looking after the patient must at least know what to do if the power which is driving the machine fails and must be able to cope with an emergency situation concerning the ventilator and artificial and controlled ventilation.

4. Patients on a ventilator must be nursed in an intensive care environment with immediate access to equipment, and additional nursing help, and where there are facilities to summon medical help. Essential equipment such as suction machine and catheters should be within reach, beside the patient. A resuscitation trolley and equipment (see p. 277) should be nearby.

5. The principles of humidification and clearance of the airways from secretions must be applied.

6. The condition of the patient, and the effectiveness of the respiration controlled by the ventilator are monitored.

7. The patient should be sedated and be made as comfortable as possible.

In particular, attention should be concentrated on preventing discomfort to the patient through heavy tubing and connector dragging and the manner in which the endotracheal tube is fixed and managed (Fig. 4.10). The prevention of injury to the trachea with consequent tracheal stenosis must be kept in mind.

SPECIAL POINTS RELATED TO ARTIFICIAL VENTILATION IN CHEST SURGERY

In patients requiring artificial ventilation, following pulmonary surgery, it is important to consider additional points which are related specifically to this type of surgery. For instance, intermittent positive pressure ventilation imposes additional strain on the bronchial stump and its suture line, with an increased risk of the development of broncho-pleural fistula. This is more likely to occur in pneumonectomy cases than in patients with partial pulmonary resection. If pleural drains are *in situ*, alteration in the rate and volume of air and fluid drainage should be noted. When the drains have been removed the expansion of the residual lung (in lobectomy cases), or alteration of the pneumonectomy space, should be checked clinically and radiologically.

There is also an increased risk of pleuro-pulmonary infection after pulmonary surgery with artificial ventilation, because of endotracheal intubation. There is higher risk of contamination and difficulty in carrying out effective physiotherapy and removal of secretions. Extra-special care should be taken in all manipulations to prevent infection in patients requiring artificial ventilation following oesophageal resection and reconstruction. In addition, the possibility of regurgitation and subsequent pulmonary aspiration must be kept in mind. It is also important to consider the metabolic demands for patients on ventilation superimposed to the nutritional requirements of oesophagectomy.

28 Cardio-respiratory Resuscitation in Cardiac Arrest

Cardiac arrest (circulatory arrest) can be defined as a sudden and unexpected cessation of cardiac action with consequent circulatory arrest.

A number of patients with cardio-respiratory arrest can survive, providing that immediate and effective measures are taken to re-establish circulation and heart action, and to re-institute ventilation and oxygenation. Recovery depends partly on the effectiveness of the treatment. The latter is dependent on careful planning in the formation of a team and the efficiency of all involved in resuscitation. Lectures, demonstrations and an educational programme should be organised in each hospital or unit for members of staff. Charge nurses must introduce their staff to the type of equipment used and its location in the ward.

It is important to consider two factors that have a considerable bearing on the success of resuscitation: (1) Equipment should be adequate and in good working order. (2) Those concerned with the patient's management must have a clear idea of the procedure.

EQUIPMENT

Each unit or ward should organise its emergency equipment according to the ward lay-out, and the type of patients accommodated. Newly appointed members of staff should be informed about the type of equipment and drugs on the trolley. The nurse in charge should instruct nurses to familiarise themselves with the equipment.

Emergency trolley
An emergency trolley (Fig. 4.11) containing the necessary apparatus and drugs should be kept in an accessible place.

The trolley should contain the following apparatus:

1. *For ECG monitoring and defibrillation:*
   (a) DC defibrillator, with external electrodes, and in some cases internal electrodes.
   (b) ECG monitor and fitting electrodes, with a recording device.
2. *For endotracheal intubation:*
   (a) Ambu bag.
   (b) Endotracheal tube and connections.
   (c) Laryngoscope in working order and a spare battery.

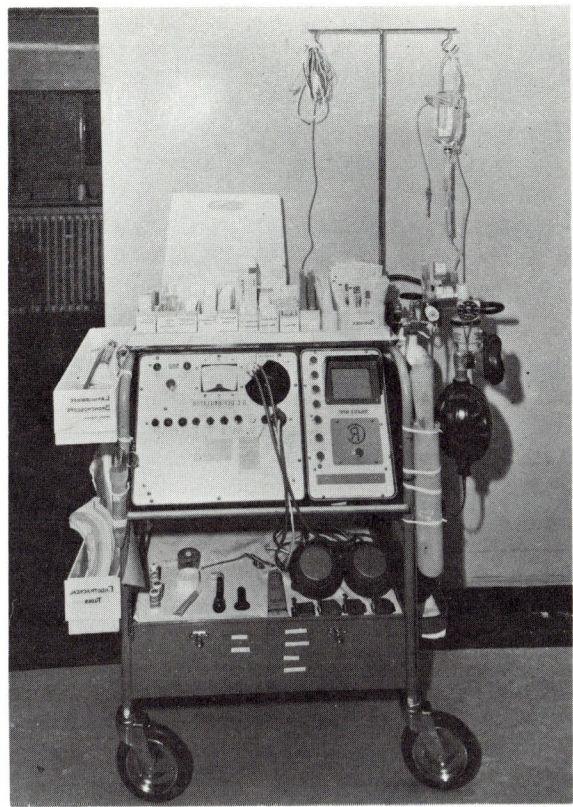

Figure 4.11 Resuscitation trolley with defibrillator, monitor, etc. (See text for details.)

3. *For airway clearing:*
   (a) Suction catheters and connector to fit the suction machine or tube of the mural central suction apparatus.
   (b) Container for disposable suction catheters.

Additional equipment

The following equipment should also be readily available and, if possible, placed on the emergency trolley:

1. Bronchoscope (portable) in working order, with a spare bulb and battery.
2. Selection of 5 and 10 ml syringes with matching needles, one of which should be fine and long for percutaneous intracardiac puncture.
3. IV cannula, IV infusion set and sodium bicarbonate 8.4%.
4. Drugs. The drugs on the trolley should consist of those primarily used in a case of cardiac arrest, together with those which may be life-saving in some situations. The latter are dependent on the type of cases in the ward or unit. The trolley must not be needlessly overcrowded. Drugs used for primary cardio-

vascular and respiratory action are of first priority. These are Adrenaline 1/1000; Adrenaline 1/10000; Isoprenaline; Calcium Chloride; Hydrocortisone; Ephedrine; Aminophyllin; An intravenous diuretic (e.g. Frusemide).

In addition other drugs may be kept on this trolley according to the type of ward and patients accommodated.

MANAGEMENT

The management of a case of cardiac arrest can best be described under the following headings:

Diagnosis
It is vital to diagnose cardiac arrest. Palpation of the carotid artery in the neck or the femoral artery in the groin are easy methods for confirming the presence or absence of pulsation (reflecting heart action). In the absence of pulsation, diagnosis is established. If the patient is connected to an ECG monitor, the tracing of ventricular fibrillation or asystole provides the diagnosis.

First-aid measures
Once diagnosis is made, circulation must be established promptly, and artificial ventilation undertaken. At the same time assistance should be summoned.

Establishment of circulation   The simplest effective method is to undertake external cardiac massage. This is based on the intermittent compression of the anterior chest wall (sternum) towards the back (vertebral column) which is placed on a firm surface. During compression the blood is squeezed out of the heart (which is pressed between the sternum and the vertebral column) and ejected into the aorta, mimicking the systolic phase of the cardiac cycle. During relaxation, the anterior chest wall regains its original position and the heart fills with blood once more, mimicking the diastolic phase of the cardiac cycle. For external cardiac massage, the following technique is used: (1) Place the patient on a firm surface such as the floor. If the patient is lying in bed a hard board is placed under the patient; (2) Place the hands over each other, with the heel of one hand on the lower part of the sternum (Fig. 4.12a), and extend the forearm to compress the sternum towards the back; (3) Allow flexion of the arm and relaxation of the chest (sternum moving upwards); (4) Repeat the procedure 50 to 60 times/minute.

Establishment of artificial ventilation   There are several methods of providing artificial ventilation. A safe, simple and effective method is by mouth to mouth, or mouth to nose breathing. The patient's lungs are inflated with the exhaled air of the operator (Fig. 4.12b). Technique is: (1) place the patient on his back; (2) clear the airways (i.e. mouth and pharynx); (3) extend the neck and pull the jaw forward with one hand in order to prevent the tongue falling back; (4) if mouth to nose breathing is applied, block the mouth with one hand, take a deep breath and breathe out into the nose of the patient, making sure that there is no air leak; (5) if mouth to mouth breathing is applied, block the nose by pinching it between the finger and thumb. Take a deep breath and breathe out into the patient's mouth; (6) watch for movement of the chest, so that the effectiveness of ventilation is monitored visually. Repeat this procedure 10 to 20 times/minute.

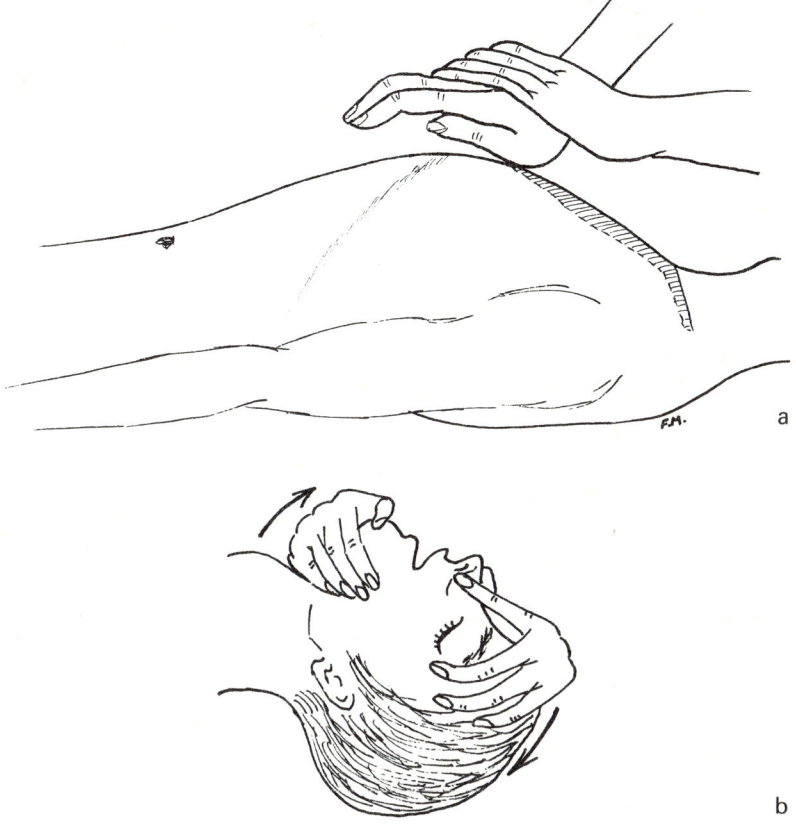

Figure 4.12 (a) External cardiac massage. (b) Mouth-to-mouth artificial ventilation.

If the operator is alone, or while assistance is on the way, and cardiac massage and artificial respiration has to be carried out single-handed, then the operator should try to carry out two or three cardiac massages to one artificial ventilation, continuing until aid arrives.

Raising the alarm to summon assistance
Whilst it is possible to keep an individual alive temporarily by external cardiac massage and artificial respiration, it is important that a complete management plan be made for the return of heart action and respiration. This involves the immediate availability of equipment and expert assistance at the scene of arrest. Each ward or department must have specific arrangements for communication, which essentially involve (1) facilities in the ward for communication with the switch-board, (2) provision of a system at the switch-board to enable the telephone operator to recognise the emergency cardiac arrest call, and (3) means of transmitting the cardiac arrest call and its location to the members of the team undertaking resuscitation.

Arrival of assistance

Whilst first-aid measures are in progress, the equipment is brought near to the patient. An ECG monitor is established as soon as possible. On the arrival of the medical staff, an endotracheal tube is inserted and artificial ventilation, using an Ambu bag (or similar device), is carried out. An IV drip for the administration of drugs and sodium bicarbonate is then established.

Arrangements are then made for the estimation of blood gases and serum potassium and a chest radiograph is taken. Further procedures and management depend on the duration and the aetiology of the circulatory arrest, and require the expertise of the medical personnel and the assistance of the nursing staff.

Diagnosis of the cause of the arrest

It is important to ascertain whether there is a complete cardiac standstill, or ventricular fibrillation (Fig. 4.13). The use of the DC defibrillator depends on this distinction, as it is effective for ventricular fibrillation only. Should the defibrillator be required (as is usually the case), the utmost care should be taken before it is applied, so that patient's or staff's lives are not endangered by its misuse. When heart action resumes, the medical staff should establish the cause of arrest and introduce effective therapeutic measures.

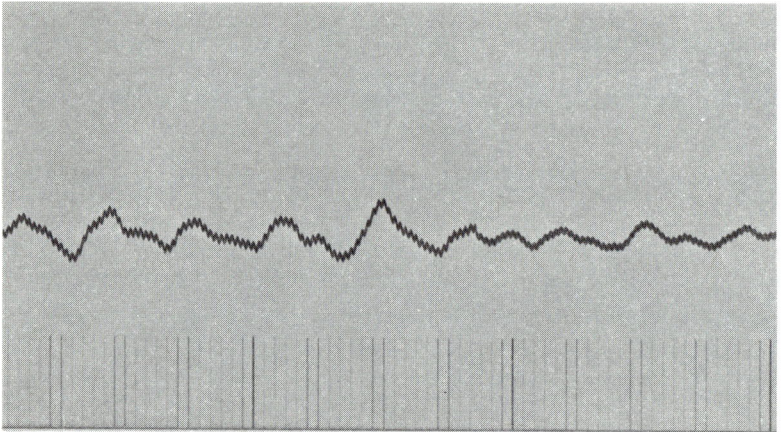

Figure 4.13   ECG of patient in ventricular fibrillation.

Maintenance of heart beat

When the heart beat and circulation are re-established with the return of the carotid and femoral pulses, the patient's colour should improve and signs of life become apparent. Recurrence of arrest should be prevented: observations of vital functions should be instituted. It is advisable to establish central venous pressure and to insert a catheter into the bladder.

Cardiac massage and artificial ventilation are continued and defibrillation attempted again until heart action resumes. When all attempts fail, the decision to abandon resuscitation should be made by a doctor.

29 Parenteral Nutrition in Thoracic Surgery

Living processes depend on metabolism which consists of two phases, namely catabolism and anabolism. The catabolic process is concerned with the breakdown of food into simpler compounds, and releases energy. The anabolic process involves building complicated storage or structural material from simpler compounds; it requires energy. Energy is the key to metabolism and is normally derived from food.

The term 'enteral feeding' applies to food taken by the alimentary tract. In the nutritional field it has come to assume the narrower meaning of artificial feeding, and is applied to naso-gastric tube feeding, gastrotomy and jejunosotomy feeding.

The term 'elemental diet' refers to high calorie and protein food preparations containing all essential requirements in a more assimilable form.

The term 'parenteral nutrition' is applied to methods of providing food stuffs and other essential requirements of the body by a route other than the alimentary tract. For practical purposes this has become synonymous with intravenous feeding. The last 25 years have seen the emergence and expansion of indications for parenteral nutrition in medicine and surgery. More advanced and safer techniques of infusion have been designed to reduce the incidence of complications and more consideration has been given to nutritional requirements in specific situations. Consequently the intravenous route has become a well-established method of feeding. For all its widespread acceptance, parenteral nutrition should not be regarded as a simple method but as a planned and well-controlled therapeutic measure.

In practice this involves selection of patients; assessment of nutritional state; assessment of nutritional requirements and selection of a solution to satisfy the patient's specific needs; technical aspects including circulatory access; care of the infusion set and the intravenous drip; monitoring the efficiency of therapy and prevention of complications.

SELECTION OF PATIENTS

Parenteral nutrition is indicated in a variety of medical and surgical cases in which the patient's nutritional requirements cannot be met by alimentary tract feeding.

In thoracic surgery parenteral feeding is indicated particularly in pre-operative preparation and post-operative management of patients with obstructive lesions of the oesophagus undergoing major reconstructive oesophageal surgery. In addition parenteral feeding is used in severe injuries and infection. Recently supplementary intravenous feeding has been recommended as an adjunct to chemotherapy in disseminated bronchial carcinoma.

ASSESSMENT OF NUTRITIONAL STATE OF PATIENTS

When an individual receives an inadequate supply of nutrients the amount necessary to cover body requirements is made up first from tissue breakdown, collectively referred to as body reserves. In extreme cases, that is in starvation, the individual has to depend entirely on body reserves. The body store of glycogen is the first source of energy to be called upon, but it is only sufficient to cover requirements at most for a few days. The main source of energy in nutritional deficiencies is derived from fat stores and tissue proteins. The latter come predominantly from muscle-mass breakdown. When this takes place there is loss of weight, loss of muscle-mass and fat. Biochemically this results in an increase of nitrogen in the urinary output and negative nitrogen balance (i.e. nitrogen loss in excess of nitrogen intake derived from food proteins). A negative nitrogen balance means that some of the body proteins, primarily those of muscular tissues, are broken down. The non-nitrogenous residue of the breakdown product is then metabolised as a source of energy, whilst the nitrogen radical is excreted in the urine, thus accounting for the increased urinary output of nitrogen.

Nitrogen balance study is therefore a good index of the contribution that the body makes to metabolism from its own reserves when supplies are inadequate.

Whilst the recognition of starvation and advanced nutritional deficiencies is not very problematic, the assessment of lesser nutritional deficiencies can be difficult. It is therefore important to consider some of the nutritional markers which are commonly used. These can be classified as clinical, biochemical and immunological.

CLINICAL MARKERS

Loss of weight
When severe, loss of weight can be shown by a simple clinical examination. In some cases of deficiencies, particularly those affecting vitamins, cutaneous and mucosal lesions may become apparent. Weight loss, even assessed by the patient, is a guideline, particularly when recorded as percentage weight change according to the following formula:

$$\% \text{ weight change} = \frac{(\text{usual weight} - \text{present weight}) \times 100}{\text{usual weight}}$$

or

$$\% \text{ weight change} = \frac{\text{loss of weight} \times 100}{\text{usual weight}}$$

Anthropometric studies

Mid-arm circumference measurement   This is the circumference of the flexed non-dominant arm in cm. This is taken with a simple tape measure and relates to protein reserves.

Triceps skinfold measurement   This is taken with skinfold calipers; the measure of the fold of skin over the lower portion of the triceps muscle relates to fat reserves.

There are normal ranges of values available for males and females with which the patient's values are compared, but the changes of values recorded in an individual over a period of time are a more reliable index of losses or gains.

BIOCHEMICAL MARKERS

Plasma proteins
These proteins only alter in very severe difficiencies. Plasma albumin reduction is a more sensitive index of deficiency. Serum transferrin (protein involved in iron binding) is an even more sensitive index of protein deficiency.

Nitrogen balance study
Reference has already been made to nitrogen balance study which is designed to calculate the nitrogen intake and output. The latter, in the absence of abnormal losses (diarrhoea, fistula), is calculated by determining the nitrogen content of the urinary output over a period of 24 hours.

The body is said to be in nitrogen equilibrium when nitrogen intake and output are equal in amount. It is said to be in negative nitrogen balance when the output is superior to the intake. Nitrogen balance is positive when intake is more than output.

IMMUNOLOGICAL MARKERS

Skin testing
These tests are based on delayed-type hypersensitivity reaction. Antigens are introduced intradermally causing localised oedema and inflammation in responsive individuals. The principle on which these tests are based is that the majority of the population react to certain antigens to which they have been previously exposed, but that in certain circumstances (e.g. cancer cachexia and malnutrition) they fail to do so. This state of unresponsiveness or anergy is associated with severe malnutrition. The two commonest antigens used in this country for this type of skin reaction are tuberculin and candida albicans.

Lymphocyte count
Lymphocytes are concerned with the body's immunological response. Both their total number and the variation of their type (T and B) can be affected in some types of malnutrition.

NUTRITIONAL REQUIREMENTS AND SELECTION OF NUTRIENTS

In assessing patients' nutritional needs both quantitative and qualitative aspects have to be considered. In order to maintain normal body composition and allow basic physiological processes to take place it is necessary to supply a balanced quantity of energy and materials for tissue synthesis, especially proteins, minerals, vitamins, and water.

ENERGY REQUIREMENTS

In planning a regime to cover the individual's needs, consideration should be given to dietary requirements as well as any additional requirements needed to cover increased metabolic needs such as trauma or operation. Also, extra allowances should be available to make good any pre-existing deficiencies such as may be encountered in patients with carcinoma of the oesophagus.

The value is expressed in kcal (or kJ) and the assessment of requirements is made in terms of kcal/kg body weight. It is also customary to express the quantity of proteins required in terms of their nitrogen content and therefore in g nitrogen/kg b.w.

The energy requirements of an adult male at rest (i.e. basic requirements) are estimated to 1700–2000 kcal/24 hrs or 26–31 kcal/kg b.w./24 hrs. Requirements are slightly lower for females and for the elderly (above 75 years of age). A higher allowance should be made for children and adolescents.

Energy requirements for patients undergoing major surgery have been variously assessed. Patients undergoing oesophageal resection and reconstruction require 40–45 kcal/kg b.w./24 hrs.

NITROGEN (AMINO-ACID) REQUIREMENTS

Based on nitrogen loss calculation (principally in urine) a basal allowance of 95–130 mg nitrogen/kg b.w./24 hrs or 0.7–1 g amino-acid mixture/kg b.w./24 hrs is estimated to cover an adult's basic requirements.

Nitrogen requirements in surgical cases have also been variously assessed. After major oesophageal operations they are estimated to be 0.20–0.25 g of nitrogen/kg b.w./24 hrs.

WATER

In assessing patients' water requirements, consideration should be given to the volume of fluid needed to cover daily requirements in water, and the volume of fluid required to contain the daily allowance in calories and nitrogen.

It is estimated that an adult at rest requires 2000–2500 ml of water per day or 30–35 ml/kg b.w./24 hrs.

In principle fluid balance should be maintained, therefore an additional allowance is made for patients with either an increased fluid loss or suffering from pathological conditions.

MINERALS

These can be classified in two groups:

1. Minerals which are electrolytes (e.g. sodium and potassium) form an important constituent of tissue fluid in the body and are vital for the exchange of fluid and for neuromuscular activities. They should be supplied daily and plasma level should be monitored regularly.

2. Other minerals which are important constituents of enzymes and proteins and participate in catalytic activities are collectively referred to as trace elements (e.g. copper, zinc, phosphorus). They should be supplied in adequate quantity in the total regime.

VITAMINS

Vitamins are classified as water-soluble (Vit. B complex and Vit. C) and fat-soluble (Vit. A, D, K, E).

The parenteral regime must contain an adequate quantity of these vitamins.

SELECTION OF NUTRIENT SOLUTIONS

Sources of energy

In normal diet the main energy sources are fats, carbohydrates and proteins. The calorie value, that is the calorie yields of these energy providers, has been calculated as:

carbohydrates   4.1 kcal/g
proteins   4   kcal/g
fats   9   kcal/g.

In intravenous feeding a variety of energy providers are used:

Carbohydrates: glucose, fructose, levulose, sorbitol.
Alcohol with a high calorie yield of 7.1 kcal/g.
Fat: soya bean oil.

Nitrogen source—Amino-acid solution

In an intravenous feeding programme a balanced quantity of amino-acid mixture is provided. The selected solution should contain essential amino acids, i.e. those which the body cannot synthesise, and the non-essential ones.

It is suggested that the optimum amino-acid mixture should resemble in proportion that of the body protein amino-acids.

Arranging intravenous nutrition regime

When arranging a 24-hour regime for intravenous feeding, consideration should be given to the following:

1. Assessment of energy requirements in terms of cal/24 hrs based on body weight and metabolic demands.

2. Assessment of nitrogen requirements based on the same criteria.

3. Type of energy providers. In this connection it is suggested that fat emulsion should form 40% of the total energy requirements unless there are definite contra-indications for using fat.

4. The ratio of provided energy (expressed as calories) to amino-acids (expressed as grams of nitrogen) is important. It is generally agreed that in most cases 200 kcal per 1 g nitrogen is the optimum ratio.

5. Minerals and vitamins are provided according to the patient's needs.

In practice, as the contents of the available intravenous feeding solutions provided by manufacturers are known, the selection of the appropriate preparation to suit the patient's needs is a matter of choice for the clinician.

The daily intravenous programme should be written up by the medical officer and it is the nurses' duty to see that the solutions are given as prescribed.

TECHNICAL ASPECTS—CIRCULATORY ACCESS

An uninterrupted supply of nutrient is dependent upon its efficient delivery into the circulation. This in turn depends on the catheter and circulatory access.

CATHETERS

There are now several suitable catheters available on the market for intravenous feeding. They fall into three types: catheter inside the needle, needle inside the catheter, and catheter without a needle.

The first two types are suitable for percutaneous vene-puncture whereas the third requires surgical introduction of the catheter by the cut-down technique. Each type of catheter can be either short (suitable for peripheral veins) or long (for catheterisation of a central vein, usually the superior vena cava).

CIRCULATORY ACCESS

Access can be gained through the peripheral veins, a long catheter placed in a central vein via a peripheral vein, or a central vein.

In each case the vein can be entered by percutaneous puncture or cut-down technique.

Peripheral vein

This route is generally unsuitable for parenteral feeding as the amino-acid and hypertonic sugar solutions in particular irritate the veins, causing thrombophlebitis. If this route is used the site has to be changed 24–48 hours later.

Long catheter

A long catheter can be placed in a central vein via a peripheral vein. Usually an ante-cubital vein is used percutaneously to introduce the catheter which is advanced into the vein and positioned in the superior vena cava.

Central vein

This means catheterisation of the superior vena cava. Several techniques are used to place the catheter. This may be achieved through percutaneous puncture of the external jugular, internal jugular or subclavian veins (Fig. 4.14).

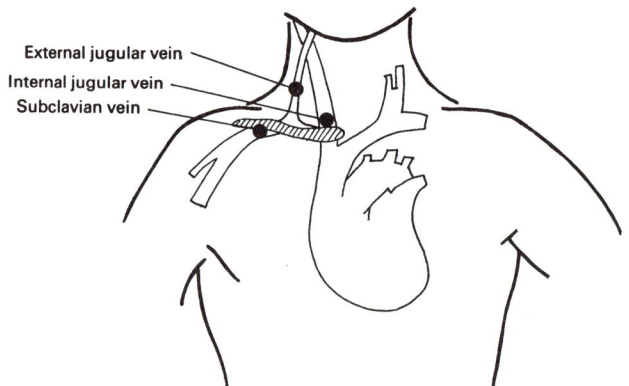

Figure 4.14   Percutaneous insertion of intravenous catheter into central vein.

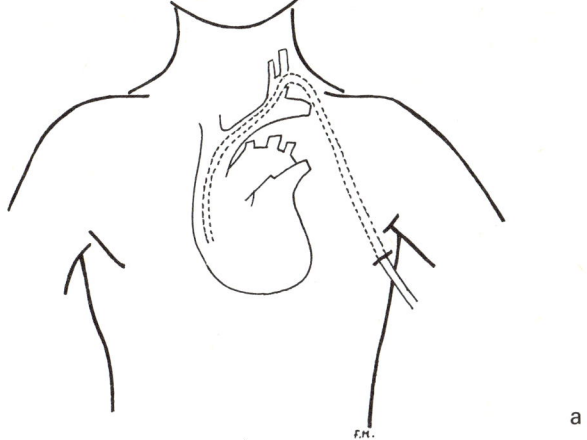

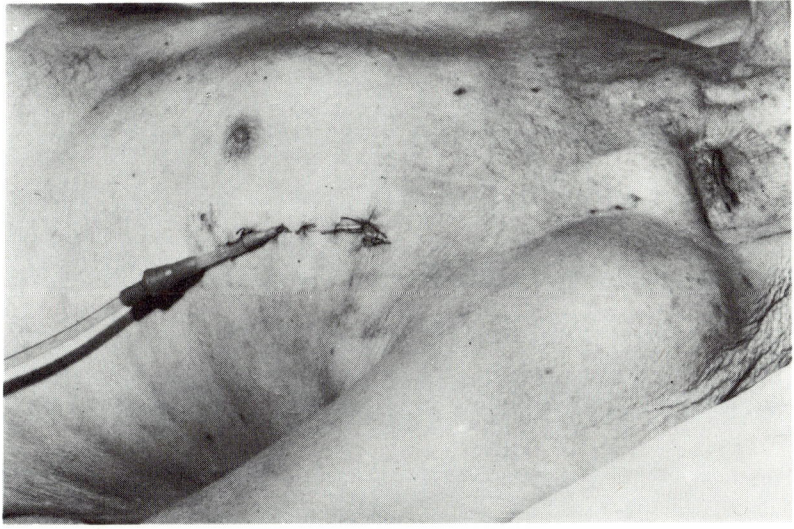

Figure 4.15 (a) *Cut-down technique of external jugular vein with tunnelling for superior vena caval catheterisation.* (b) *Photograph of same.*

In all cases the position of the tip of the catheter in the central vein is checked radiologically.

In the cut-down technique an incision is made over the selected tributary of the central vein. The catheter is then introduced and its connecting (giving set) end is brought out at, or near, the incision. A variation of the cut-down technique is to insert the catheter as above, then to pass the drip end of the catheter through a subcutaneous tunnel, bringing it out via another skin incision some distance away from the site of the catheter entry into the vein (Fig. 4.15a,b).

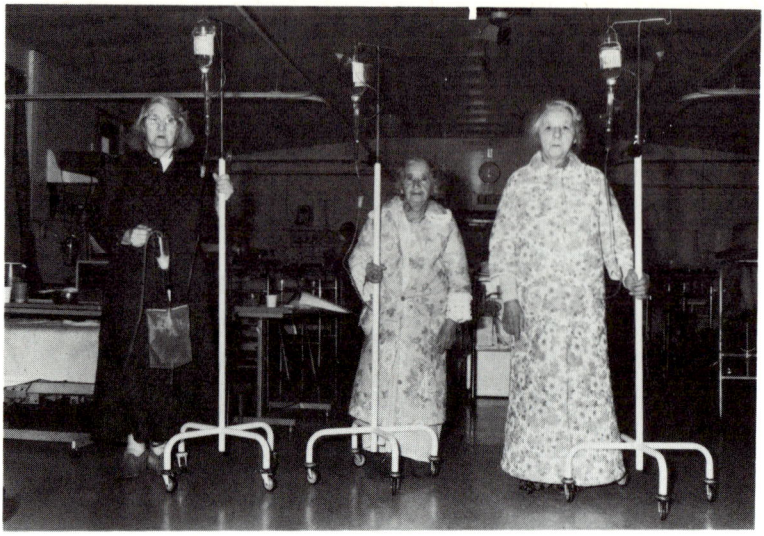

Figure 4.16   Patients receiving intravenous nutrition through central venous catheter; out of bed, independent and mobile.

This technique reduces the hazard of catheter and venous infection and allows mobilisation of the patient whilst infusion is in progress (Fig. 4.16).

CARE OF INFUSION SET AND INTRAVENOUS DRIP

Once the intravenous drip for parenteral nutrition is established, its care remains in the hands of the nursing staff. It is of paramount importance to look after the intravenous drip in order to maintain nutrition. This is even more important in patients after oesophageal resection and reconstruction who cannot receive nutrition by any other route. Certain points should be emphasised:

1. Daily requirements should be written by the medical officer and should be administered by the nursing staff just as any other drug.

2. The nurse in charge or a nurse who is in the nutritional team should take the responsibility of administration.

3. In all manipulations concerned with the change of giving sets and nutrient solutions strict antiseptic techniques must be observed.

4. Inflammation around the intravenous catheter must be reported to the medical staff.

5. Drugs and electrolyte solutions should not be added to nutrient solutions.

MONITORING PATIENTS AND PARENTERAL NUTRITION

It is important to monitor the patient, the effectiveness of the nutritional therapy, and that the intravenous drip is running safely.

CLINICAL MONITORING

Patients receiving parenteral nutrition must be clinically observed so that any complications may be prevented, or early treatment given should they arise. Therefore the patients' temperature and pulse should be recorded every 6 to 8 hours and, if their condition allows it, they should be weighed daily—ideally this weighing should be carried out at the same time each day. Fluid retention and oedema should be checked for, as well as any untoward reactions and complication.

The site of the catheter entry, and the integrity of the catheter and the three-way tap, should also be regularly checked for inflammation, leaks and breaks in the plastic. Such findings should be reported to the medical officer.

CHARTING

The volume intake and type of intravenous nutrition should be charted, and the fluid output recorded.

BIOCHEMISTRY MONITORING

Serum electrolytes and blood urea levels are estimated daily for guidance on the next day's regime, particularly when a concentrated solution of carbohydrate is used. It should be noted that the sample of blood for biochemical analysis must be withdrawn by venous puncture and not from the 'line'. The sample is not taken whilst fat solutions are in progress, or when they have just been completed.

URINE COLLECTION AND ANALYSIS

Urine should be collected over 24 hours in a special container with preservatives. An analysis of urine over 24 hours for electrolyte and nitrogen contents is carried out when required, particularly for nitrogen balance studies. Additionally, an analysis for sugar and acetone is carried out every 24 hours.

COMPLICATIONS OF PARENTERAL NUTRITION

These complications may be described as metabolic, vascular and infective.

METABOLIC COMPLICATIONS

Metabolic acidosis, hyperammoniaemia and hypophosphataemia have been recorded in some cases.

VASCULAR AND CATHETER COMPLICATIONS

Thrombo-phlebitis is a common complication when a peripheral vein is used for more than 24–48 hours. .Blocking of the catheter of a peripheral vein can be avoided if the running of the intravenous drip is uninterrupted and a fast flowing vein is used.

Catheter complications are mainly due to faults with the equipment. The majority of catheters for IV feeding can develop faults after a short or long period. Faults such as breaks or cracks at the junction of the catheter with the hub, can be due to mishandling.

INFECTIVE COMPLICATIONS

Local inflammation and infection at the site of the catheter insertion is not uncommon when a peripheral vein is used and when the intravenous drip is not cared for. More serious generalised infection and septicaemia have been recorded. Extreme care and attention to asepsis prevent these complications. An unexplained swinging temperature should draw attention to the vein, the site of the catheter and the technique of changing the infusion bottles and sets. If an infection is suspected blood culture should be carried out, the catheter removed and the tip cultured.

30 Care of Patients with Disseminated Thoracic Neoplasia

One of the essential roles of a nurse is to participate in the total management and care of patients, and nowhere is this more applicable than in cases of individuals suffering from disseminated cancer. The frequency of neoplasms within the thorax is such that inevitably some patients with widespread cancer will have to spend their last days in a hospital ward.

The inevitability of death in patients with carcinomatosis should not detract the medical and nursing staff's attention from the care they require and yet the fact that these patients are in hospital, or indeed, in an acute surgical or medical ward, should not let the routine of life-saving machinery override their privilege to die peacefully. Patients with disseminated growth should be helped mentally and physically to an acceptable death, which is free from pain, fear and suffering. The philosophy and the attitude of 'nothing can be done for these patients' should be condemned. The aim of the treatment is obviously not to cure but to reduce suffering and to offer the patient a better quality of life. With this in mind, a lot can be done for them. Active resuscitative measures in a terminal cancer case should not be pursued, as there is no more horrifying spectacle than to witness the eager nursing and medical team jumping on the chest of such patients for the purpose of cardiac massage in cases of cardiac arrest, nor is artificial ventilation justifiable when their respiration is failing. It is clear, therefore, that there must be a balance between treatment to relieve pain and agony on the one hand, and on the other, disturbing procedures and exhaustive invasive examinations which can induce unnecessary suffering.

It is appropriate to describe the management of a terminal cancer patient under medical management and nursing care.

MEDICAL MANAGEMENT

This is discussed under specific cancer therapy, and symptomatic therapy and psychological treatment.

SPECIFIC THERAPY
Chemotherapy consists of single or combination drug therapy which adversely affects the cancer cells and their rate of growth. All cytotoxic drugs have side-effects which have to be considered when the decision is taken to include them in the therapy of these patients.

They affect to varying degrees blood corpuscles, the gastro-intestinal tract and general metabolism. They can induce anaemia, leucopenia, thrombo-cytopenia, leading to infection and bleeding tendencies respectively. Some drugs affect hair follicles, with resulting baldness, others suppress appetite and add to malnutrition.

In spite of advances, radiotherapy can be of use in only some cases of widespread malignancy of the thorax. Side-effects, particularly those related to the gastro-intestinal tract, should also be considered.

NON-SPECIFIC SYMPTOMATIC THERAPY

In many cancer patients, specific therapy may be unhelpful or even responsible for producing unpleasant side-effects. Therefore, in order to provide as good a quality of life as possible, it becomes necessary to withhold specific therapy and concentrate on alleviation of the patient's symptoms.

Pain

The most important aspect of the care of terminal cancer patients must be the elimination or suppression of pain. As pain is a sensation with strong emotional components varying with individuals, so patients' response and tolerance to analgesics are similarly subject to variations. Therefore, great care and patience are required to select the appropriate analgesic and the correct dose for the individual. Additional consideration should be given to the influence that some analgesics may have on the gastro-intestinal tract. Nausea and uncomfortable constipation are often present in patients with carcinomatosis receiving analgesics in frequent daily doses. When oral analgesics become ineffective or impracticable intramuscular injections of strong analgesics and opiate should be introduced.

Sedatives

Fear of death in patients aware of their condition, and anxiety and depression in those who do not know their diagnosis but see themselves deteriorating, should concern doctors and nurses looking after terminal cancer patients. Nurses should draw the doctor's attention to the need for sedatives and their effectiveness or ineffectiveness.

Anti-emetics

Many patients are nauseated because of side-effects of drugs, or gastro-intestinal and metabolic disturbances resulting from growth dissemination. Nausea and vomiting must be stopped by appropriate drugs given intra-muscularly or intravenously.

Other symptomatic treatment

There are a variety of symptoms which may appear and have to be recognised and treated. For instance, coughing, sputum expectoration.

Cough   In many cases coughing, particularly at night, may be troublesome. It is important to suppress persistent coughing in cases of incurable cancer when the patient is deteriorating fast. In some cases incessant cough is due to sticky and tenacious secretions and it may be advisable to use a mucolytic and expectorant agent.

Sputum   Expectoration of purulent or haemorrhagic material can be frightening to the patient. In some cases there is some infecting element which responds to antibiotic therapy.

Psychological treatment

It is very difficult to categorise the different mental attitudes that will exist among cancer patients. Many patients in this country choose to remain ignorant of their condition, and in spite of a great deal of publicity surrounding cancer, they are not prepared to recognise and come to terms with a disease which is 'mainly for other people'. Some cancer sufferers suspect their diagnosis but do not like to talk about it and, therefore, choose to keep their thoughts to themselves. Other patients would like to know everything about their case; they try to organise their mind and life accordingly and accept the ordeal with resignation and courage. A few go further than that; not only do they want to know, but they discuss their condition openly, and fight to remain active and useful members of society up to near the end. It is difficult to appreciate and understand the psychology of every patient, but time should be spent by everyone involved in the management to try and help them with maximum compassion and understanding. Patients who know they are dying may pass through several types of attitudinal reaction. These have been described as 'stages' by Elisabeth Kubler-Ross in her book *On Death and Dying* (Tavistock Publications, London, 1969). She has labelled these stages as denial and isolation, anger, bargaining, depression and acceptance.

NURSING CARE

Nursing is the most important aspect of management of patients with disseminated neoplasia in its terminal stage, and the following is set out to provide the nurse with useful guidelines.

OBSERVATIONS

As long as the patient is in a ward, a series of relevant observations must be made and recorded to indicate progress or deterioration. It must be realised that some patients can temporarily improve and be discharged home. The nature and frequency of observations such as temperature and pulse rate have to be discussed with the medical staff. The occurrence of new signs or symptoms must be recorded and brought to the attention of the medical staff.

HYGIENE

It is important to attend to the patient's hygiene (e.g. cleanliness and comfort). Different patients require different levels of help in personal hygiene according to the progress of their disease. It is the duty of the nurse to assess this and attend to it as required.

BOWEL ACTION

Constipation may present a constant source of discomfort in some. In others, diarrhoea, partial or total incontinence can occur because of neurological involvement.

There are many ways to make a patient comfortable. A good relationship should exist between nurses and such patients in order to make them feel at ease and not embarrassed because of their helplessness.

MICTURITION
Micturition can be difficult in terminal cases. Urinary retention, overflow incontinence or true incontinence can be present in patients with disseminated cancer. The insertion of a urinary catheter is helpful in the majority of cases.

BED SORES
Careful nursing of the pressure areas is necessary if bed sores are to be prevented as much as possible. In some instances, patients have more pain and discomfort from sores than from a surgical wound or bony metastases. Pain should be alleviated by the introduction of strong analgesics and bed sores should be attended to.

PERSONAL APPEARANCE
Some patients, particularly young females, are most concerned about their appearance and it is part of the terminal care to see that patients remain happy in this respect.

COMMUNICATION WITH RELATIVES
It is very important to communicate with the next of kin and explain the condition of the patient. It is also necessary to give reports on progress to the family and enquire from the patient's relatives if the patient is satisfied with the care he is receiving. It is important to realise that the patient may feel that treatment is deficient in some respects and expresses this only to relatives.

Relatives must be made aware that the patient is looked after and not neglected because of the nature of his condition. Many relatives are under great emotional stress and may misinterpret some aspects of the patient's care and the attitude of the establishment.

PRESENCE AT DEATH
It is important to make certain that a relative (if they so wish) or a member of the nursing staff who is known to and liked by the patient, remains with the patient during his last hours.

31 Discharge from the Hospital

GOING HOME

In the absence of complications and when post-operative progress has been entirely satisfactory the patient is discharged from hospital. The decision to discharge a patient is the responsibility of the medical staff, but the nursing staff share in the decision in several ways.

In the first place it is the nurse's duty to bring to light any fact which may influence the decision.

Secondly the nursing staff are in a good position to evaluate the family situation and the environment to which the patient is returning on discharge.

It should be remembered that although patients are discharged when it is safe to do so, particularly in thoracic surgery, for economic and psychological reasons this may be earlier than the ideal time. Therefore, part of their convalescence takes place outside the hospital.

Two aspects of 'going home' arrangements need special emphasis. They are discharge of patients, and continuing treatment and management at home.

DISCHARGE OF PATIENTS

The majority of patients are sent to their own home, others have to be sent to a convalescent home, a remaining few may have to be transferred to other departments or another hospital for specific treatment. When possible, patients are sent to their own home to be looked after by their relatives. This has the great advantage of patients being in their own surroundings and progressively adapting themselves to the type of life and degree of independence consistent with their milieu.

Nurses should acquire information on the patient's home conditions and its facilities. They should also evaluate discreetly the type of psychological and physical help that patients are likely to receive from their immediate family. This information should be passed to the doctors in charge for an adequate decision to be reached. Both relatives and patients should be taught about the continuing care of the patient before his discharge.

A convalescent home accommodates different types of people who have completed active hospital treatment but are unable to go home on discharge for social or medical reasons. Such homes have the advantage of providing supervision and preparation for ultimate return home. Their disadvantage is that, as institutions, they have rules and regulations that limit the patient's freedom and may undermine self confidence.

CONTINUING TREATMENT AND MANAGEMENT AT HOME

Going home should be regarded as a stage in the post-operative recovery period in which the patient can be managed outside the hospital under the care of the family practitioner. It is essential to appreciate that, unless proper communication exists between the hospital and the family practitioner, continuity of management will not be achieved. It is therefore important to prepare the patient for discharge from the hospital unit, and to communicate with the medical services concerned with the patient's care outside the hospital. In practice the following points are relevant:

1. The patient is examined before going home. The surgical wound in particular is inspected. Should the wound require regular dressing, then appropriate arrangements are made through the family practitioner's service for this to be carried out by the district nurse.

2. The patient's medications are checked and a few days' supply of every item is given to the patient to take home. Clear written instructions concerning the dosage and mode of taking should be given.

3. Explicit information and instructions are given regarding the amount of activity he can safely undertake and dietary or other restrictions (smoking, alcohol) he should observe.

4. Many female patients, particularly younger ones, have queries about sexual intercourse and contraceptives. They should be given the required information in consultation with the medical officer.

5. A note containing essential information about the patient's condition, type of operation and all drugs is given to the patient. This is handed over to the family doctor by the patient at the earliest moment possible, in order to provide the doctor with adequate information before he receives the formal discharge letter.

6. The patient is told about follow-up procedures in the out-patients' clinic.

Follow-up procedures should be explained to the patient when they attend the out-patients' clinic.

Glossary

Aetiology   Cause of disease.

Anastomosis   Operative union of the divided ends of two hollow or tubular structures.

Anthropometrics   Measurements of parts of the body.

Antibiotics (broad spectrum)   Antibiotics having a wide range of activity against Gram-positive and Gram-negative organisms.

Anti-emetic   Medication which tends to control nausea and vomiting.

Approximation   Bringing together. In surgery, bringing one structure to another by suturing.

Actinomycosis   Disease, or swelling, commonly found in the cervico-facial area, abdomen or thorax. Caused by *Actinomyces israelii*, a species of bacteria.

Aspergillus   Genus of fungi of the *Ascomycetes* class which is characterised by the presence of a sac-like structure containing ascospores (spores). Caused by *Aspergillus fumigatus*, the commonest type of fungus found in man.

Bolus   Masticated volume of food ready to be swallowed.

Bougie   Cylindrical instrument—usually flexible and yielding—used in the dilation of strictures.

Bouginage   Passage of a bougie.

Bronchotomy   Incision of a bronchus (to inspect the lumen).

Cachexia   General malnutrition and wasting occurring in the course of a chronic disease.

Calorie   Unit of heat quantity. 1 Cal. is the quantity of heat required to raise the temperature of 1 kg of water by 1°C.

Cancer/Carcinoma   Malignant epithelial tumour.

Congenital   Existing at birth (not necessarily hereditary).

Crus of the diaphragm (pl. Crura)   Muscular origin of the diaphragm arising from the bodies of the lumbar vertebrae.

Cyst   Abnormal sac containing gas, fluid or a semi-solid material.

Diffusion   Movement of gases, according to the gradient of pressure, through a membrane.

Dyspepsia   Indigestion.

Electrolyte   Compound which, in solution, conducts a current of electricity and is decomposed by it (e.g. sodium Na$^+$, potassium K$^+$).

Empyema   Pus in the pleural cavity.

Endoscopy   Visual examination of the interior of a canal or hollow internal organ.

Enucleation   Removal of a tumour or cyst entire, with rupture.

Extrinsic   Developing or having its origin from without, not internal.

Fascia   Sheet of fibrous tissue which envelops the body beneath the skin and also encloses the muscles and groups of muscles.

Fibroptic (instrument)   Instrument used from the visual examination of an organ in which the light is carried through fibres.

Fissure   Furrow, cleft or slit.

Fistula   Abnormal passage leading from an abscess cavity or hollow organ to the surface, or from the one abscess cavity or organ to another.

Flatulence   Presence of an excessive amount of gas in the stomach and intestines.

Fungus   Vegetable organism feeding on organic matter.

Gastrostomy   Establishment of an artificial opening into the stomach.

Gastrotomy   Incision into the stomach.

Glossitis   Inflammation of the tongue.

Granulation tissues   Minute, rounded, fleshy projections on the surface of a wound in the process of healing.

Granuloma   Indefinite term applied to nodular inflammatory lesions, usually small or granular, firm, persistent and containing proliferated macrophages.

Haematemesis   Vomiting of blood.

Heterogeneous   Composed of parts having various and dissimilar characteristics.

Histoplasmosis   Commonest pulmonary fungal disease in the USA. Caused by *Histoplasma capsulatum*, a genus of yeast-like fungus.

Homeostasis   State of equilibrium in the living body with respect to various functions, and to the chemical compositions of the fluids and tissues.

Homogeneous   Uniform structure or composition throughout.

Iatrogenic   Produced by doctors (or nurses), in a patient, by inadvertent or erroneous treatment.

Ileus   Mechanical or adynamic (paralytic) obstruction of the bowels.

Infection   Invasion of a part of the body by living pathogenic micro-organisms with injurious effect on the tissues.

Intrathoracic   Within the cavity of the chest.

Intrinsic   Inherent, belonging to a part, from within.

Intubation   Insertion of a tube into a canal or other part of the body.

Isotopes   Alternative forms of an element which are chemically identical; have the same atomic number, but yet a different mass number.

Laparotomy   Surgical opening of the abdomen.

Lavage   Washing out of a hollow organ by injections and rejections of water.

Lumen (pl. Lumina)   Space in the interior of a tubular structure.

Macroscopically   Examined with the naked eye.

Manometer   Instrument for indicating the pressure of gases or vapour, or tension of the blood.

Mastication   Chewing.

Membrane   Thin layer of pliable tissue serving as a covering of a part, the lining of a cavity, as a partition or to connect two structures.

Metastasis (pl. Metastases)   In cancer, the appearance of neoplasms in parts of the body remote from the site of the primary tumour.

Moniliasis   Infection caused by *Candida Albicans*; commonly an infection of the oropharynx, vagina and gastro-intestinal tract.

Monitoring   Gauging the patient's progress by repeated measurements.

Myotomy   Surgical division of a muscle.

Necrosis   Death of cells.

Occult   Hidden, concealed, not easily recognisable.
Oesophagoplasty   Reconstruction of the oesophagus.

Parenchyma   Specific tissue of an organ carrying out a specialised function.
Pathogenesis   Origin or development of a disease.
Peristalsis   Wave of contraction and relaxation of a tubular organ by which the contents are propelled onward.
Pleural effusion   Collection of fluid, blood or pus within the pleural space.
Pleurodesis   Creation of adhesion between the visceral pleura and chest wall.
Plication   Operation for reducing the size of a hollow organ by making folds in its walls.
Prophylactic   Preventing disease.
Prosthesis   Artifical replacement of a lost part of the body.

Regurgitation   Return of gas or small amounts of food from the stomach.
Residue diet (high)   Diet containing foods which are mostly excreted.
Residue diet (low)   Diet containing foods which are mostly absorbed, and leave little to be excreted.

Scolex (pl. Scoleces)   Head by which a worm is attached to the wall of a host organ. It is formed in the interior of the daughter cyst.
Sphincter   Orbicular muscle which serves—when in a state of normal contraction—to close one of the orifices of the body.
Stenosis   Narrowing of a canal (stricture).
Subphrenic   Subdiaphragmatic (under the diaphragm).
Syndrome   Group of signs and symptoms associated with a disease.

Therapeutic   Relating to the treatment of diseases.
Transthoracic   Passing through the thoracic cavity.

Vascular   Relating to or containing blood vessels.
Vascular arcade   Arrangement of blood vessels of an organ resembling a series of arches (e.g. intestinal, colonic).
Vascularisation   The acquisition of a blood supply. The process of becoming vascular.

Index